James Cornelius Wilson, Henry Tucker

The Complete Medical Pocket-Formulary and Physician's

Vade-Mecum

James Cornelius Wilson, Henry Tucker

The Complete Medical Pocket-Formulary and Physician's Vade-Mecum

ISBN/EAN: 9783742830005

Manufactured in Europe, USA, Canada, Australia, Japa

Cover: Foto ©Lupo / pixelio.de

Manufactured and distributed by brebook publishing software
(www.brebook.com)

James Cornelius Wilson, Henry Tucker

The Complete Medical Pocket-Formulary and Physician's Vade-Mecum

THE

Complete Medical Pocket-Formulary

AND

PHYSICIAN'S VADE-MECUM:

CONTAINING UPWARDS OF 2500 PRESCRIPTIONS, COL-
LECTED FROM THE PRACTICE OF PHYSICIANS
AND SURGEONS OF EXPERIENCE, AMERICAN
AND FOREIGN, ARRANGED FOR READY
REFERENCE UNDER AN ALPHABET-
ICAL LIST OF DISEASES;

Also a Special List of New Drugs, with their Dosage,
Solubilities, and Therapeutical Applications;

TOGETHER WITH

A TABLE OF FORMULÆ FOR SUPPOSITORIES; A TABLE OF FOR-
MULÆ FOR HYPODERMIC MEDICATION; A LIST OF DRUGS
FOR INHALATION; A TABLE OF POISONS, WITH THEIR
ANTIDOTES; A POSOLOGICAL TABLE; A LIST OF
INCOMPATIBLES; A TABLE OF METRIC EQUIV-
ALENTS; A BRIEF ACCOUNT OF EXTERNAL
ANTIPYRETICS, DISINFECTANTS, MED-
ICAL THERMOMETRY, THE URI-
NARY TESTS; AND MUCH
OTHER USEFUL IN-
FORMATION.

COLLATED FOR THE USE OF PRACTITIONERS

BY

J. C. WILSON, A.M., M.D.,

Physician to the German Hospital, Philadelphia, etc., etc.

REVISED BY

HENRY TUCKER, M.D.

PREFACE.

NO apology is offered for presenting to the profession The Complete Medical Pocket-Formulary. The value of such a manual for ready reference at all times has been fully established, and is understood not only by the oft-referred-to busy practitioner, but also by every physician at the outset of his professional labors. Nor, indeed, will those who are more experienced and critical in all instances deny the immediate value of suggestions found between its covers.

This little book is not intended to take the place either of treatises on practice or of hand-books of therapeutics. Nor is it designed to eke out the defects of an imperfect medical education.

Its true office will consist in bringing to the attention of the practitioner, when most needed, the results of the experience of the profession at large, in rendering available a wider range of therapeutic knowledge than most possess, and in refreshing the memory with facts which from disuse are often difficult to recall at once. Those who use it rightly will avoid the error of forcing their individual cases to fit the requirements of formal recipes ; they will, on the contrary, so modify the suggestive formulæ as to render them available for each case in turn, and will find throughout its pages, often usefully referred to in haste, the starting-point for valuable reading and investigation at leisure.

PHILADELPHIA, July 4, 1891.

CONTENTS.

AUTHORITIES.

Abadie.
Abercrombie.
Abernethy.
Acton.
Adams.
Agnew.
Ainslie.
Aitken.
Aldridge.
Alibert.
Allan.
Andeer.
Anderson.
Andrew, James.
Andrews.
Anglada.
Annacker.
Annual Universal
  Medical Sciences.
Anstie.
Antony.
Antzman.
Armaignac.
Arthaud and Ray-
  mond.
Aschenbach.
Ashwell.
Atkinson.
Atlee, W.
Atthill.
Aubergier.
Aubert.
Audhoui.
Ayer.

Baccelli.
Bachen.
Baer.
Bailey.
Baillie.
Baker.
Balfour.
Ball.
Balzer.
Banyer.
Baratoux.
Barbacci.
Bareges.
Barker.
Barlow.
Barnes, Robert.
Barnsfather.
Barthez.
Bartholow.
Bartlett.
Barwell.
Basham.
Bazin.
Bean.
Beard.
Beasley.
Beauperthuy.
Bedard.
Beddoes.
Bedoin.
Begbie.
Bellevue Hospital,
  N.Y.
Beneké.
Bennett.
Bérenger-Féraud.
Berezovsky.
Berry.
Bertarelli.
Besnier.
Bethune.
Bevan.
Bezold.

Bibron.
Biett.
Billington.
Billroth.
Bird, George.
Bird, Golding.
Bishop.
Blachez.
Black.
Blair.
Blanc.
Blasius.
Blaud.
Boeck.
Bonjean.
Bosley.
Botler.
Bouchard.
Bouchut.
Bourdeaux.
Bourdon.
Boys.
Bradley.
Brande.
Brera.
Brinton.
Brockes.
Brocq.
Brodie.
Brondel.
Brown.
Brown-Séquard.
Browne, Crichton.
Bruce.
Brunäuer.
Bruns.
Brunton.
Bryce.
Buck.
Bucknill.
Budd.
Bulkley.
Bumstead.
Bumstead and Tay-
  lor.
Burgess.
Burman.
Burnett, C. H.
Busch.

Cammann.
Campbell.
Campi.
Canali.
Cane.
Canquoin.
Capitan.
Carmichael.
Carpenter.
Carré.
Carson.
Casovati.
Cazeaux.
Cazenave.
Chambers.
Chandler.
Channier.
Channing.
Chapman.
Charity Hospital,
  N.Y.
Charovin.
Charteris.
Chassaignac.
Chaves.
Cheatham.
Chennevière.
Chéron.

Chilton.
Chrestien.
Christie.
Churchill.
Cividale.
Clark, Alonzo.
Clark, H. M.
Clarke, Andrew.
Clarus.
Clouston.
Comstock.
Corfc.
Condie.
Cooper, Sir Astley.
Cooper, Bransby.
Copland.
Cordes.
Cornillon.
Correa.
Corrigan.
Corry.
Corvisart.
Coster.
Coulson.
Cousot.
Coxe.
Credé.
Crewcour.
Creyx et Jarry.
Cruice.

Da Costa.
Da Costa, J. C.
Dalton.
Danet.
D'Ardenne.
Darrach, J.
Darrach, Wm.
Darwall.
Date.
Davidson.
Davis.
Davis, E. P.
Day.
De Bleyer.
Deboué.
Debove.
Debreyne.
De Lacaille.
Delafield.
Delapert.
Dellenbaugh.
Delthil.
Demange.
Demarquay.
Demiéville.
Demme.
De Mussy.
De Renzi.
Dervieux.
De Schweinitz.
Descroizilles.
De Smet.
Dessau.
Devay.
Devergie.
Dewar.
Dewees.
Dick.
Diday.
Diederichs.
Dovell.
Dobronravoff.
Dochmann.
Donavan.
Donnelly.
Dowell.
Doyon.

Drasche.
Drescher.
Druitt.
Dubief.
Du Castel.
Duchenne.
Duckworth.
Duguet.
Duhring.
Dujardin-Beaumetz.
Dukes.
Dumas.
Duncan.
Dunglison.
Dunn.
Duparc.
Dupasquier.
Dupont.
Dupuytren.
Duraud.

Easby.
Eberle.
Ebstein.
Echeverria.
Eillard.
Eisenhart.
Eitelberg.
Elleaume.
Eller.
Elliott.
Ellis.
Elsberg.
Embleton.
Emmet.
Endler.
Erichsen.
Erlenmeyer.
Eshner.
Eulenburg.
Evans.
Ewald.

Fahnestock.
Fairbank.
Faust.
Fenn.
Fenwick.
Ferguson.
Fernald.
Ferrier.
Fischer.
Fisher.
Flanagan.
Fleischmann.
Fleming.
Fliesburg.
Fordyce.
Foster.
Fothergill.
Fournier.
Fowler.
Fox, G. H.
Fox, L. W.
Fox, Tilbury.
Foy.
Fraipont.
Fräntzel.
Fraser.
Free.
Frerichs.
Frey.
Froumueller.
Frost.
Frühwald.
Fuller.
Furey.
Furlonge.

Gabre.
Galezowski.
Garageorgiades.
Gardner.
Garretson.
Garrod.

Georgi.
Getchell.
Gilles de la Tourette.
Gimbert.
Giné.
Giordano.
Girard.
Girwood.
Glover.
Goelet.
Gola.
Goldberg.
Golding-Bird.
Gooch.
Goodell.
Goodfellow.
Goodman.
Goolden.
Gottschalk.
Graefe.
Graham.
Graudin.
Grandmout.
Grant (Bey).
Granville.
Grasset.
Graves.
Green.
Greenhalgh.
Gregory.
Grieve.
Gross, S. D.
Gross, S. W.
Grossich.
Gsell-Fels.
Gubler.
Guibout.
Guichon.
Guild.
Guitéras.
Guthrie.
Guttmann.
Guy.
Guy's Hospital.

Habershon.
Haden.
Halford.
Hallopeau.
Hamilton.
Hammerschlag.
Hammond.
Hannay.
Haunon.
Hardy.
Hare.
Harkin.
Harley.
Hartmann.
Hartshorne.
Hasterlik.
Haughton.
Hausmaun.
Hawack.
Hawack and Arboe.
Hawkins.
Hay.
Hazard.
Headland.
Hearn.
Heath.
Hebersmith.
Hebra.
Hecket.
Heder.
Heinzelmann.
Henry.
Henson.
Hering.
Herrmann.
Heuter.
Hicks.
Higginbottom.
Higgins.
Hildenbrand.

Hildreth.
Hill.
Hillier.
Hinsberg and Kast.
Hirsch.
Hirst.
Hirtz.
Hitchman.
Hodgson, A. L.
Hodgson, G. F.
Hogg.
Hogner.
Holloway. ·
Holt.
Hood.
Hooper.
Hope.
Hôpital St. Louis.
Horwitz.
Hôtel-Dieu.
Housman.
Howard.
Howe.
Huchard.
Hufeland.
Hull.
Hulse.
Hunter.
Hutchinson.
Hyde.

Icard.
Ihle.
Ingals.
Ingraham.

Jaccoud.
Jackson.
Jacobi.
Jamieson.
Janeway.
Jefferson Hospital, Phila.
Jenner.
Joffroy.
Johnson.
Johnston.
Jolly.
Jones, Wharton.
Jordan.
Joret et Homolle.
Jorie.
Jorissenne.
Joy.
Judkins.

Kaposi.
Kappesser.
Kassowitz.
Kennard.
Kennedy.
Kentish.
Kerner.
Kesteven.
Keyes.
Keyser.
Kilgour.
King.
Kingdon.
King's College Hospital.
Kinney.
Kinnicutt.
Kirk.
Klapp.
Knaggs.
Knoll.
Kobert.
Kobler.
Koebner.
Kolover.
Kopp.
Kortüm.
Kossobudski.
Krafft-Ebing.

Riggs.
Ringer.
Rivas.
Rivière.
Robert.
Robinson, Beverley.
Roche.
Rodet.
Rodgers.
Rodier.
Rolland.
Romanovsky.
Romberg
Roosa.
Roosevelt Hospital, N.Y.
Rosenbach.
Rosenberg.
Rosenthal.
Rothe.
Rouquette.
Roussel.
Runult.
Rudermacher.
Rudolphi.
Ruschenberger.
Rush.
Rust.
Ryan.

Saalfeld.
Sabbitine.
Saerbs.
Sajous.
Salter.
Sands.
Sansom.
Sarzance.
Sawyer.
Scarenzio.
Schafhirt.
Schenker.
Schilling.
Schmidiger.
Schmidt.
Schneck.
Schnitzler.
Schott
Schubarth.
Schwarz.
Scott and McCormac.
Scudamore.
Sedgwick.
Sée.
Seguin.
Seifert.
Seiler.
Selkirk.
Selldén.
Selwyn.
Semmola.
Seymour.
Shapter.
Shaw.
Shillitoe.
Shinn.
Shoemaker, J. V.
Silverthorn.
Simon.
Simpson.
Sinéty.
Skoda.
Smith, A. A.
Smith, A. H.
Smith, Charles.
Smith, Eustace.
Smith, F. A. A.
Smith, F. G.
Smith, H. H.
Smith, Hugh.
Smith, J. Lawrence.
Smith, J. Lewis.
Smith, Tyler.
Sobernheim.

Soden.
Sollard.
Solon.
Sonneberg.
Sonnenberger.
Soubeiran.
Soulez.
Sozinsky.
Spillmann.
Spitzka.
Squibb.
Squire, B.
Squire, P.
Starr.
Startin.
Stekoulia.
Stelwagon.
Stetter.
Stewart.
Stillé.
St. Luke's Hospital, N.Y.
Stokes.
Stone.
Stowell.
Strother.
Stroud.
Stubbs.
Stuckley.
Sturgis.
Styrap.
Suckling.
Sullivan.
Sully.
Sundelin.
Swediaur.
Sweringen.
Sylvestrini and Picchini.
Symonds.
Szadek.

Tait.
Tanner.
Tauret.
Tanturri.
Tardieu.
Taylor, R. W.
Teale.
Teixeira.
Terrillon.
Testivin.
Theiry.
Thibierge.
Thiersch.
Thomas.
Thomas, T. G.
Thompson, A. T.
Thompson, J. A.
Thomson, W. H.
Thor.
Thornton.
Thuries.
Todd.
Tortunl.
Tournie.
Troilius.
Trousseau.
Trousseau et Reveil.
Truman.
Trussewitsch.
Tucker.
Tuke.
Turnbull.
Tutt.
Tweedy.
Tyrell.
Tyson, J.

L'Union Médicale.
University Hospital.
Unna.
Ure.
Uspenski.

Valleix.
Van Buren.
Van Buren and Keys.
Van den Corput.
Van Goidtsnoven.
Van Harlingen.
Van Mons.
Vanoye.
Vecchizetti.
Velpeau.
Venot.
Vetlesen.
Vian.
Vidal.
Vigier.
Villate.
Villemin.
Vieminckx.
Vogt.
Von Mering.
Von Ziemssen.
Vulpian.

Waakes.
Walker.
Wallace.
Walsh.
Walshe.
Walter and Blundell.
Ward's Island Insane Asylum, N.Y.
Ware.
Warfinge.
Waring.
Waring-Curran.
Waterhouse.
Waters.
Watson.
Waugh.
Webb.
Weber.
Weir.
Weiss.
Weller.
Wells.
Wende.
West.
White, J. W.
Wicherkiewicz.
Wiehmann.
Widerhofer.
Widowitz.
Wils.
Wigan.
Wiglesworth.
Wilcox, R. W.
Wilde.
Wilkes.
Wilks.
Willard.
Williams.
Willis.
Wilson, Ellwood.
Wilson, Erasmus.
Wilson, J. C.
Winzar.
Woakes.
Wolf.
Wolfenden.
Wood, G. B.
Wood, H. C.
Wood, James.
Wooster.
Wright.
Wulfsberg.
Wyeth.

Young.
Yvon.

Zakrzhevski.

A

I.

FORMULÆ.

ABORTION, THREATENED.

1—℞ Tinct. opii . . . . ℥xx–xxx.
Sig. Mix with two or three tablespoonfuls of boiled starch
and inject into the rectum.   PARVIN.

2—℞ Ext. viburni prunif. fld. . . . . f℥iij.
Sig. A teaspoonful in a sherryglassful of water every four
hours.   JENKS.

3—℞ Tinct. opii deod. . . . . ℥lx.
Sodii bromidi . . . . ℥iij.
Chloral. hydrat. . . . . ℥iss.
Syr. acaciæ. . . . . f℥j.
Aquæ . . . . q. s. ad f℥iij.—M.
Sig. A dessertspoonful in water every four hours. E. WILSON.

4—℞ Ext. gland thyroid. . . . . ℥ij.
Fiant in tabellæ compressæ no. xl.
Sig. One three times daily. (*For threatened abortion with
hemorrhage.*)   CHÉRON.

5—℞ Potassii iodidi . . . . ℥j.
Aquæ . . . . f℥j.—M.
Sig. Twenty to forty drops in water or milk two or three
times a day. (*Habitual abortion. When due to syphilis.*)
                                                       J. C. WILSON.

6—℞ Mist. asafœtidæ . . . . ℥viij.
Sig. A tablespoonful several times daily. (*In habitual abortion.*)   NEGRI.

7—℞ Tinct. ferri chlor. . . . . ℥ss.
Potassii chloratis . . . . ℈iv.
Syr. simplicis . . . . ℥j.
Aquæ menth. pip. . . . . ad ℥iv.—M.
Sig. A dessertspoonful in a wineglassful of water after meals.
                                                       STROTHER.

ABSCESSES

8—℞ Iodoformi . . . . ℥iss–℥v.
Ætheris . . . . ℥vj.—M.
Inject three to five ounces after aspirating the abscess. (*In
tubercular abscess.*)   MOSETIG-MOORHOF.

9—℞ Iodoformi . . . . gr. xlviij.
Liq. petrolati . . . . f℥j.—M.
Sig. Inject into abscess cavity after washing out with H_2O_2
and bichloride solution 1–2000.

10—℞ Calcii sulphureti . . . . gr. vj.
Pulveris glycyrrhizæ . . . . q. s.
Fiat massa, in pilulas no. xii dividenda.
Sig. One pill every three hours.   WAUGH.

11—℞ Calcii sulphidi. . . . . gr. j.
Sacchari lactis . . . . gr. x.
Misce et fiant chartulæ no. x.
Sig. One powder every two hours.   RINGER.

12—℞ Sodii hypophosphitis . . . . ℈iv.
Calcii hypophosphitis . . . . ℈viij.
Syrupi simplicis . . . . f℥iss.
Aquæ fœniculi . . . . q. s. ad f℥iv.—M.
Sig. A dessertspoonful four times a day.   CHURCHILL.

ACIDITY. (See also Pyrosis.)

13—℞ Tinct. nucis vomicæ . . . . f3j.
Sig. Five drops a quarter of an hour before food
three times daily. RINGER.

14—℞ Infusi rhei . . . . f3iss.
      Sodii bicarb. . . . . 3iiss.
      Syr. aurantii cort. . . . . f3vj.—M.
Sig. A teaspoonful twice daily. EWALD.

15—℞ Pulv. Ipecac. . . . . gr. ss.
      Pulv. rhei . . . . gr. ij.
      Sodii bicarb. . . . . gr. xij.—M.
In chartulas no. xii. dividenda.
Sig. One powder every four to six hours to an infant one year
old. J. LEWIS SMITH.

16—℞ Sodii bicarb. . . . . 3j.
      Pulv. rhei . . . . 3ss.
      Spts. menth. pip. . . . . f3ij.
      Aquæ. . . . . q. s. ad f3iv.—M.
Sig. A tablespoonful after meals. (*For acidity combined with
constipation.*) *Bellevue Hosp.*

17—℞ Sodii bicarb. . . . . 3iij.
In pulveres no. xii dividenda.
Sig. A powder in a wineglassful of water after meals.
 ALONZO CLARK.

18—℞ Hydrargyri cum cretâ . . . . gr. iij.
      Bismuthi subnitratis . . . . gr. xij.
      Pulveris nucis myristicæ . . . . gr. iij.
Misce et divide in chartulas no. vi.
Sig. One powder morning and night. BARTHOLOW.

19—℞ Sodium sulphate . . . . 3j.
      Potassium sulphate . . . . 3iss.
      Sodium chloride . . . . 3j.
      Sodium carbonate . . . . 3vj.
      Sodium borate . . . . 3iiss.—M.
Sig. Half a teaspoonful in half a glassful of water before
breakfast and two hours before the other two meals. WOLFF.

20—℞ Spiritus ammoniæ aromatici . . . . f3iss.
      Spiritus ætheris compositi . . . . f3j.
      Syrupi zingiberis . . . . f3ij.
      Aquæ anisi . . . . f3iiiss.—M.
Sig. The one-third part, frequently repeated. DRUITT.

ACNE. (See also Skin Diseases.)

21—℞ Sulphuris iodidi . . . . 3ss.
      Adipis . . . . 3j.—M.
Sig. Use freely over the eruption night and morning. (*In acne
indurata and rosacea.*) RINGER.

22—℞ Naphthol β . . . . 3iiss.
      Sulphur. præcip. . . . . 3ss.
      Vaselin. vel lanolin.,
      Sapon. viridis . . . . ãã 3ij.—M.
Leniter terendo fiat pasta.
Sig. Spread a thin layer on affected skin and leave for fifteen
to twenty minutes; then rub off the ointment and dust with
powdered talc. LASSAR.

23—℞ Hydrarg. protoiodid. . . . . gr. v-xv.
      Hydrarg. ammon. . . . . gr. x-xxx.
      Ung. simplicis . . . . 3j.—M.
Sig. Externally. DUHRING.

24—℞ Liq. potassæ . . . . f3j.
      Aquæ rosæ . . . . f3iv.—M.
Sig. Apply with a soft sponge twice daily. BARTHOLOW.

25—℞ Acidi nitrohydrochlorici diluti . . . . . f3iss.
      Syrupi simplicis . . . . f3iss.
      Aquæ aurantii florum . . . . . . q. s. ad f3iv.—M.
Sig. A dessertspoonful three times a day. DA COSTA.

ACNE (Continued).

26—℞ Syrupi hypophosphitum compositi . . . f ℥iv.
Sig. A dessertspoonful thrice daily. DA COSTA.

ADENITIS.

27—℞ Syr. ferri iodidi . . . . f ℥j.
Sig. Ten to thirty drops in water thrice daily. J. C. WILSON.

28—℞ Ichthyol. . . . . ℨij.
Adipis . . . . ℥j.—M.
Sig. Apply twice daily. COHEN.

AGALACTIA.

29—℞ Ext. pilocarpi fld. . . . . f ℥ij.
Sig. A teaspoonful two or three times daily. BARTHOLOW.

30—℞ Ext. gland thyroid. . . . . ℨij.
Fiant in tabellæ compressæ no. xl.
Sig. One twice daily. CHÉRON.

31—℞ Ricinis communis fol. . . . . ℨij.
Aquæ bullientis . . . . f ℥vilj.—M.
Sig. Make an infusion and apply as a fomentation to the
breasts. TANNER.

ALBUMINURIA (Bright's Disease).

32—℞ Liq. trinitrin. (1 per cent.) . . . . f ℥j.
Sig. Three drops in water three times a day. BARTHOLOW.

33—℞ Auri et sodii chlor. . . . . gr. ij.
Hydrarg. chlor. corr. . . . . gr. v.
Ext. gentian. . . . . q. s.—M.
Ft. massa et in pil. no. lx div.
Sig. One pill morning and evening. BARTHOLOW.

34—℞ Methylene blue . . . . gr. xxiv.
Pone in capsulas no. xxiv.
Sig. One three times daily. H. TUCKER.

35—℞ Potassii iodidi . . . . ℨiss.
Syrupi simplicis . . . . f ℥ss.
Aquæ cinnamomi . . . . q. s. ad f ℥ij.—M.
Sig. A teaspoonful three times a day. GOLDBERG.

36—℞ Tincturæ ferri chloridi . . . . f ℥iij.
Acidi acetici diluti . . . . f ℥lj.
Syrupi simplicis . . . . f ℥iss.
Liquoris ammonii acetatis . . . . q. s. ad f ℥iv.—M.
Sig. A dessertspoonful every six hours. BASHAM.

37—℞ Spiritus ammoniæ aromatici . . . . . . f ℥j.
Sig. Half teaspoonful in water before meals.

38—℞ Acidi gallici . . . . ℨj-ij.
Acidi sulphurici dil. . . . . f ℥ss.
Tinct. lupuli . . . . f ℥j.
Infusi lupuli . . . . ad f ℥vj.—M.
Sig. A tablespoonful thrice daily. (*If urine is smoky.*)
AITKEN.

39—℞ Ferri sulphat. . . . . ℈j.
Ext. nucis vom. . . . . gr. x-℈j.
Pil. galbani co. . . . . ℈ij-iij.—M.
Ft. massa et in pil. no. xx div.
Sig. A pill twice or thrice daily. (*When dyspeptic symptoms
arise.*) GOODFELLOW.

40—℞ Tinct. strophanthi hisp. (1-20) . . . . . . f ℥ss.
Sig. Five to ten drops in water three times daily. (*When
there is a weak rapid pulse, scanty secretion, and dyspnœa.*)
PINS.

41—℞ Ol. erigerontis . . . . f ℥ss.
Sig. Five drops on a lump of sugar every three or four hours.
(*In the chronic forms.*) BARTHOLOW.

ALBUMINURIA (Continued).

42—℞ Sparteine sulphat. . . . . gr. iij.
Caffeine citrat. . . . . gr. xxiv.
Infusion digitalis . . . . f3vj.—M.
Sig. ½ ounce three times daily.   H. Tucker.

ALCOHOLISM.

43—℞ Hydrarg. chl. mitis . . . . gr. j.
Sacch. lactis . . . . gr. iij.
M. et in chtt. no. vi div.
Sig. One powder every hour.   J. C. Wilson.

44—℞ Codeinæ . . . . gr. iij.
Camphor. monobrom. . . . . gr. xij.
M. et in pil. no. xii div.
Sig. One pill every two or three hours.   J. C. Wilson.

45—℞ Paraldehydi . . . . f3vj.
Mucilag. acaciæ,
Spts. vini gallici . . . . āā f3ij.—M.
Sig. Shake the vial. A tablespoonful to induce quiet and
sleep; repeat in an hour if necessary.   J. C. Wilson.

46—℞ Spts. ammon. aromat. . . . . f3ij.
Tinct. camphoræ . . . . f3iss.
Tinct. hyoscyami . . . . f3iiss.
Spts. lavandulæ co. . . . . q. s. ad f3ij.—M.
Sig. A teaspoonful every hour till relieved. Then give—

47—℞ Pulv. capsici . . . . gr. ij.
Quininæ sulph. . . . . gr. iij.—M.
Ft. pulv. no. i.
To be taken before each meal for several days. If sleepless-
ness, then give—

48—℞ Tincturæ nucis vomicæ . . . . f3j.
Acidi hydrochlorici diluti . . . . f3jv.
Tincturæ capsici . . . . f3j.
Tincturæ gentianæ compositæ . . q. s. ad f3ij.—M.
Sig. Two teaspoonfuls in water before meals. (*To improve ap-
petite and digestion after an alcoholic debauch.*)

49—℞ Tinct. gentianæ co.,
Tinct. calumbæ co. . . . . āā f3ij.
Tinct. nucis vom. . . . . ℳxxx.—M.
Sig. A dessertspoonful before each meal.   Loomis.

50—℞ Strychninæ sulph. . . . . gr. j.
Aquæ font. . . . . 3j.—M.
Sig. Five minims, increased cautiously to twenty minims,
hypodermically twice daily. (*In both acute and chronic
forms.*)   Dobronravoff.

51—℞ Zinci oxidi . . . . 3j.
Piperinæ . . . . 3j.
Misce et fiant pilulæ no. xx.
Sig. One pill three or four times a day.   Chapman.

52—℞ Sol. nitro-glycerin. (1 per cent.) . . . . . f3ij.
Sig. One drop every two hours. (*In acute form, with cerebral
anæmia and intense depression.*)   Van Goidtsnoven.

ALOPECIA.

53—℞ Spts. æther. 110.00
Tinct. benzoin. . . . . 15.00.—M.
Sig. Apply once a day.   Hebra

54—℞ Tinct. capsici . . . . f3ss.
Tinct. saponariæ quill. . . . . f3j.
Glycerini . . . . 3ij.
Tinct. cantharidis . . . . f3iij.
Spiritus rosmarini . . . . f3iss.
Aquæ rosæ . . . . ad f3viij.—M.
Sig. Drop on the hair night and morning.   Shoemaker.

55—℞ Quininæ sulphatis . . . . gr. xl.
    Tincturæ cantharidis . . . . f3j.
    Spiritus ammonii aromatici . . . . f3j.
    Olei ricini . . . . f3iss.
    Spiritus myrciæ . . . . f3vss.
    Olei rosmarini . . . . gtt. vj.
Fiat mistura.
Sig. Shake well. Apply once a day.   J. C. WILSON.

56—℞ Chrysarobin . . . . gr. xlviij.
    Lanolin . . . . 3j.—M.
Fiant in ungt.
Sig. Rub into affected area.   H. TUCKER.

57—℞ Tinct. cantharidis . . . . f3iss.
    Tinct. capsici . . . . Mlxx.
    Glycerini . . . . f3ss.
    Spts. odoratæ . . . . ad f3vj.—M.
Sig. Apply to the head two or three times daily.   GROSS.

58—℞ Tinct. macis . . . . f3iss.
    Olei olivæ . . . . ad f3ij.—M.
Sig. Apply two or three times daily to affected spots. HEBRA.

59—℞ Quininæ sulphat. . . . . 9iv.
    Spiritus vini rectif. . . . . f3iv.
    Tinct. capsici,
    Tinct. cantharidis,
    Spts. ammon. arom. . . . . āā f3ss.
    Glycerini . . . . f3iv.
    Aquæ. . . . . q. s. ad ft. Oj.—M.
Sig. Apply locally.   BRINTON.

60—℞ Tinct. cantharidis . . . . f3ss.
    Olei ricini . . . . f3iv.—M.
Sig. Rub well into roots of hair night and morning. WARING.

61—℞ Acidi acetici,
    Chloroformi . . . . āā f3j.—M.
Sig. Shake and apply to affected area two or three times a
week. (*For chronic cases of alopecia areata.*)

62—℞ Hydrarg. sulphat. flav.,
    Sulphuris loti . . . . āā 3j.
    Vaselini . . . . 3x.—M.
Ft. ungt.
Rub in the affected spots, after washing with soap and warm
water, thrice daily. When nearly well, use the following :

63—℞ Acidi boracici . . . . 3ij.
    Spts. camphoræ,
    Olei terebinthinæ . . . . āā f3xiiss.
    Aquæ coloniensis . . . . f3iv 3vj.-M.
Ft. lotio.
Rub in locally morning and evening.   ROUQUETTE.

AMAUROSIS (Functional).

64—℞ Strychninæ sulphatis . . . . gr. j.
    Confectionis rosæ . . . . q. s.
Fiat massa, in pilulas no. xxx dividenda.
Sig. One pill after each meal.   MAGENDIE.

65—℞ Aloini . . . . gr. vj.
    Ferri sulphatis exsiccati . . . . gr. xxiv.
    Asafœtidæ . . . . gr. xxiv.
Misce et fiant pilulæ no. xxiv.
Sig. One pill after meals.

66—℞ Potassii iodidi . . . . 3j.
    Aquæ . . . . f3j.—M.
Sig. Twenty to forty drops in water three times a day. LEVIS.

67—℞ Pilocarpinæ muriatis . . . . gr. j.
In pil. no. viii div.
Sig. One pill every three hours.   LEVIS.

68—℞ Manganesii binoxidi . . . . ℨj.
Fiat massa et in pil. no. xxx div.
Sig. One pill three times daily after meals.　　F. Barker.

69—℞ Ext. aloë aq. . . . . ℨj.
　　Ferri sulph. exsic. . . . . ℨij.
　　Asafœtidæ . . . . ℨiv.—M.
Ft. massa et in pilulæ no. c div.
Sig. One pill after each meal, gradually increased to three.
　　　　　　　　　　　　　　　　　　　　　　Goodell.

70—℞ Tinct. ferri muriat. . . . . ℨiij.
　　Tinct. cantharidis . . . . ℨj.
　　Tinct. guaiaci ammon. . . . . ℨiss.
　　Tinct. aloës. . . . . ℨss.
　　Syrupi . . . . q. s. ad ℨvj.—M.
Sig. A tablespoonful thrice daily.　　　　Dewees.

71—℞ Myrrhæ . . . . gr. viij.
　　Pulveris jalapæ . . . . gr. xv.
　　Ferri sulphatis exsiccatæ,
　　Pulveris aloës et canellæ . . . . . . āā ℨj.
　　Syrupi simplicis . . . . q. s.
Fiat massa et divide in pilulas l.
Sig. Two or three pills at bedtime, for several nights succes-
　　sively.　　　　　　　　　　　　　　　Chapman.

72—℞ Potassii carbonatis . . . . ℨss.
　　Myrrhæ . . . . ℨj.
Tere simul, dein adde—
　　Ferri sulphatis,
　　Sacchari albi. . . . . āā ℨss.
Fiat massa et divide in pilulas xl.
Sig. Two or three pills three times a day.　　Hulse.

73—℞ Apiolis . . . . ℨj.
Pone in capsul. no. xx.
Sig. One three times a day.　　　　H. A. Hare.

74—℞ Pulveris sabinæ,
　　Pulveris zingiberis . . . . āā gr. vj.
　　Sodii biboratis . . . . gr. xv.
Misce et fiat pulvis.
Sig. Two powders daily, morning and evening.　　Thomson.

75—℞ Iodi . . . . ℈ij.
　　Spiritus lavandulæ compositi . . . . . . f'ℨij.
　　Spiritus vini . . . . f'ℨj.
Fiat tinctura.
Sig. From five to ten drops in sweetened water twice a
　　day, gradually and cautiously increasing the dose.
　　　　　　　　　　　　　　　　　S. G. Morton.

76—℞ Tabellas extracti thyroidei no. xxiv . āā gr. v.
Sig. One tablet after meals.

77—℞ Acidi oxalici . . . . gr. xx.
　　Syr. aurantii cort. . . . . ℨij.
　　Aquæ ferv. . . . . ad ℨviij.—M.
Sig. A tablespoonful every hour at the time of the usual men-
　　strual period.　　　　　　　　　　Poulet.

78—℞ Tinct. aconiti radicis . . . . ℨss.
Sig. One drop every hour. (*When checked by cold.*)　Ringer.

79—℞ Salicini . . . . gr. xv.
　　Pulv. rhei . . . . gr. viiss.
　　Confect. rosæ . . . . q. s. ut ft. massa.—M.
Ft. massa et in pil. no. x div.
Sig. One thrice daily.　　　　　　　De Mussy.

80—℞ Terebinthinæ alb.,
　　Pulv. aloës,
　　Ferri sulph. exsic. . . . . āā ℈j.—M.
Ft. massa et in pil. no. xx div.
Sig. One thrice daily.　　　　　　　Parvin.

81—℞ Ferri sesquibromidi . . . . ℨj.

Fiant capsulæ no. xii.
Sig. A capsule after meals.   HECKET.

82—℞ Hydrarg. chlor. corr. . . . . gr. i-ij.
    Liq. arsenici chlor. . . . . ℨj.
    Tinct. ferri chlor. . . . . ℨiv.
    Acidi hydrochlor. dil. . . . . ℨiv.
    Syrupi . . . . ℨiij.
    Aquæ . . . . ad ℨvj.—M.

Sig. A dessertspoonful in a wineglassful of water after
    meals.   A. H. SMITH.

83—℞ Strychninæ sulphatis . . . . gr. j.
    Acidi arseniosi . . . . gr. ij.
    Extracti belladonnæ . . . . gr. v.
    Quininæ sulphatis,
    Pulveris ferri . . . . āā ℈ij.
    Extracti taraxaci . . . . ℨss.
Misce et fiant pilulæ no. xl.
Sig. One pill after each meal.   FRANCIS GURNEY SMITH.

84—℞ Sodium bicarbonate,
    Calcium phosphate,
    Sodium chloride,
    Sugar . . . . āā gr. iiiss.
    Reduced iron . . . . gr. iij.—M.
Make one cachet.
Sig. From four to six daily.   LUTAUD.

85—℞ Syrupi ferri iodidi . . . . fℨij.
    Syrupi zingiberis . . . . fℨj.
    Aquæ destillatæ . . . . fℨv.—M.
Sig. A tablespoonful three times a day.   R. M'GREGOR.

86—℞ Quininæ sulph. . . . . gr. xx.
    Ferri sulph. exsiccat. . . . . gr. xl.
    Strychninæ sulph. . . . . gr. ss.—M.
Ft. massa et in pilulas no. xx div.
Sig. One pill thrice daily.'   BARTHOLOW.

87—℞ Ferri sulph. exsiccat.,
    Potassii carbonat. . . . . āā ℨj.
    Syrupi . . . . q. s. ut ft. massa.—M.
Ft. massa et in pil. no. xxiv div.
Sig. One pill after meals.   BLAUD.

88—℞ Tincturæ ferri chloridi . . . . fℨiiss.
    Acidi phosphorici diluti . . . . fℨiiiss.
    Syrupi acidi citratis . . . . . . q. s. ad fℨiv.—M.
Sig. A dessertspoonful in water three times a day. GOODELL.

89—℞ Tabellas ferratini no. c . . . . āā gr. v.
Sig. One to two tablets after meals.

90—℞ Pulveris ipecacuanhæ . . . . gr. vj.
    Hydrargyri cum cretâ . . . . gr. xij.
    Ferri subcarbonatis . . . . gr. xlviij.
Misce et divide in pulveres vi.
Sig. One powder twice a day.   S. ASHWELL.

91—℞ Extracti glandulæ suprarenalis . . . . ℨij.
Pone in capsulas no. xxiv.
Sig. One capsule after meals.   (In pernicious anæmia.)

92—℞ Emuls. amygdalæ amar. . . . . ℨx.
    Pulpæ spleniæ . . . . ℨiv.
    Spts. vini gallici . . . . ℨij.—M.
Sig. To be given in the twenty-four hours.   MARAGLIANO.

ANEURISM.

93—℞ Potassii iodidi . . . . ℨj. (!)
    Syrupi simplicis . . . . fℨj.
    Aquæ destillatæ . . . . q. s. ad fℨiij.—M.
Sig. A teaspoonful three or four times a day, largely diluted.
                                               BALFOUR.

ANEURISM (Continued).

94—℞ Antipyrin. . . . . ʒiss.
    Syr. tolutan. . . . . ʒiss.
    Aquæ. . . . . ad ʒiij.—M.
Sig. A tablespoonful at intervals of one to four hours until relieved. (*For cardiac pains.*)   GERMAIN SÉE.

95—℞ Tincturæ veratri viridis . . . . fʒj.
    Tincturæ opii deodoratæ. . . . . fʒiss.
    Syrupi simplicis . . . . fʒvss.
    Aquæ destillatæ . . . . fʒj.—M.
Sig. A teaspoonful every two, three, or four hours, cautiously.
    DA COSTA.

96—℞ Tincturæ digitalis . . . . fʒss.
    Extracti ergotæ fluidi . . . . fʒiiiss.—M.
Sig. A teaspoonful three times a day.   DA COSTA.

ANGINA PECTORIS.

97—℞ Amyli nitritis . . . . fʒj.
Sig. From two to five drops to be inhaled from a clean handkerchief.   BRUNTON.

98—℞ Methylal . . . . ʒix.
    Amyli nitritis . . . . ʒj.—M.
Sig. Drop thirty or forty drops on a handkerchief and inhale. Repeat if necessary.   RICHARDSON.

99—℞ Antipyrin. . . . . ʒj.
    Syr. tolutan. . . . . ʒj.
    Aquæ. . . . . ad ʒij.—M.
Sig. A tablespoonful at intervals of one to four hours until relieved.   GERMAIN SÉE.

100—℞ Pyridin. . . . . ʒss.
Sig. Six to ten drops daily, increasing to twenty-five drops, well diluted with water. Or five to ten drops may be inhaled.
    DE RENZI.

101—℞ Zinci cyanidi. . . . . gr. iv-v.
    Confect. rosæ. . . . . q. s.—M.
In pilulas no. xl div.
Sig. One pill three times daily.   LASHKEVITCH.

102—℞ Sol. nitro-glycerin. (1 per cent.) . . . . ʒss.
Sig. One to two drops internally. (*When pallor of face exists.*)
    WM. PEPPER.

103—℞ Nitro-glycerin. . . . . grs. iij.
    Tinct. capsici . . . . ʒss.
    Spir. rectificat.,
    Aq. menth. pip. . . . . āā ʒiij.
Sig. Two to ten drops.   SCHOTT.

104—℞ Tincturæ digitalis . . . . fʒiiss.
    Spiritus chloroformi . . . . fʒvj.
    Extracti buchu fluidi . . . . fʒj.
    Spiritus juniperi compositi . . . q. s. ad fʒiv.—M.
Sig. A dessertspoonful three times a day.   FOTHERGILL.

105—℞ Quininæ muriatis . . . . ʒj.
In pilulas no. xx div.
Sig. Four pills daily.   J. C. WILSON.

ANTHRAX.

106—℞ Acidi carbolici . . . . ♏xx-xxv.
    Aquæ. . . . . ʒj.—M.
Sig. Inject a few drops into and around the pustule. USPENSKI.

107—℞ Cresol-antolis . . . . gr. v.
    Aquæ . . . . fʒj.—M.
Sig. Shake well and inject a few drops in several places, from the border of the infiltration towards the centre of the patch.

APHTHÆ.

108—℞ Mel. boracis . . . . ʒj.
Sig. Apply to patches with a brush.   RINGER.

APHTILÆ (Continued).

109—℞ Formaldchydi (40 per cent. sol.) . . . . gtt. xv.
    Aquæ hydrogeni dioxidi . . . . f ʒvj.
Sig. Two teaspoonfuls in half-glass of water every two or three hours.

110—℞ Potassii chloratis . . . . Ðij.
    Tincturæ ferri chloridi : . . . . f ʒj.
    Syrupi simplicis . . . . f ʒvj.
    Aquæ cinnamomi . . . . . . q. s. ad f ʒij.—M.
Sig. A teaspoonful e ery two hours for a child two years old.
                      STUBBS.

111—℞ Tinct. myrrhæ . . . . f ʒij.
    Aquæ. . . . . q. s. f ʒij.—M.
Sig. A teaspoonful in wineglassful of water when needed for mouth-wash.
                      BRINTON.

112—℞ Zinci chloridi . . . . gr. iij-xv.
    Alcohol diluti . . . . f ʒviij.—M.
Sig. Gargle and mouth-wash. (*The weakest strength for infants; the strongest for adults.*)
                      JULES SIMON.

113—℞ Argenti nitratis . . . . gr. xlv.
    Aquæ . . . . f ʒj.—M.
Sig. Use locally.
                      STELWAGON.

114—℞ Acidi hydrochlorici diluti . . . . ℳxx.
    Syrupi simplicis . . . . f ʒss.
    Aquæ destillatæ . . . . q. s. ad f ʒij.—M.
Sig. Two teaspoonfuls every two hours.
                      J. C. WILSON.

115—℞ Acid. pyrolig. . . . . ʒj
    Aquæ . . . . f ʒviij.—M.
Sig. Wash the mouth every four hours. (*For mucous patches.*)
                      HORWITZ.

116—℞ Papain. . . . . gr. xxx.
    Glycerini . . . . f ʒiiss.
    Aquæ destillatæ . . . . ad f ʒv.—M.
Sig. Apply four or five times daily with a brush on the white patches.
                      SCHMIDIGER.

117—℞ Sodii salicylat. . . . . ʒiss.
    Aquæ destillatæ . . . . f ʒj.—M.
Sig. Apply five or six times daily.
                      HIRTZ.

ASTHENIA.

118—℞ Quininæ sulphat. . . . . gr. xxx.
    Acidi sulphur. dil. . . . . q. s.
    Aquæ . . . . ʒij.
    Tinct. ferri mur. . . . . ʒss.
    Spts. chloroformi . . . . ʒvj.
    Glycerini . . . . ad ʒiv.—M.
Sig. A teaspoonful three times daily.
                      LOOMIS.

119—℞ Elixiris phosphori . . . . f ʒij.
Sig. Teaspoonful in water two hours after meals.

120—℞ Vini cocæ . . . . f ʒviij.
Sig. A tablespoonful three times a day.   J. C. WILSON.

121—℞ Tinct. nucis vomicæ . . . . f ʒj.
Sig. Ten to fifteen drops in wine of coca three or four times a day.
                      J. C. WILSON.

ASTHMA.

122—℞ Syrupi hypophosphitum comp. . . . . f ʒiss.
    Syrupi acidi hydriodici . . . . . . f ʒvj.
    Extr. euphorbiæ piluliferæ fluid. . . . . f ʒvj.
    Extr. nucis vomicæ fluid. . . . . . . f ʒj.
    Syrupi simplicis . . . . f ʒj.
    Aquæ destillatæ . . . . f ʒij.—M.
Sig. A tablespoonful every three hours. Shake well.
                      JOHNSON.

ASTHMA (Continued).

123—℞ Infusi quebracho. . . . . 3iij–3iij.
  Potassii iodidi . . . . ℈ij.
  Tinct. opii camphorati . . . . f3ij.—M.
Sig. A tablespoonful every two hours.   KRUTOVSKI.

124—℞ Ext. euphorbiæ piluliferæ fluid. . . . . 3j.
Sig. Thirty to sixty drops as required.   PAYNE.

125—℞ Tinct. sanguinariæ,
  Tinct. lobeliæ,
  Ammonii iodidi . . . . āā 3j.
  Syr. tolutani . . . . 3vj.—M.
Sig. A teaspoonful every two to four hours.   (In humid asthma.)   BARTHOLOW.

126—℞ Tinc. lobeliæ æthereæ . . . . ♏xv.
  Spirit. ætheris . . . . ♏xx.
  Tinc. chlorof. comp. . . . . ♏v.
  Aquæ camphoræ . . . . ad 3j.—M.
Sig. To be taken when breathing is difficult.

127—℞ Antipyrin . . . . gr. xv.
  Pyridine . . . . 3j.
  Sodium nitrate . . . . 3ij.
  Tincture belladonna,
  Tincture lobelia,
  Tincture stramonium,
  Tincture ipecac . . . . āā 3v.
  Glycerin . . . . q. s. ad 3iv.—M.
Sig. Nebulized and inhaled.   F. T. RODGERS.

128—℞ Potassii iodidi . . . . 3ss.
  Tinct. gentian. co. . . . . 3iij.—M.
Sig. One teaspoonful, gradually increased to two teaspoonfuls, three times daily for several months. ALONZO CLARK.

129—℞ Chloral. hydratis . . . . 3vj.
  Syrupi tolutani . . . . f3j.
  Aquæ fœniculi . . . . q. s. ad f3ij.—M.
Sig. A teaspoonful every half-hour or hour, until relieved.   S. WEIR MITCHELL.

130—℞ Ammonii bromidi . . . . 3viij.
  Ammonii chloridi . . . . 3iss.
  Tinct. lobeliæ . . . . 3iij.
  Spts. ætheris eo. . . . . 3j.
  Syr. acaciæ . . . . ad 3iv.—M.
Sig. A dessertspoonful in water every hour or two during paroxysm.   PEPPER.

131—℞ Amyli nitritis . . . . 3j.
Sig. Inhale three to five drops from a handkerchief. FRASER.

132—℞ Pyridin. . . . . 3j.
Sig. Put on a hot plate in a small room, and send patient to inhale the vapor several times.   GERMAIN SÉE.

133—℞ Potassii iodidi,
  Chloral. hydrat. . . . . āā 3j.
  Syr. aurantii cort. . . . . 3j.
  Aquæ aurantii flor. . . . . ad 3ij.—M.
Sig. A tablespoonful once or twice during the attack.   LAZARUS.

134—℞ Foliorum belladonnæ,
  Foliorum hyoscyami . . . . āā gr. iij.
  Extracti opii aquosi . . . . gr. ¼.
  Aquæ laurocerasi . . . . q. s.
Sig. Moisten the leaves with a solution of the opium extract in the cherry-laurel water. Let them dry thoroughly and roll into a cigarette. Two to four of these cigarettes may be smoked every day.   TROUSSEAU.

135—℞ Potassii iodidi . . . . 3viiss.
  Tinct. lobeliæ . . . . 3viiss.
  Aquæ destillatæ . . . . 3xvss.—M.
Sig. From a teaspoonful to a tablespoonful in a glass of beer before meals.   DUJARDIN-BEAUMETZ.

B

BERI-BERI.

136—℞ Pilocarpinæ mur. . . . . gr. iij.
Aquæ font. . . . . ℥iv.—M.
Sig. Ten to twenty minims hypodermically.　LODEWYKS.

BILIOUSNESS.

137—℞ Podophyllin.,
Pulv. zingiberis . . . . āā gr. xij.
Mellis . . . . q. s. ut ft. massa.—M.
Ft. massa et in pil. no. xxxvi div.　C. PAUL.

138—℞ Ammonii chloridi . . . . gr. xxiij.
Sig. To be taken thrice daily in a glass of fresh milk.
MURCHISON.

139—℞ Acidi nitromuriat. dil. . . . . f℥j.
Sig. Ten or fifteen drops, well diluted, before meals.
BARTHOLOW.

140—℞ Massæ hydrargyri,
Ext. colocynth. co. . . . . āā ℈ij.
Ext. hyoscyami . . . . ℈ss.—M.
Ft. massa et in pil. no. xx div.
Sig. Two pills at bedtime, followed by a saline cathartic be-
fore breakfast.　DARRACH.

141—℞ Ext. chiratæ . . . . gr. xl.
Podophyllin . . . . gr. iv.
Euonymin . . . . gr. viij.
Leptandrin . . . . gr. viij.
Creasoti . . . . gr. x.
M. et fiant in pill. no. xx.
Sig. One at night.　H. A. HARE.

142—℞ Pulveris ipecacuanhæ . . . . gr. iij.
Massæ hydrargyri . . . . gr. viij.
Extracti colocynthidis compositi . . . . gr. xvj.
Misce et divide in pilulas no. viii.
Sig. One pill night and morning.　PENDLETON TUTT.

143—℞ Fellis bovini purificati . . . . ℨj.
Manganesii sulphatis exsiccati . . . . . ℈ij.
Resinæ podophylli . . . . gr. v.
Misce et fiant pilulæ no. xx.
Sig. One pill three times a day.　(In catarrhal jaundice.)
DA COSTA.

144—℞ Extracti hydrastis fluidi . . . . f℥iss.
Tincturæ rhei . . . . f℥viss.
Tincturæ cinchonæ compositæ. . . . . f℥iij.—M.
Sig. A dessertspoonful two or three times a day.　NIEMEYER.

145—℞ Saloli . . . . ℈iv.
Fiant chartulæ no. xxiv.
Sig. One powder before meals.

BITES OF SNAKES.

146—℞ Potassii permanganat. . . . . ℨj.
Aquæ. . . . . f℥vi.—M.
Sig. Apply freely to the wound, and inject hypodermically
above the seat of the wound.　HAWACK.

147—℞ Strychninæ . . . . gr. j.
Glycerini . . . . ♏xx.
Aquæ . . . . f℥ss.
Sig. ♏xx hypodermically every ten or twenty minutes till
slight muscular spasms result.　MUELLER.

148—℞ Aquæ ammoniæ . . . . ♏xxx.
Aquæ. . . . . f℥iss.—M.
To be injected into the vein with hypodermic syringe.
HALFORD.

149—℞ Tinct. iodi . . . . f℥j.
Sig. Apply freely to the wound.　S. WEIR MITCHELL.

BLADDER, AFFECTIONS OF. (See Catarrh.)

BOILS. (See Abscess.)

BRIGHT'S DISEASE. (See Albuminuria.)

BROMIDROSIS.

150—℞ Ext. geranii mac. fld. . . . . ʒij.
   Sig. For external use.   PEPPER.

151—℞ Pulv. acid. salicylici . . . . gr. x-xx.
   Pulv. acid. borici . . . . ʒij.
   Pulv. amyli . . . . ʒvj.—M.
   Sig. Dusting powder.   STELWAGON.

152—℞ Sodii biborat. . . . . ʒss.
   Resorcin. . . . . ʒj.—M.
   Sig. Use as a dusting-powder.   J. C. WILSON.

153—℞ Tinct. belladonnæ . . . . f ʒss.
   Sig. Three drops three times a day in water; gradually increase to six drops.   J. C. WILSON.

BRONCHITIS.

154—℞ Terpin. hydrat. . . . . ʒj.
   In pil. no. xxx div.
   Sig. Two or three pills every three or four hours.
                        J. C. WILSON.

155—℞ Sol. hydrogen. dioxidi (10 vol.) . . . . . ʒij.
   Sig. A teaspoonful in a glassful of water three times daily.
   (*In chronic bronchitis with dyspnœa.*)   DE BLEYER.

156—℞ Codeinæ . . . . gr. iv.
   Acid. hydrocyanic. dilut. . . . . gtt. xlv.
   Ammonii chloridi . . . . gr. xlv.
   Syrupæ pruni virginiani . . . . f ʒiss.—M.
   Sig. Dose, a teaspoonful every three or four hours.
               Amer. Medico-Surg. Bulletin.

157—℞ Potassii cyanidi . . . . gr. j.
   Syrupi limonis . . . . f ʒss.
   Aquæ destillatæ . . . . f ʒiliss.—M.
   Sig. A tablespoonful every two hours. (*In spasmodic cough with vomiting.*)   DONOVAN.

158—℞ Syrupi lactucarii . . . . f ʒij.
   Syrupi acaciæ . . . . f ʒiss.
   Syrupi aurantii florum . . . . f ʒss.—M.
   Sig. A teaspoonful every three hours. (*In senile catarrh.*)
                  AUBERGIER.

159—℞ Pulveris scillæ,
   Extracti conii . . . . āā ʒss.
   Ammoniaci . . . . ʒj.
   Fiat massa et divide in pilulas no. xxx.
   Sig. One pill every four hours.   PARISET.

160—℞ Pulveris ipecacuanhæ . . . . gr. vj.
   Pulveris myrrhæ. . . . . gr. xij.
   Potassii nitratis . . . . ʒss.
   Misce et divide in partes vi.
   Sig. One every fourth hour. (*For elderly persons.*)   PARIS.

161—℞ Tincturæ veratri viridis . . . . ♏xv.
   Syrupi ipecacuanhæ,
   Spiritus ætheris nitrosi . . . . āā f ʒss.—M.
   Sig. Fifteen drops every three hours. (*For a child one to two years old.*)   B. F. SCHNECK.

162—℞ Morphinæ acetatis . . . . gr. iij.
   Tincturæ sanguinariæ . . . . f ʒij.
   Vini antimonii,
   Vini ipecacuanhæ . . . . āā f ʒiij.
   Syrupi pruni virginianæ . . . . f ʒiij.—M.
   Sig. A teaspoonful.   J. C. AYER.

163—℞ Ammonium chloride . . . . ʒij.
　　　Fluid extract grindelia,
　　　Fluid extract quebracho,
　　　Fluid extract lobelia . . . . āā fʒss.
　　　Comp. licorice mixture . . . . f ʒiss.—M.
　　Sig. The mixture is to be well shaken and a teaspoonful ad-
　　ministered every three hours. ESHNER.

164—℞ Aquæ laurocerasi . . . . fʒij.
　　　Extracti glycyrrhizæ fluidi . . . . . . fʒj.
　　　Syrupi althææ . . . . fʒij.
　　　Decocti althææ . . . . .q. s. ad fʒvj.—M.
　　Sig. A tablespoonful every two or three hours. LIEBREICH.

165—℞ Olei santali . . . . fʒj.
　　Pone in capsulas no. xx.
　　Sig. One capsule every four hours.

166—℞ Vini ipecac. . . . . fʒij.
　　　Vini antimonialis . . . . fʒj.
　　　Vini xerici . . . . fʒiij.—M.
　　Sig. Three drops every hour to a child six months old.
　　(*Where larger tubes only are affected*) DESSAU.

167—℞ Terebene . . . . fʒss.
　　Sig. Two to five drops on sugar every four hours, according
　　to child's age. (*In chronic form.*) CARMICHAEL.

168—℞ Tinct. aconiti rad. . . . . fʒss.
　　Sig. One or two drops every hour. (*In severe cases with fever,
　　where medium and small tubes are affected.*) DESSAU.

169—℞ Pulveris ipecacuanhæ et opii . . . . . . gr. x.
　　Pone in capsulas no. iv.
　　Sig. Take the capsules upon going to bed, also lemonade with
　　hot whiskey.

170—℞ Ergotini . . . . ʒss-j.
　　　Glycerini . . . . fʒj.
　　　Aquæ . . . . ad fʒij.—M.
　　Sig. A teaspoonful at night. (*For violent and persistent cough.*)
　　　ALLAN.

171—℞ Capsulæ morrhuol. . . . . no. xxiv.
　　Sig. One capsule after meals and at bedtime. (*In chronic
　　form of adults.*) LAFARGUE.

172—℞ Vini ipecac. . . . . fʒj.
　　　Tinct. scillæ . . . . fʒij.
　　　Syr. tolutani . . . . fʒv.
　　　Aquæ . . . . fʒj.—M.
　　Sig. A teaspoonful every three or four hours. DELAFIELD.

173—℞ Vini ipecac. . . . . fʒij.
　　　Liq. potass. citratis . . . . fʒiv.
　　　Tinct. opii camph.,
　　　Syr. acaciæ . . . . āā fʒj.—M.
　　Sig. A tablespoonful three times daily. (*In first stage of ordi-
　　nary acute bronchitis.*) DA COSTA.

174—℞ Acidi salicylici . . . . ʒij.
　　　Ammonii carbonatis . . . . ʒvj.
　　　Syrupi simplicis . . . . fʒij.
　　　Aquæ . . . . ad fʒvij.—M.
　　Sig. A dessertspoonful every hour or two to an adult.
　　　FLIESBURG.

175—℞ Liq. ammonii acetat. . . . . fʒss.
　　　Syr. ipecac. . . . . fʒj.
　　　Liq. morph. sulph. (U.S.P.) . . . . . . ℥xl.
　　　Syr. acaciæ . . . . fʒj.
　　　Aquæ . . . . fʒiss.—M.
　　Sig. A teaspoonful every two hours for a child two years old.
　　(*In capillary bronchitis.*) MEIGS AND PEPPER.

176—℞ Terpinol . . . . gr. ij.
　　　Benzoate of sodium . . . . gr. ij.
　　　Sugar, sufficient quantity.
　　Sig. Make into one pill and give six to twelve a day.

BRONCHITIS (Continued).

177—℞ Tinct. sanguinariæ . . . . f ʒj. -
    Tinct. lobeliæ . . . . f ʒj.
    Vini ipecac. . . . . f ʒij.
    Syr. tolutan. . . . . f ʒss.—M.
Sig. A teaspoonful every three hours.   BARTHOLOW.

178—℞ Acidi hydrocyanici dil. . . . . ℔xvj.
    Syr. pruni virginianæ,
    Aquæ camphoræ . . . . āā f ʒj.—M.
Sig. A teaspoonful every two or three hours. (*In violent,
troublesome cough.*)   HARTSHORNE.

BUBO.

179—℞ Tinct. iodi . . . . f ʒj.
Sig. Apply with brush every other day till skin becomes
tender.   VAN BUREN.

180—℞ Acidi carbolici . . . . gr. viij.
    Aquæ destillatæ . . . . f ʒj.—M.
Sig. Inject ℔xx deep into the enlarged gland.

181—℞ Cadmii iodidi . . . . ʒss.
    Ætheris . . . . ℔xl.
Tere simul, et adde—
    Adipis . . . . ʒj.
Misce et fiat unguentum.
Sig. Once or twice daily.   A. B. GARROD.

182—℞ Ichthyol,
    Lanolin . . . . āā ʒij.
M. et fiant ungt.
Sig. Apply twice daily.   H. TUCKER.

183—℞ Unguenti hydrargyri . . . . ʒij.
    Ammonii chloridi . . . . ʒj.
Misce bene.
Sig. Apply twice daily.   DUPUYTREN.

184—℞ Sol. hydrogen. peroxidi (10 vol.) . . . . f ʒviij.
Sig. Apply after suppuration has begun.   RINGER.

BUNIONS.

185—℞ Tinct. iodi,
    Tinct. belladonnæ . . . . āā f ʒij.—M.
Sig. Apply twice daily.   J. C. WILSON.

186—℞ Acidi tannici,
    Cosmolini . . . . āā ʒss.—M.
Sig. Apply to joint after the skin has been removed by
blister.   GROSS.

BURNS AND SCALDS.

187—℞ Acid. picric. . . . . ʒjⁿ½.
    Spirit. vini . . . . : . . . ʒiss.
    Aquæ destillatæ . . . . Oij.—M.
Ft. sol.
Sig. A gauze bandage saturated with this solution is laid on
the parts, which have previously been disinfected.
   THIERY.

188—℞ Acidi tannici . . . . ʒj.
    Spts. vini rectif. . . . . f ʒj.
    Ætheris sulphur. . . . . f ʒviiss.—M.
Sig. Apply locally. (*In burns of the first degree.*)   NIKOLSKI.

189—℞ Sodii bicarb. . . . . ʒij.
    Aquæ . . . . Oj.—M.
Sig. Apply freely on lint or linen.   LEVIS.

190—℞ Ol. lini,
    Liq. calcis . . . . āā f ʒiv.
    Acidi carbolici . . . . gtt. xxx.—M.
Sig. Apply freely.   *Charity Hospital, N.Y.*

24

BURNS AND SCALDS (Continued).

191—℞ Cocaini . . . . gr. x-xx.
    Boroglyceridi . . . . 3ij.—M.
Sig. Apply locally on absorbent cotton.   ELLER.

192—℞ Cocaini . . . . gr. v-xx.
    Lanolini . . . . 3j.—M.
Sig. Apply locally.   WENDE.

193—℞ Aristol . . . . 5j to 5ij.
    Dissolve in olive oil . . . . f 3ss.
    Add vaseline, lanolin . . . . āā 5ij.—M.
Sig. Apply topically.

194—℞ Acidi salicylici . . . . 5j.
    Olei olivæ . . . . f 3viij.—M.
Sig. Apply to burn, covering with linen or lint. BARTHOLOW.

195—℞ Cerati resinæ . . . . 3ij.
    Olei terebinthinæ . . . . f 5ij.
Fiat unguentum.
Sig. Apply on linen or lint.   KENTISH.

196—℞ Plumbi carbonatis . . . . 3iv.
    Olei lini . . . . q. s.
Tere simul et fiat pinguentum.
Sig. Apply liberally on linen or lint.   GROSS.

CALCULI, BILIARY.

197—℞ Sodii succinat. . . . . 3j.
In pilulas (compressas) no. xcvj div.
Sig. One pill three times a day, fifteen minutes before food.
                     J. C. WILSON.

198—℞ Sodii phosphatis . . . . 3ss.
Divide in partes vi.
Sig. One before each meal, continued for several months.
                    BARTHOLOW.

199—℞ Olei olivæ optim. . . . . Oj.
Sig. To be taken in divided doses before breakfast.

200—℞ Sodii bicarb. . . . . 3v.
In chartulas no. xx div.
Sig. One powder three times daily for several months. (Prophylactic.)   ALONZO CLARK.

201—℞ Chloroformi . . . . 3iv.
Sig. To be inhaled, a small quantity at a time, until paroxysm
ceases.   RINGER.

202—℞ Morphinæ sulphat. . . . . gr. vj.
    Atropinæ sulphat. . . . . gr. ⅛.
    Aquæ destillatæ . . . . 3ss.—M.
Sig. Ten minims to be injected hypodermically during paroxysm, and repeated if necessary. BARTHOLOW.

203—℞ Olei terebinthinæ,
    Ætheris . . . . āā f 3ss.—M.
Sig. A large teaspoonful on sugar every half-hour until relief is obtained.   DURAND.

CALCULI, RENAL AND VESICAL, WITH ACID URINE.

204—℞ Sodii benzoatis,
    Lithii carbonatis,
    Ext. stigmat. maydis . . . . āā 3j.
    Olei anisi . . . . gtt. iv.—M.
Ft. massa et in pil. no. lxxx div.
Sig. Four pills daily.   HUCHARD.

205—℞ Magnesii carbonatis . . . . ℥j.
Sodii biboratis,
Acidi citrici . . . . āā ℥ij.
Aquæ bullientis . . . . ad f℥viij.—M.
Sig. A tablespoonful three or four times daily. BARTHOLOW.

206—℞ Magnesii carbonatis . . . . ℥j.
Infusi gentianæ compositi . . . . f℥vj.
Fiat mistura.
Sig. A wineglassful to be taken three times daily. BRANDE.

207—℞ Liquoris potassæ . . . . f℥ij.
Infusi buchu . . . . f℥viij.—M.
Sig. Three tablespoonfuls an hour after meals. REECE

208—℞ Liquoris potassæ . . . . f℥ss.
Tincturæ humuli . . . . f℥iss.
Infusi calumbæ . . . . f℥iv.
Syrupi aurantii corticis . . . . f℥ij.
Fiat mistura.
Sig. A tablespoonful three times daily. H. GREEN.

209—℞ Lithii citratis . . . . ℥ss.
Syrupi aurantii corticis . . . . f℥j.
Aquæ . . . . ad f℥ij.—M.
Sig. A teaspoonful in a wineglassful of water three times
daily. GUY.

210—℞ Piperazini . . . . ℥j.
Pone in phialas no. xl.
Sig. Dissolve the contents of one of the phials in a pint of
water and administer after each meal.

211—℞ Urea,
Sodium bicarbonate,
Calcium carbonate . . . . aa ℥j.
Sig. Half a teaspoonful four or five times daily.

CALCULI, RENAL AND VESICAL, WITH ALKA-
LINE URINE.

212—℞ Acidi phosphorici diluti . . . . f℥ss.
Tincturæ cardamomi compositæ . . . . f℥ss.
Infusi calumbæ . . . . f℥vij.
Fiat mistura.
Sig. A tablespoonful in sweetened water every four hours.
NELIGAN.

213—℞ Acidi hydrochlorici diluti . . . . f℥j.
Decocti hordei . . . . f℥viij.—M.
Sig. A tablespoonful, largely diluted, three times a day.
ELLIS.

214—℞ Acidi nitrici dil.,
Acidi hydrochlor. dil. . . . . āā ℳxl.
Infusi serpentariæ . . . . f℥viij.—M.
Sig. A half-wineglassful three times daily. GOLDING-BIRD.

215—℞ Acidi nitrici dil.,
Acidi hydrochlor. dil. . . . . āā f℥ij.
Syrupi aurantii corticis,
Aquæ aurantii flor. . . . . āā f℥j.
Aquæ destillatæ . . . . f℥xiiiss.—M.
Sig. A wineglassful three or four times daily. DRUITT.

216—℞ Strychninæ . . . . gr. j.
Acidi nitrici dil. . . . . f℥j.
Aquæ . . . . f℥xij.—M.
Sig. Two tablespoonfuls three times daily. GOLDING-BIRD.

217—℞ Condurango corticis contusæ . . . . . . ℨiiss.
Syrupi simplicis . . . . f℥v.
Aquæ bullientis . . . . ad f℥vj.—M.

Fiat infusio.
Sig. A tablespoonful every hour or two, the whole to be taken
during the day. To be continued for several months. (*In
gastric cancer.*)   L. RIESS.

218—℞ Bismuthi subnitratis . . . . ℨij.
Acidi hydrocyanici diluti . . . . f℥ss.
Mucilaginis acaciæ,
Aquæ menthæ piperitæ . . . . . . āā f℥ij.—M.
Sig. A tablespoonful three times a day in milk. (*In cancer of
stomach.*)   BARTHOLOW.

219—℞ Formaldehydi (40 per cent. sol.) . . . . gtt. viij.
Aquæ hydrogenii dioxidi . . . . f℥xvj.—M.
Sig.—Use as wash every two hours.

220—℞ Ext. conii fructus fld. . . . . f℥ss.
Sig. Take ten minims every half-hour till sleep comes on.
(*For pain and insomnia.*)   MADIGAN.

221—℞ Liquoris potassii arsenitis . . . . f℥ss.
Mucilaginis acaciæ . . . . f℥vliss.
Aquæ cinnamomi . . . . f℥j.—M.
Sig. A teaspoonful three times a day. (*In gastric and uterine
cancer.*)   WASHINGTON ATLEE.

222—℞ Antifebrin. . . . . ℨj.

In capsules no. xii div.
Sig. Take a capsule, and repeat in twenty minutes if required.
(*For lancinating pains and insomnia of cancer.*) DEMIÉVILLE.

223—℞ Acetanilid . . . . ℨj.
Aristol . . . . : . . . . . ℨij.
Acid. boric. . . . . ℨj.—M.
Sig.—Locally as a dusting powder.   ATKINSON.

224—℞ Acidi chromici. . . . . ℨij.
Aquæ destillatæ . . . . q. s. ut. fiat magma.
Sig. Apply to affected part as an escharotic.   BUSCH.

225—℞ Liquoris ferri subsulphatis . . . . f℥j.
Aquæ destillatæ . . . . f℥ij.—M.
Sig. To inject into the uterus, in hemorrhage from cancer.
BARNES.

226—℞ Methylene blue . . . . gr. xv.
Alcohol,
Glycerin . . . . āā ♏lxxv.—M.
Sig. Apply locally.   DU CASTEL.

227—℞ Acidi arseniosi,
Pulv. acaciæ . . . . āā ℨj.
Aquæ . . . . f℥v.—M.
Sig. Paint over the tumor night and morning, not more than
one square inch at a time. Aid sloughs by poulticing. (*For
epithelioma.*)   MARSDEN.

228—℞ Iodoformi. . . . . gr. xv.
Ext. opii . . . . gr. viij.
Essentiæ menthæ (vel bergamottæ) . . gtt. x.
Butyr. cacao . . . . ℨiiss.
Ft. supp. no. xii.
Sig. A suppository to be introduced into the vagina in cases
of cancer of the cervix uteri.   SINÉTY.

229—℞ Iodoformi. . . . . ℨj.
Sig. Use as a dusting-powder to the broken surface and cover
with lint soaked in glycerin.   RINGER.

CARBUNCLE.

230—℞ Tinct. ferri mur. . . . . f℥j.
 Potassi chloratis . . . . ℥j.
 Glycerini . . . . f℥j.
 Aquæ. . . . . ad f℥iv.—M.
Sig. A teaspoonful in a wineglassful of water every two
 hours. RINGER.

231—℞ Calcii sulphidi . . . . gr. iij.
 Ext. glycyrrhizæ . . . . . . q. s. ut ft. massa.—M.
In pil. no. xxx div.
Sig. One pill every hour or two. RINGER.

232—℞ Quininæ hydrochloratis . . . . gr. xxiv.
 Acidi hydrochlorici dil. . . . . ℞xl.
 Tincturæ cardamomi . . . . f℥iss.
 Aquæ. . . . . q. s. ad f℥vj.—M.
Sig. A tablespoonful three times a day after food.
 J. C. WILSON.

233—℞ Lini farinæ,
 Aquæ bullientis . . . . āā q. s.
Misce et fiat cataplasma.
Sig. Apply as hot as bearable, cover with oil-silk, and renew
 every four hours. ELLIS.

234—℞ Argenti nitratis. . . . . ℈iv.
 Aquæ destillatæ . . . . f℥iv.—M.
Sig. To be applied two or three times on the inflamed sur-
 face, and beyond it, on the healthy skin. HIGGINDOTTOM.

235—℞ Resorcin. . . . . ℈iss-℈iss.
 Lanolini . . . . ℥j.—M.
Ft. ungt.
Sig. Apply after making multiple parallel incisions into
 carbuncle. (*Abortive.*) L. WEISS.

236—℞ Pulveris opii,
 Unguenti hydrargyri,
 Saponis duræ . . . . āā ℥ss.—M.
Sig. Apply spread on thick leather. BUXTON SHILLITOE.

237—℞ Extracti opii . . . . ℥ss.
 Glycerini . . . . q. s. ut fiat magma.—M.
Sig. Smear thickly over the swelling three or four times a
 day ; then apply—

238—℞ Tincturæ iodi . . . . f℥j.
Sig. Apply so as to encircle the carbuncle until it produces
 vesication. FURNEAUX JORDAN.

CARIES.

239—℞ Elixiris phosphori,
 Syrupi calcis . . . . āā f℥ij.—M.
Sig. Teaspoonful in water two hours after meals. (*For caries
 of teeth in pregnant and nursing women.*)

240—℞ Guaiacoli . . . . ℥j.
Pone in capsulas no. xxx.
Sig. One capsule after meals and increase to two. (*Used in
 caries in tuberculous subjects.*)

241—℞ Cupri sulphatis,
 Zinci sulphatis . . . . āā partes xv.
 Liquoris plumbi subacetatis . . . . . . partes xxx.
 Aceti . . . . partes cc.—M.
Sig. Inject thoroughly into sinus. VILLATE.

CATARRH, BRONCHO-PULMONARY.

242—℞ Tinct. opii . . . . gtt. iij.
 Spts. frumenti . . . . f℥j.
 Aquæ bullientis . . . . f℥iv.
 Sacchari albi . . . . q. s.—M.
Sig. Take at bedtime. (*Incipient catarrh.*) RINGER.

243—℞ Morphinæ sulphatis . . . . gr. ss.
   Quininæ sulphatis . . . . gr. xx.

Misce et fiant chartulæ no. ii.
Sig. At bedtime, *in incipient catarrh.* BARTHOLOW.

244—℞ Morphinæ acetatis . . . . gr. ij.
   Acidi acetici diluti . . . . f3j.
   Syrupi pruni virginianæ,
   Syrupi ipecacuanhæ,
   Syrupi tolutani . . . . āā f3j.—M.
Sig. A teaspoonful every three hours. ELLIS.

245—℞ Syr. tolutani,
   Syr. pruni virgin.,
   Tinct. hyoscyami,
   Spts. ætheris co.,
   Aquæ . . . . āā] f3j.—M.
Sig. A teaspoonful three times daily. (*Chronic form.*)
              JANEWAY.

246—℞ Ol. santal. . . . . ℳv.
In capsules.
Sig. One every three hours. (*Chronic offensive bronchorrhœa.*)
             J. C. WILSON.

247—℞ Ammonii carbonatis . . . . gr. xxxij.
   Ext. senegæ fld.,
   Ext. scillæ fld. . . . . āā f3j.
   Tinct. opii camph. . . . . f3vj.
   Aquæ . . . . f3iv.
   Syr. tolutani . . . . q. s. ad f3iv.—M.
Sig. A teaspoonful every three or four hours. (*Chronic form.*)
             STOKES.

248—℞ Syr. ferri iodidi . . . . 3j.
Sig. Twenty drops in water three times daily. H. TUCKER.

249—℞ Tincturæ eucalypti,
   Syrupi simplicis . . . . āā f3j.—M.
Sig. A teaspoonful every three hours. (*In the more chronic
cases.*)   GUBLER.

CATARRH OF GALL-DUCTS.

250—℞ Sodii phosphatis . . . . 3ij.
In chartulas no. xvi div.
Sig. A powder every four hours. (*For children, one-third to
one-sixth the quantity.*)   BARTHOLOW.

251—℞ Ammonii iodidi . . . . 3j.
   Liquoris potassii arsenitis . . . . . . f3ss.
   Tincturæ calumbæ . . . . f3ss.
   Aquæ destillatæ . . . . f3iss.—M.
Sig. A teaspoonful three times a day, before meals. (*With
jaundice.*)   BARTHOLOW.

252—℞ Ext. hydrastis fld. . . . . f3j.
Sig. Five to fifteen drops before meals daily for some weeks.
             BARTHOLOW.

253—℞ Ammonii chloridi . . . . 3ss.
   Ext. taraxaci fld. . . . . f3iij.—M.
Sig. A teaspoonful three times daily. BARTHOLOW.

254—℞ Potassii carbonatis . . . . 3j.
   Vini ipecacuanhæ . . . . f3j.
   Extracti rhei fluidi . . . . f3ij.
   Aquæ destillatæ . . . . q. s. ad f3iij.—M.
Sig. One fluidrachm in boiling water before each meal.
             WAUGH.

255—℞ Hydrargyri chloridi mitis . . . . gr. v.
   Sodii bicarbonatis . . . . 3ij.
Misce et fiant chartulæ no. x.
Sig. One powder every three hours. N. CHAPMAN.

CATARRH OF GALL-DUCTS (Continued).

256—℞ Ammonii chloridi .... ʒij.
    Extracti hydrastis fluidi .... f ʒss.
    Syrupi sarsaparillæ compositi ..... f ʒiss.
    Aquæ destillatæ .... f ʒij.—M.
Sig. A dessertspoonful every three hours.   NOTHNAGEL.

CATARRH, GASTRO-INTESTINAL.

257—℞ Liq. potass. arsenitis .... f ʒss.
Sig. One or two drops before meals. (*Vomiting of drunkards.*)
    BARTHOLOW.

258—℞ Tinct. capsici .... f ʒvj.
    Tinct. nucis vomicæ .... f ʒij.—M.
Sig. Twenty drops every four hours.   RINGER.

259—℞ Ext. hydrastis fld. .... f ʒss.
Sig. Five to fifteen drops before meals, in water.
    BARTHOLOW.

260—℞ Argenti nitratis .... gr. x.
    Ext. hyoscyami .... ʒii-iv.—M.
In pilulas no. xx div.
Sig. A pill every night for six or eight weeks. SYMONDS.

261—℞ Copper arsenite .... gr. $\frac{1}{50}$.
    Milk-sugar .... ;gr. lxxv.—M.
Divide into sixteen powders.
Sig. At the commencement of the attack, one powder every
hour; in case of amelioration, one every two or three hours
(*Acute gastric catarrh in infants.*)   H. KRUEGER.

262—℞ Acidi tannici .... ʒss.
    Aquæ destillatæ .... f ʒilj.
Fiat mistura.
Sig. A teaspoonful every two hours. (*In acute cases with
purging.*)   NIEMEYER.

263—℞ Zinci oxidi .... ʒj.
    Sodii bicarbonatis .... ʒiiss.
    Piperinæ .... ʒj.
Misce et fiant chartulæ xx.
Sig. One powder three or four times a day. (*In drunkards.*)
    REVILLOUT.

264—℞ Caffeinæ citratis .... ʒss.
    Syrupi aurantii florum .... f ʒiss.
    Aquæ destillatæ .... f ʒiiss.—M.
Sig. A dessertspoonful every two hours. (*With migraine.*)
    AUBERT.

265—℞ Bismuth. subnitrat. .... gr. x.
    Potass. bromid. .... gr. xv-xx.
    Acid. hydrocyanic. dilut. .... ♏v.
    Spirit. chloroform. .... ♏x.
    Mucilag. acaciæ .... ʒij.
    Aquæ .... q. s. ad ʒj.—M.
Sig.—To be taken every three hours, about ten minutes before food. (*Acute gastric catarrh.*)

266—℞ Carbonei bisulph. puri .... gr. xxv.
    Essentiæ menthæ .... gtt. xxx.
    Aquæ .... f ʒxv.—M.
The mixture is placed in a large bottle, shaken, and allowed
to settle; eight to twelve tablespoonfuls are to be given
daily in half a tumblerful of water and wine, or in milk.
    DUJARDIN-BEAUMETZ.

267—℞ Argenti nitratis .... gr. ¼.
    Aquæ destillatæ .... f ʒij.
    Gummi acaciæ .... ʒij.
    Sacchari albi .... ʒij.—M.
Sig. A teaspoonful every two hours. (*When evacuations are
frequent. For child one year old.*) HIRSCH.

268—℞ Bismuthi subnitratis .... ʒij.
    Pulv. ipecac. co. .... gr. ix.—M.
In chartulas no. xii div.
Sig. Once every three hours. (*For child one year old.*)
    J. LEWIS SMITH.

269—℞ Tinct. opii deodorat. . . . . gtt. xvj.
Bismuth. subnitrat. . . . . ℥ij.
Syr. simplicis . . . . f℥iv.
Aquæ cinnamomi . . . . f℥iss.—M.

Sig. Shake bottle. Give one teaspoonful every two to four
hours. (*For child one year old.*) J. LEWIS SMITH.

270—℞ Hydrarg. chlorid. mit. . . . . gr. iii-iv.
Magnes. calc. . . . . gr. xxxvj.
Pulv. ipecac. . . . . gr. ii-iij.
Ext. hyoscyami. . . . . gr. iv-vj.—M.

Ft. chart. no. xii.
Sig. One every three hours. (*In chronic forms in children.*)
CONDIE.

CATARRH, GENITO-URINARY.

271—℞ Fol. hyoscyami. . . . . ℥ss.
Aquæ bullientis . . . . Oj.—M.

Ft. infusio.
Sig. A tablespoonful every half-hour for one forenoon, unless
throat becomes dry or patient drowsy. DIDAY.

272—℞ Urotropin. . . . . ℥vj.
Aquæ. . . . . f℥ij.—M.

Sig. Teaspoonful in a glass of lithia water three times daily.
(*Cystitis.*) H. TUCKER.

273—℞ Atrophiæ sulph. . . . . gr. j.
Acidi acetici . . . . gtt. xx.
Alcoholis,
Aquæ. . . . . āā f℥ss.—M.

Sig. Four drops in a wineglassful of water before each meal.
(*In acute cystitis.*) GOODELL.

274—℞ Copaibæ,
Spts. lavand. co. . . . . āā f℥ij.
Mucil. acaciæ. . . . . f℥ss.
Syrupi simp. . . . . f℥ij.
Aquæ. . . . . f℥iv.—M.

Sig. A tablespoonful twice daily. WOOD.

275—℞ Infusi buchu . . . . f℥vij.
Potassii bicarb. . . . . ℥j.
Tinct. hyoscyami . . . . f℥iss.
Ext. sarsæ fld. . . . . f℥iv.—M.

Sig. Two tablespoonfuls three times daily. (*In irritable bladder, with acid urine.*) COULSON.

276—℞ Cubebæ. . . . . ℥j.
Sodii bicarbonatis,
Potassii bitartratis . . . . āā ℥ij.

Misce et divide in partes æquales xii.
Sig. One powder three times a day. DRUITT.

277—℞ Chimaphilæ . . . . ℥ij.
Aquæ bullientis . . . . Oj.
Coque . . . . ad f℥vj.
Cola et adde—
Spiritus juniperi compositi . . . . f℥ij.—M.

Sig. A tablespoonful every two or three hours, with demulcent drinks. PROCTOR.

278—℞ Potassii citrat. . . . . ℥ss.
Spts. chloroformi . . . . f℥iss.
Tinct. digitalis . . . . ℳlxxx.
Infusi buchu . . . . f℥viij.—M.

Sig. Two tablespoonfuls three or four times daily.
FOTHERGILL.

279—℞ Pulveris uvæ ursi . . . . ℥iss.
Sodii bicarbonatis ! . . . . ℥j.

Misce et divide in chartulas xii.
Sig. One powder three times a day, in sugar and water.
ELLIS.

280—℞ Resinæ copaibæ . . . . ℨiij.
    Alcoholis . . . . f ℥v.
    Spiritus chloroformi . . . . f ℨj.
    Mucilaginis acaciæ . . . . f ℨij.
    Aquæ destillatæ . . . . q. s. ad f ℥xij.—M.
Sig. A tablespoonful three times a day. WILKES.

281—℞ Extracti grindeliæ fluidi . . . . f ℨj.
    Elixiris simplicis,
    Spiritus juniperi compositi . . . . . āā f ℨiss.—M.
Sig. A dessertspoonful every four hours. C. J. RADEMAKER.

282—℞ Fol. uvæ ursi . . . . ℨj.
    Aquæ fervid. . . . . f ℥xviij.—M.
Sig. Macerate for two hours and boil down to one pint and
strain. A wineglassful every two to four hours. BRODIE.

283—℞ Olei cubebæ,
    Olei santali . . . . āā ℨj.—M.
Pone in cap. no. xii.
Sig. One every four hours. H. TUCKER.

284—℞ Olei terebinthinæ. . . . . f ℨiss.
    Syrupi simplicis . . . . f ℨj.
    Aquæ cinnamomi . . . . f ℨij.
    Olei limonis . . . . ℳviij.—M.
Sig. A teaspoonful every three hours. MAUNSELL.

285—℞ Argenti nitratis . . . . gr. vij.
    Aquæ destillatæ. . . . . f ℨiiiss.—M.
Sig. Inject into the bladder, every third or fourth day, after
washing it out with warm water. RICORD.

286—℞ Iodoformi . . . . gr. xij.
    Ext. hyoscyami . . . . gr. vilj.
    Olei theobromæ . . . . ℨvj.—M.
In suppositoria no. viii div.
Sig. Introduce one into the rectum twice daily, one hour
after giving the patient a lukewarm-water enema.
RELIQUET.

CATARRH, NASAL AND FAUCIAL.

287—℞ Iodoformi pulv.,
    Pulveris acaciæ . . . . āā gr. xxx.
    Cocainæ hydrochloratis . . . . gr. j.
Sig. Use as a snuff. GARAGEORGIADES.

288—℞ Resorcin. . . . . gr. v-x.
    Aquæ destillatæ . . . . f ℨij.—M.
Sig. Use with atomizer twice daily, four minutes each time.
MASINI AND MASSEI.

289—℞ Acidi boracici . . . . gr. lx.
    Glycerini . . . . ℳxx.
    Aquæ . . . . f ℨvj.—M.
Dissolve with heat and saturate cotton-wool, with a thin sheet
(℥j), with the solution, and dry. Pack the upper part of
· nose with the prepared cotton, leaving a space below for
breathing. (Rhinitis.) WOAKES.

290—℞ Acidi carbolici liq. . . . . ℳxxx.
    Sodii biborat.,
    Sodii bicarb. . . . . āā ℨj.
    Glycerini . . . . f ℨiiiss.
    Aquæ . . . . q. s. ad f ℨiv.—M.
Sig. To be used with atomizer. (Simple chronic rhinitis.)
DOBELL.

291—℞ Chloroformi . . . . f ℨij.
    Glycerini,
    Spts. vini gallici . . . . āā f ℨj.—M.
Sig. One teaspoonful in water every three hours. (For acute
coryza.) SAJOUS.

292—℞ Sodii salicylat. . . . . ℨij.
   Sodii biborat. . . . . ℨij.
   Glycerini . . . . f℥iv.
   Aquæ . . . . q. s. ad f℥vj.—M.
Sig. A dessertspoonful in a pint of water, used with spray or douche.   BEAN.

293—℞ Sodii bicarbonatis . . . . ℨj.
Sig. Insufflate or apply with finger to the inflamed tonsil. (*Tonsillitis.*)   GINE.

294—℞ Cocainæ muriatis . . . . gr. vj.
   Bismuthi subcarb. . . . . ℨss.
   Talci . . . . ℨiss.—M.
Sig. Enough to cover a silver five-cent piece insufflated into each nostril every two hours. (*For acute coryza.*)   SAJOUS.

295—℞ Tinct. aconiti radicis . . . . f℥j.
   Tinct. belladonnæ . . . . f℥ij.—M.
Sig. Three drops every hour. (*Pharyngitis and acute tonsillitis.*)   RINGER.

296—℞ Cocainæ hydrochloratis . . . . partes ij.
   Pulveris sacchari albi . . . . partes c.—M.
Sig. Use as a snuff.   WYETH.

297—℞ Pulveris cubebæ . . . . partem j.
   Pulveris sacchari albi . . . . partes ij—M.
Sig. Use by insufflation.   J. C. WILSON.

298—℞ Tincturæ aconiti radicis . . . . f℥ij.
   Tincturæ opii deodoratæ . . . . f℥vj.—M.
Sig. Eight drops in water every hour or two.   BARTHOLOW.

CHANCRE.

299—℞ Dithymol-diiodidi . . . . ℨiv.
Sig. Use freely as dusting powder.

300—℞ Iodoformi . . . . ℨij.
   Unguenti petrolei . . . . ℨj.
   Olei cinnamomi . . . . gtt. v.
Misce et fiat unguentum.
Sig. Apply twice daily.   IZARD.

301—℞ Hydrargyri biniodidi . . . . ℈j.
   Adipis . . . . ℨiss.—M.
Sig. Apply on lint. (*For inveterate chancres and indolent vene-real ulcers.*)   RATIER.

302—℞ Hydrarg. chlorid. mit. . . . . gr. xv.
   Liq. calcis . . . . f℥ij.—M.
Sig. Shake and apply as a wash.   BARTHOLOW.

303—℞ Hydrarg. chlorid. mit. . . . . ℨss.
Sig. Dust on and cover with dry lint.   VAN BUREN AND KEYES.

304—℞ Hydrarg. chlorid. corros. . . . . gr. j.
   Liq. calcis . . . . f℥viij.—M.
Sig. Shake and apply on lint.   JAS. L. LITTLE.

305—℞ Formaldehydi (40 per cent. sol.) . . . . f℥j.
Sig. Apply to sore with cotton swab.

306—℞ Hydrogen. peroxidi . . . . partem j.
   Aquæ destillatæ . . . . part. iij.—M.
Sig. Wash three times a day, and keep covered with lint moistened with it. (*Also for open buboes.*)   RINGER.

307—℞ Aristol. . . . . ℨss.
Sig. Use as a dusting-powder.   J. C. WILSON.

CHANCROID.

308— ℞ Acidi nitrici . . . . f ʒss.
Sig. After cleaning the surface, apply with a match or glass
rod, exposing the surface until nearly dry or painless ; then
dry the surface and reapply acid in same way.   Dry-lint
dressing.   VAN BUREN AND KEYES.

309— ℞ Acidi sulphurici,
Pulv. carbonis ligni . . . . . . āā q. s. ut ft. magma.
Sig. Dry the sore and apply evenly with wooden spatula.
                                                  RICORD.

310— ℞ Pulv. acidi salicylici . . . . ʒij.
Sig. Dust on sore and cover with dry dressing.   ANGLADA.

311— ℞ Iodoformi . . . . ʒij.
Sig. Dust on sore and cover with lint dipped in glycerin.
                                                  RINGER.

312— ℞ Hydrarg. chlorid. mit. . . . . ʒiij.
Sig. Use as a dusting-powder.   J. C. WILSON.

.**313—** ℞ Bismuthi subiodidi . . . . ʒiv.
Sig. Dust on sore and use dry dressings.   CHASSAIGNAC.

314— ℞ Succi limonis . . . . ʒiss.
Vini opii . . . . ♏xlv.
Liq. plumbi subacet. . . . . ʒj.
Aquæ destillatæ . . . . ʒv.—M.
Ft. lotio.
Sig. Soak pledgets of lint in the solution and apply locally.
(*In phagedæna.*)   RODET.

CHILBLAINS.

315— ℞ Collod. flexil. . . . . ʒiv.
Olei ricini . . . . ʒiv.
Spts. tereb. . . . . ʒiv.—M.
Use two or three times daily.   *British Med. Journal.*

316— ℞ Lin. belladonnæ . . . . ʒij.
Lin. aconiti. . . . . ʒj.
Acidi carbolici . . . . ♏vj.
Collod. flexil. . . . . ad ʒj.—M.
Sig. Apply every night with a camel's-hair pencil.
                                        British Med. Journal.

317— ℞ Bismuthi salicylat. . . . . ʒij.
Pulv. amyli . . . . ʒxviij.—M.
Sig. First bathe the chilblains in a decoction of walnut-
leaves, then rub with spirits of camphor and cover with
the powder. To quiet the itching use the following:

318— ℞ Ichthyol.,
Resorcin.,
Acid. tannic. . . . . āā ʒj.
Aquæ. . . . . f ʒv.—M.
Sig. Paint the parts.   BOECK.

319— ℞ Acidi carbolici . . . . gr. x.
Cosmolini,
Olei terebinthinæ . . . . āā ʒj.—M.
Sig. Apply to affected part.   DAVIDSON.

320— ℞ Camphoræ . . . . gr. lxxv.
Spts. vini rectif. . . . . f ʒiij.
Glycerini . . . . f ʒv.—M.
Ft. linimentum.
Use locally several times daily.   FOY.

321— ℞ Linimenti chloroformi . . . . f ʒij.
Sig. Apply to part with gentle friction. (*Early stage.*)
                                                  DAVIDSON.

322— ℞ Tinct. iodi . . . . f ʒj.
Apply to parts with brush.   DAVIDSON.

323—℞ Creolin . . . . ♏xl.
Aquæ . . . . f ℥viij.—M.
Sig. A dessertspoonful at short intervals.　　GRONEMAN.

324—℞ Emplastri cantharidis . . . . 2 in. × 4 in.
Sig. Apply from back of right ear downwards and forwards.
　　　　　　　　　　　　　　　　　　　　　　HECKIN.

325—℞ Magnesia sulphate . . . . ℥ij.
Sulphurous acid,
Water . . . . of each ℥xvj.
Tinct. capsicum . . . . ℥iv.—M.
Dissolve perfectly.
Sig. Teaspoonful night and morning. (*Prophylactic.*) BEVAN.

326—℞ Sulphurous acid,
Water . . . . of each ℥xvj.
Tinct. capsicum . . . . ℥iv.
Morphine sulphate . . . . gr. ij.—M.
Dissolve perfectly.
Sig. Teaspoonful every half-hour until relieved. (*Therapeutic.*)
　　　　　　　　　　　　　　　　　　　　　　BEVAN.

327—℞ Dilute hydrochloric acid . . . . ♏xv.
Pure pepsin essence,
Wine of opium . . . . āā ♏xx.
Peppermint water . . . . ℥iv.
Syrup of orange flower . . . . ℥j.—M.
Sig. A teaspoonful each hour.　　　　　　CHAUVIN.

328—℞ Tinct. opii,
Tinct. capsici,
Spts. camphoræ . . . . āā f℥j.
Chloroformi . . . . f℥ij.
Alcoholis . . . . q. s. ad f℥v.—M.
Sig. Twenty to forty minims, diluted.　　SQUIBB.

329—℞ Tincturæ opii deodoratæ . . . . f℥ij.
Acidi sulphurici aromatici . . . . . . f℥iij.—M.
Sig. Twenty drops every hour or two in ice-water.
　　　　　　　　　　　　　　　　　　　　　　BARTHOLOW.

330—℞ Acidi nitrosi . . . . f℥j.
Tincturæ opii . . . . gtt. xl.
Aquæ camphoræ . . . . f℥viij.— M.
Sig. One-fourth to be taken every three or four hours. HOPE.

331—℞ Strychninæ sulphatis . . . . gr. ¼.
Acidi sulphurici diluti . . . . f℥ss.
Morphinæ sulphatis . . . . gr. ij.
Aquæ camphoræ . . . . f℥iiiss.—M.
Sig. A teaspoonful every hour or two, well diluted. *(In threat
ened collapse. Also as a prophylactic, given less frequently.)*
　　　　　　　　　　　　　　　　　　　　　　BARTHOLOW

332—℞ Acidi tannici . . . . ℥j.
Fiant chartulæ no. iv.
Sig. Dissolve one powder in two pints of warm water, and
with soft rubber catheter and fountain syringe inject slowly
and gently into colon every two or three hours.

333—℞ Acidi sulphurici diluti . . . . f℥j.
Sig. Fifteen to thirty drops in ice-water every fifteen to thirty
minutes until vomiting and purging are arrested. (*This
and ferri sulph. are prophylactic.*)　　S. T. CHANDLER.

334—℞ Acidi phosphorici diluti . . . . f℥j.
Sig. A half-fluidrachm in ice-water. (*In cholerine and early
stage of confirmed cholera.*)　　WILLIAM SEDGWICK.

335—℞ Sodii chloridi . . . . ℥iv.
Aquæ ferventis . . . . cong. j.—M.
Sig. For injection into colon by means of soft rubber catheter.
About one to two quarts very gently introduced every two
or three hours. (*Used to control diarrhœa and prevent col-
lapse.*)

336—℞ Creasoti . . . . gt. j.
    Aquæ camphoræ,
    Infusi gentianæ compositi . . . . . āā f ʒvj.—M.
Sig. One dose every two hours.   J. T. JONES.

337—℞ Chloroformi . . . . ℳvj.
    Aquæ destillatæ . . . . f ʒj.—M.
Fiat haustus.
Sig. To be given after five grains of calomel and two grains
of opium, and to be repeated if necessary.   OATES.

338—℞ Morphinæ sulph. . . . . gr. ij.
    Spts. camphoræ . . . . f ʒj.—M.
Sig. Fifteen minims every three or four hours by mouth, or
hypodermically, in severe cases. (In initial stage.) Also—

339—℞ Morphinæ sulph. . . . . gr. x.
    Atropinæ sulph. . . . . gr. j.
    Aquæ destillatæ . . . . f ʒx.—M.
Sig. Five to ten minims hypodermically, as required. (In
stage of collapse.)   NAKAMURA.

340—℞ Plumbi acetatis . . . . gr. xij.
    Liquoris morphinæ acetatis . . . . . . ℳxij.
    Acidi acetici diluti . . . . f ʒj.
    Aquæ destillatæ . . . . f ʒiij.—M.
Sig. A teaspoonful every five, six, or eight hours to a child
one year old. (Choleraic diarrhœa.)   FLEMING.

CHOLERA INFANTUM.

341—℞ Argenti nitratis . . . . gr. j.
    Acidi nitrici diluti . . . . ℳviij.
    Tincturæ opii deodoratæ . . . . ℳviij.
    Mucilaginis acaciæ . . . . f ʒss.
    Syrupi simplicis . . . . f ʒss.
    Aquæ cinnamomi . . . . f ʒj.—M.
Sig. A teaspoonful every three, four, or six hours. (For a
child one year old.)   BARTHOLOW.

341bis.—℞ Creasoti . . . . gtt. viij.
    Aquæ chloroformi . . . . f ʒij.—M.
Sig. A teaspoonful every hour or two.   BUTTERFIELD.

342—℞ Potassii bromidi . . . . ʒij.
    Syrupi simplicis . . . . f ʒss.
    Aquæ menthæ piperitæ . . . . f ʒiss.—M.
Sig. A teaspoonful every hour or two. (With irritable nervous
system.)   BARTHOLOW.

343—℞ Hydrarg. cum cretâ . . . . gr. j.
    Sacchari lactis . . . . gr. x.—M.
In pulv. no. xii div.
Sig. A powder every hour.   RINGER.

344—℞ Hydrarg. chlorid. mit. . . . . gr. j.
    Sodii bicarb. . . . . ʒj.
    Pulv. zingiberis . . . . gr. xij.—M.
In pulv. no. xii div.
Sig. One powder three or four times daily. (In incipient
stage.)   HARTSHORNE.

345—℞ Hydrarg. chlorid. mit. . . . . gr. j.
    Cretæ præp. . . . . gr. xxxvj.
    Plumbi acetat. . . . . gr. xij.
    Pulv. ipecac. . . . . gr. iij.—M.
In chart. no. xii div.
Sig. One every three hours.   CONDIE.

346—℞ Calomel,
    Sugar of milk,
    Benzonaphthol . . . . āā gr. iij.—M.
Sig. To be made into one powder and given every three hours
in the milk.   GRASSET.

347—℞ Saloli . . . . gr. xxiv.
Bismuthi subnitratis . . . . ℈iv.
Aquæ camphoræ . . . . q. s. ad f ℥iij.—M.
Sig. Shake and give teaspoonful every two hours.

348—℞ Plumbi acetatis . . . . gr. ii.
Acidi acetici diluti . . . . gtt. vj.
Tincturæ opii deodoratæ . . . . gtt. iv.
Syrupi simplicis,
Aquæ menthæ piperitæ . . . . . . āā f℥ss.—M.
Sig. A teaspoonful every two or three hours. (*For a child two years old.*)
DA COSTA.

349—℞ Acidi carbolici . . . . gr. ij.
Bismuthi subnitratis . . . . ℈j.
Syrupi acaciæ . . . . f℥ss.
Aquæ menthæ piperitæ . . . . f℥iss.—M.
Sig. A half-teaspoonful every two to four hours. (*For a child one to two years old.*)
ROTHE.

350—℞ Hydrargyri chloridi mitis,
Plumbi acetatis . . . . āā gr. j.
Misce et fiant pulveres no. iv.
Sig. One powder every three hours. (*For a child from ten to twenty months old.*)
T. D. MITCHELL.

351—℞ Ol. ricini . . . . f℥ij.
Pulv. acaciæ,
Sacch. albi . . . . āā ℈ij.
Tinct. opii . . . . ℳxxj.
Aq. cinnam. . . . . q. s. ad f℥iv.—M.
Sig. A teaspoonful every two or three hours. WEST.

352—℞ Tinct. opii deodoratæ . . . . gtt. xvj.
Spts. ammon. aromat. . . . . f℥j.
Bismuthi subnitratis . . . . ℈ij.
Syrupi simplicis . . . . f℥iv.
Mist. cretæ . . . . f℥iss.—M.
Sig. Shake well and give a teaspoonful every two or three hours to a child eight to twelve months old. (*Six months old, half the dose.*)
J. LEWIS SMITH.

353—℞ Tinct. cocæ (1-5) . . . . f℥j.
Sig. Four to six drops every two hours at three months of age. Fifteen to twenty drops in older children.
DIEDERICHS.

354—℞ Resorcin. . . . . gr. viij-xl.
Syr. aurantii cort. . . . . f℥j.
Aquæ aurantii flor. . . . . ad f℥ij.—M.
Sig. A teaspoonful every two hours. FLIESBURG.

355—℞ Naphthalini . . . . gr. xx-lxx.
Ol. bergamli . . . . gtt. j-ij.—M.
In pulv. no. xii div.
Sig. A powder every two or three hours. HOLT.

356—℞ Saloli . . . . gr. vj.
Sacchari lactis . . . . gr. x.—M.
In pulv. no. xii div.
Sig. A powder every two hours. (*For a child aged six months. Between five and ten years old, three grains of salol may be taken every two hours.*)
GOELET.

356bis.—℞ Pulv. opii . . . . gr. ss.
Bismuthi subnitratis . . . . gr. lx.
Iodoformi . . . . gr. iv.—M.
In chartulas no. xvi div.
Sig. One powder every two or three hours. SANDERS.

CHORDEE.

357—℞ Plumbi bromidi,
Lupulinæ,
Ext. belladonnæ . . . . āā gr. xv.—M.
Ft. massa et in pil. no. xxx div.
Sig. Two or three pills daily. VAN DEN CORPUT.

CHORDEE (Continued).

358—℞ Camphorœ,
Ext. lactucarii . . . . āā ʒj.
Misce et fiant pilulæ no. xxx.
Sig. One, two, or three pills at bedtime.   RICORD.

359—℞ Cannabis indicæ . . . . gr. j.
Pulveres opii . . . . gr. ss.
Camphorœ . . . . gr. ij.
Misce et fiat pilula.
Sig. At bedtime.   LOMBE ATTHILL.

360—℞ Ext. opii aquosi . . . . gr. ij.
Pulv. camphoræ . . . . gr. iv.—M.
In pil. no. ii div.
Sig. One or both on retiring.   VAN BUREN AND KEYES.

361—℞ Liq. morph. sulph. (Magendii) . . . . . f ʒlv.
Atropinæ sulph. . . . . gr. j.
Acidi acetici . . . . q. s.
Aquæ destillatæ . . . . ad f ʒj.—M.
Sig. Five to eight minims at bedtime, hypodermically.
    STURGIS.

362—℞ Extracti hyoscyami . . . . gr. vj.
Extracti opii . . . . gr. vj.
Olei theobromatis . . . . q. s.
Misce et fiant suppositoria no. vi.
Sig. One by rectum at bedtime. Repeat once during night if required.

363—℞ Ext. opii . . . . gr. iss.
Ol. theobromæ . . . . gr. xxx.—M.
Ft. suppositor. no. i.
Sig. Introduce into rectum on going to bed.
    VAN BUREN AND KEYES.

364—℞ Vini colchici seminis,
Syrupi simplicis . . . . āā f ʒss.—M.
Sig. A teaspoonful at bedtime.   BRODIE.

CHOREA.

365—℞ Chloralamid. . . . . ʒss.
In chartulas no. xii div.
Sig. One powder twice a day.   J. C. WILSON.

366—℞ Chloral. hydratis . . . . ʒij.
Syr. aurantii cort. . . . . f ʒij.—M.
Sig. A teaspoonful three times daily for one or two months.
(Child ten years old.)   JOFFROY.

367—℞ Succi conii . . . . f ʒij.
Sig. One teaspoonful, increased gradually to two or three, once daily before dinner.   J. HARLEY.

368—℞ Succi conii . . . . f ʒvj.
Syrupi simplicis,
Aquæ destillatæ . . . . āā f ʒix.—M.
Sig. A dessertspoonful three times a day.   JAMES ANDREW.

369—℞ Morphinæ sulphatis . . . . gr. j.
Aquæ destillatæ . . . . f ʒj.
Solve.
Sig. A teaspoonful or more, pro re nata.   TROUSSEAU.

370—℞ Ext. cimicifugæ fld. . . . . f ʒij.
Sig. A half-teaspoonful, increased to one teaspoonful, three times daily. (Six to ten years old.)   JESSE YOUNG.

371—℞ Extracti cimicifugæ fluidi,
Elixiris simplicis . . . . āā f ʒiss.—M.
Sig. A dessertspoonful four times a day.   BARTHOLOW.

372—℞ Lobelinæ hydrobrom. . . . . gr. j.
Aquæ . . . . f ʒv.—M.
Sig. Three to fifteen minims hypodermically.   BARTHOLOW.

CHOREA (Continued).

373—℞ Zinci valerianat.,
Ext. hyoscyami,
Bismuthi subnitrat. . . . . āā gr. xv.—M.
In pil. no. xxx div.
Sig. Three to six pills daily.   DESCROIZILLES.

374—℞ Ferri citratis . . . . ʒij.
Syr. simplicis. . . . . f ʒiv.
Aq. aurantii flor. . . . . : . . fʒiss.—M.
Sig. A teaspoonful before or after meals.   (*In anæmic cases.*)
HARTSHORNE.

375—℞ Zinci sulphatis . . . . gr. ij.
Extracti conii . . . . gr. iij.
Misce et fiat pilula.
Sig. To be taken every night.   JAMES ANDREW.

376—℞ Zinci valerianatis . . . . gr. viij.
Tincturæ valerianæ,
Tincturæ calumbæ . . . . āā f ʒij.
Aquæ aurantii florum . . . . f ʒilj.—M.
Sig. A tablespoonful every six hours.   NELIGAN.

377—℞ Sulphonalis . . . . ʒj.
Fiant chartulæ no. xii.
Sig. One powder in glass of hot water as required.   (*For child of six years.*)

378—℞ Liquoris potassii arsenitis . . . . f ʒij. (!)
Syrupi simplicis . . . . f ʒvj.
Aquæ destillatæ . . . . f ʒij.—M.
Sig. A dessertspoonful immediately after meals. (*For a child five to twelve years of age.*)   EUSTACE SMITH.

379—℞ Escrinæ sulphatis . . . . gr. j.
Aquæ destillatæ . . . . f ʒvj.—M.
Sig. Six minims hypodermically twice daily; with tonics.
RIESS.

380—℞ Strychninæ sulphatis . . . . gr. j.
Syr. simplicis. . . . . f ʒiiss.—M.
Sig. Fifty minims three times daily, increased to seventy-five minims, or until itching of the scalp and muscular stiffness are observed.   TROUSSEAU.

COLIC.

381—℞ Tinct. opii deodoratæ . . . . gtt. xij.
Magnesii calcinat. . . . . gr. xij–xxiv.
Sacchari albi . . . . ʒj.
Aquæ anisi . . . . f ʒiss.—M.
Sig. Shake well. One teaspoonful to a child one year old.
J. L. SMITH.

382—℞ Aquæ menthæ viridis,
Aquæ camphoræ,
Aquæ . . . . āā f ʒiv.—M.
Sig. Teaspoonful as required.

383—℞ Morphinæ sulphatis . . . . gr. ij.
Aquæ destillatæ . . . . f ʒj.—M.
Sig. Five to ten minims hypodermically, repeated in fifteen minutes.   RINGER.

384—℞ Spiritus chloroformi . . . . f ʒvj.
Aquæ camphoræ . . . . q. s ad f ʒiv.—M.
Sig. A tablespoonful every hour or two.   G. P. OLIVER.

385—℞ Tinct. lobeliæ . . . . gtt. j.
Aquæ destillatæ . . . . f ʒj.—M.
Sig. Dose, a half-teaspoonful, warmed. (*For infantile colic.*)
Practitioner.

386—℞ Tinct. stramonii . . . . f ʒj.
Tinct. hydrastis can. . . . . f ʒj.
Aquæ laurocerasi . . . . f ʒv.—M.
Sig. A teaspoonful in water every four hours for an adult.
DE MUSSY.

COLIC (Continued).

387—℞ Chloroformi . . . . f3iss.
    Tinct. opii deodorat. . . . . f3j.
    Camphoræ . . . . gr. xv.
    Olei cajeputi . . . . 3j.
    Aquæ. . . . . q. s. ad f3ij.—M.
Sig. A teaspoonful every hour or two.

388—℞ Aquæ camphoræ . . . . f3j.
    Spiritus ætheris compositi . . . . f3ij.
    Tincturæ cardamomi compositæ . . . . f3ss.
    Spiritus anisi . . . . f3vj.
    Olei carui . . . . ℔xij.
    Syrupi zingiberis . . . . f3ij.
    Aquæ menthæ piperitæ . . . . f3vss.
Fiat mistura.
Sig. Two tablespoonfuls.   JOY.

389—℞ Extract. zingiberis fluid. . . . . f3iss.
    Tinct. asafœtidæ . . . . f3iij.
    Aquæ menthæ piperitæ,
    Aquæ cinnamomi . . . . āā f3j.
    Syrup. simpl. . . . . f3iv. —M.
Sig. A teaspoonful in water three times a day before meals.
(*In the flatulent colic of infants.*)   *Practitioner.*

390—℞ Naphthalini . . . . gr. viiss.
    Iodoformi . . . . gr. iij.
    Acidi tannici,
    Antipyrin. . . . . āā gr. xv.—M.
Ft. massa et in pil. no. x div.
Sig. Three or four pills in succession until relieved. (*In violent colic.*)   CAPITAN.

391—℞ Atropinæ sulphatis . . . . gr. j.
    Zinci sulphatis . . . . gr. xxx.
    Aquæ destillatæ . . . . f3j.—M.
Sig. Three to five drops two or three times daily. BARTHOLOW.

392—℞ Magnesii carb. . . . . gr. xlv.
    Sacch. albi . . . . 3iss.
    Tinct. asafœtidæ . . . . f3iss.
    Tinct. opii . . . . f3ss.
    Aquæ . . . . f3iss.—M.
Sig. Five to sixty drops, according to age. (*In infantile colic.*)
                     DEWEES.

393—℞ Spiritus ætheris compositi . . . . . . f3j.
    Tincturæ cardamomi compositæ . . . . f3ij.
    Aquæ camphoræ . . . . f3j.
Misce et fiat haustus.
Sig. At once, and repeat if necessary.   NELIGAN.

394—℞ Syr. rhei aromat.,
    Tinct. cardamomi co.,
    Tinct. opii camph.,
    Aquæ cinnamomi . . . . āā f3j.—M.
Sig. Two to four teaspoonfuls.   HARTSHORNE.

COLICA PICTONUM.

395—℞ Olei tiglii . . . . gtt. vj.
    Micæ panis . . . . q. s. ut ft. massa.—M.
In pil. no. xii div.
Sig. A pill every three or four hours until free evacuations are produced.   WARING.

396—℞ Pulv. opii . . . . gr. xij.
    Ext. belladonnæ . . . . gr. ij.
    Olei tiglii . . . . gtt. xij.—M.
Ft. massa et in pil. no. xii div.
Sig. A pill every two hours until relieved.   LOOMIS.

397—℞ Magnesii sulphatis . . . . 3j.
    Acidi sulphurici dil. . . . . f3j.
    Aquæ . . . . f3iv.—M.
Sig. A tablespoonful three times daily, preceded by five to ten grains of potassium iodide.   BRUNTON.

COLICA PICTONUM (Continued).

398—℞ Morphinæ sulphatis . . . . gr. iv.
Aquæ destillatæ . . . . f3ij.—M.
Sig. Five to ten minims hypodermically, repeated every
fifteen minutes till relieved.   BARTHOLOW.

399—℞ Aluminis . . . . 3ij.
Magnesii sulphatis . . . . 3j.
Syrupi simplicis . . . . f3iij.
Aquæ rosarum . . . . f3v.—M.
Sig. Two tablespoonfuls in two wineglassfuls of water daily,
early in the morning.   ALDRIDGE.

400—℞ Aluminis . . . . 3ij.
Acidi sulphurici dil. . . . . 3j.
Syr. limonis . . . . f3j.
Aquæ. . . . . f3iij.—M.
Sig. Tablespoonful every hour or two.   BARTHOLOW.

401—℞ Acidi sulphurici . . . . f3j.
Syrupi acidi citrici . . . . f3iv.
Aquæ. . . . . f3xxx.—M.
Sig. To be taken in small cupfuls twice or thrice daily. (As
a preventive.)   MARTIN SOLON.

402—℞ Strychninæ sulphatis . . . . gr. j.
Confectionis rosæ . . . . 3ss.
Misce et fiant pilulæ xx.
Sig. One pill three times a day.   (*In lead palsy.*)

403—℞ Potassii iodidi . . . . 3j.
Aquæ destillatæ . . . . f3iij.—M.
Sig. A teaspoonful three times a day. (*In chronic poisoning.*)

CONDYLOMATA, COMMON.

404—℞ Acidi nitrici . . . . f3ss.
Sig. App.y to wart with match or glass rod three or four
times a week.   LEVIS.

405—℞ Formaldehydi (40 per cent. sol.) . . . . f3j.
Sig. Apply locally with small swab twice daily.

406—℞ Acidi acetici glacialis f3j
Sig. Apply locally.   J. C. WILSON.

407—℞ Acidi chromici . . . . 9v.
Aquæ destillatæ . . . . f3j.—M.
Sig. Apply with a small stick of wood every other day.
(*Also for syphilitic warts.*)   WOOSTER.

CONDYLOMATA, VENEREAL.

408—℞ Hydrargyri chloridi mitis . . . . 3ij.
Sig. First wash with solution of chlorinated soda, then dust
with the calomel.   RICORD.

409—℞ Hydrarg. chlor. mit. . . . . 3vj.
Acidi boracici . . . . 3iij.
Acidi salicylici . . . . 3j.—M.
Sig. Dust over the vegetations.   GREGORY.

410—℞ Acidi carbolici . . . . 3j.
Sig. Apply locally once every day or two.   BARTHOLOW.

411—℞ Pulv. sabinæ,
Pulv. aluminis . . . . āā 3j.—M.
Sig. Dust on the parts every evening. (*In condylomata of the
vulva.*)   BLACHEZ.

412—℞ Olei terebinthinæ . . . . f3j.
Sig. Paint vegetation well with brush daily.

413—℞ Tinct. ferri mur.,
Acidi muriatici dil. . . . . āā f3ij.—M.
Sig. Apply night and morning.   BULKLEY.

414—℞ Acidi boracici . . . . 3ss.
Aquæ destillatæ . . . . f̃ʒx.—M.
Sig. Use to cleanse the eyes after washing away all discharges, and then use—

415—℞ Hydrargyri oxidi flavi . . . . gr. xvj.
Acidi boracici . . . . gr. xx.
Cocainæ muriatis . . . . gr. v-x.
Vaselini . . . . ʒj.—M.
Sig. Apply to surface.   HIGGINS.

416—℞ Acidi tannici . . . . 3ss.
Sig. Evert the eyelids, and insufflate. (*In the granular form.*)
HAMILTON.

417—℞ Aquæ dest. . . . . ʒj ℳvij.
Zinci sulph. . . . . gr. iiss.
Acidi borici . . . . gr. ix.—M.
Fiat collyrium.
Sig. Drop in the eye three or four times daily.

418—℞ Acidi boracici . . . . ʒj.
Aquæ rosæ . . . . f̃ʒiv.—M.
Sig. Bathe the lids freely. (*Early in measles as prophylactic.*)
TROUSSEAU.

419—℞ Hydrarg. chlorid. corr. . . . . gr. j.
Aquæ . . . . f̃ʒviij.—M.
Sig. Bathe the eyelids freely inside and out several times daily. (*Later in measles.*)   TROUSSEAU.

420—℞ Acidi boracici . . . . gr. vj.
Aquæ camphoræ,
Aquæ destillatæ . . . . āā f̃ʒj.—M.
Sig. Bathe the eyelids and drop two drops in the eye three or four times daily. (*In simple conjunctivitis.*)   L. W. FOX.

421—℞ Neutral acetate of lead . . . . gr. ij.
Hydrochlorate of cocaine . . . . . . gr. iij.
White vaseline . . . . gr. xlv.—M.
Sig. Apply to the edges of the inflamed lid. (*For blepharitis.*)

422—℞ Hydrargyri oxidi flavi . . . . gr. ¼-j.
Adipis benzoati . . . . ʒj.
Misce et fiat unguentum exactum.
Sig. Apply in the eye daily. (*For phlyctenular conjunctivitis.*)
KEYSER.

423—℞ Hydrargyri oxidi flavi . . . . gr. j-iij.
Vaselini . . . . ʒj.—M.
Sig. A piece the size of a pin-head placed between the lids. (*In the phlyctenular form.*)   PAGENSTECHER.

424—℞ Muc. acaciæ . . . . f̃ʒss.
Tinct. capsici . . . . f̃ʒj.
Glycerini . . . . q. s. f̃ʒj.
Sig. Locally. (*For black eye.*)   J. DA COSTA.

425—℞ Cadmii sulphatis . . . . gr. iij.
Vini opii . . . . f̃ʒj.
Aquæ rosæ . . . . f̃ʒij.—M.
Sig. Use twice daily. (*In the chronic form, and for opacities of the cornea.*)   FRONMUELLER.

426—℞ Ichthyol . . . . ʒj.
Aquæ sambuci,
Aquæ destillatæ . . . . āā ʒvj.—M.
Sig. Locally.   BERRY.

427—℞ Cupri sulphatis . . . . gr. iij.
Aquæ camphoræ . . . . f̃ʒiv.
Solve.
Sig. To be dropped in the eye. (*In the purulent form.*)   WARE.

428—℞ Sodii biboratis . . . . gr. v.
Acidi carbolici puri . . . . gtt. j.
Aquæ destillatæ . . . . f̃ʒj.—M.
Sig. Instil into the eye frequently, and then use—

42

CONJUNCTIVITIS (Continued).

429—℞ Acidi boracici . . . . gr. xv.
Petrolati . . . . ℥ij.—M.
Sig. Apply to lids. (*In purulent cases.*)   OLDHAM.

430—℞ Zinci sulphatis . . . . gr. ij.
Aquæ destillatæ . . . . f℥j.—M.
Sig. Two drops in eye three or four times daily.   ROOSA.

CONSTIPATION.

431—℞ Tinc. nuc. vom. . . . . ℳ︁ss.
Tinc. belladonnæ . . . . ℳ︁v.
Inf. sennæ . . . . ℳ︁xx.
Inf. gentianæ comp. . . . . ad f℥j.—M.
Ft. haustus.
Sig. To be taken three times a day before meals by a child
from eight to twelve months old.   EUSTACE SMITH.

432—℞ Mannæ . . . . gr. vj.
Aquæ bullientis . . . . ℥x.—M.
Ft. infusum.
Sig. When cool, give a teaspoonful to a new-born child.
      WIDERHOFER.

433—℞ Hydrargyri chloridi mitis . . . . gr. j.
Sodii bicarbonatis . . . . gr. xij.
Sacchari lactis . . . . gr. xx.
Misce et fiant chartulæ no. xii.
Sig. One every three hours until the bowels are freely
moved. (*For infants.*)   WAUGH.

434—℞ Ext. aloes . . . . gr. vj.
Pulv. rhei . . . . gr. vj.
Benzosol . . . . gr. ix.
Ext. hyoscyami . . . . gr. vj.
M. et ft. caps. xii.
Sig. One after meals.   T. H. STUCKEY.

435—℞ Ext. nucis vomicæ,
Pulv. piper. nig. . . . . āā ǝj.
Pil. colocynth. co. . . . . gr. l.—M.
In pil. no. xx div.
Sig. One every night or second night.   FOTHERGILL.

436—℞ Ext. cascaræ sagrad. fld.,
Elixiris simplicis. . . . . āā f℥ij.—M.
Sig. Two teaspoonfuls at bedtime.   BARTHOLOW.

437—℞ Extracti stillingiæ fluidi . . . . f℥v.
Tincturæ belladonnæ,
Tincturæ nucis vomicæ,
Tincturæ physostigmatis . . . . . . āā f℥j.—M.
Sig. Twenty drops in water, three times a day, before meals.
(*In habitual constipation.*)   BARTHOLOW.

438—℞ Extracti hydrastis fluidi . . . . f℥j.
Syrupi simplicis,
Elixiris simplicis. . . . . āā f℥iss.—M.
Sig. A dessertspoonful three times a day. (*In deficient secre-
tion with dry hard stools.*)   PORCHER.

439—℞ Glycerini . . . . ℥j.
Sig. Inject twenty to thirty minims into the rectum.
      ANNACKER.

440—℞ Sulphuris loti . . . . ℥j.
Potassii bitartratis . . . . ℥ss.
Misce et pone in cachetas no. xxiv.
Sig. One cachet night and morning. (*To produce mushy stools
in strictures of bowels or in hemorrhoids.*) H. A. HARE.

441—℞ Pulv. aloes socot. . . . . gr. vij.
Pulv. rhei. . . . . gr. xxiv.
Ext. belladonnæ . . . . gr. j.—M.
In pil. no. xii div.
Sig. One or two pills as required.   DA COSTA.

CONSTIPATION (Continued).

442—℞ Bicarbonate of sodium . . . . ʒiij.
Powdered rhubarb . . . . ʒij.
Sulphate of sodium . . . . ʒj.
Oil of peppermint . . . . gtt. xx.—M.
Sig. Half to one teaspoonful before breakfast. (*For children.*)

443—℞ Podophyllin . . . . gr. j.
Spts. vini rectif. . . . . ʒiss.
Syr. althææ . . . . ad ʒiv.—M.
Sig. A half-teaspoonful daily. (*For infants.*)   BOUCHUT.

444—℞ Antimonii oxidi . . . . ʒss.
Extracti colocynthidis compositi . . . ʒiss.
Misce et divide in pilulas xxx.
Sig. One or two pills at bedtime.   FOTHERGILL.

CONVULSIONS.

445—℞ Chloral. hydratis . . . . gr. xv-xxx.
Syrupi acaciæ . . . . fʒj.
Aquæ . . . . ad fʒiv.—M.
Sig. Inject a tablespoonful into the rectum, and repeat in fifteen or twenty minutes if required.   WIDERHOFER.

446—℞ Chloral. hydratis . . . . gr. i-v.
Syrupi simplicis . . . . fʒj.—M.
Sig. One dose. (*For infants and small children.*) WATERHOUSE.

447—℞ Ammonii bromidi . . . . ɘiv.
Potassii bromidi . . . . ʒvj.
Tincturæ calumbæ . . . . fʒj.
Aquæ destillatæ . . . . q. s. ad fʒiv.—M.
Sig. A dessertspoonful every hour or two.   ECHEVERRIA.

448—℞ Moschi . . . . gr iij.
Camphoræ . . . . gr. xv.
Chloral. hydratis . . . . gr. viiss.
Vitell. ovi . . . . no. j.
Aquæ destillatæ . . . . fʒiv ʒvj.-M.
Sig. Wash out the rectum with a simple enema, and then use above as an injection.   J. SIMON.

449—℞ Moschi . . . . gr. xij.
Sacchari . . . . ɘij.
Spiritus ammoniæ . . . . ℳxxx.
Infusi lini compositi . . . . fʒiv.
Fiat enema.
Sig. An injection for infantile convulsions.   ELLIS.

450—℞ Olei ricini . . . . fʒj.
Sig. A teaspoonful or two, according to age.
MEIGS AND PEPPER.

451—℞ Mist. asafœtidæ . . . . fʒij.
Sig. A tablespoonful as an enema.   WARING.

452—℞ Ætheris fort. . . . . fʒiv.
Sig. As an inhalation until paroxysm is broken. J. L. SMITH.

CORYZA. (See also Catarrh and Influenza.)

453—℞ Acidi carbolici . . . . ɘj.
Sodii boratis,
Sodii bicarbonatis . . . . āā ʒj.
Glycerini,
Aquæ rosæ . . . . āā fʒj.
Aquæ . . . . q. s. ad Oj.—M.
Sig. Use as a spray.   LEFFERTS.

454—℞ Morphinæ hydrochlor. . . . . gr. ij.
Bismuthi subnitratis . . . . ʒij.
Pulveris acaciæ . . . . ʒiss.—M.
Sig. Use as a snuff.   J. C. WILSON.

44

CORYZA (Continued).

455—℞ Cocain. hydrochlor. . . . . gr. ix.
    Aquæ . . . . ℥ss.
Ft. solutio et adde—
    Olei petrolei . . . . ℨj.
    Olei eucalypti. . . . . gtt. vj.
    Olei gaultheriæ . . . . gtt. iij.—M.
Sig. Nasal spray. Shake thoroughly before using. STOWELL.

456—℞ Menthol. . . . . gr. viij.
    Camphoræ . . . . gr. v.
    Albolene . . . . ℥ij.—M.
Sig. Use as a spray for nose. H. A. HARE.

457—℞ Sodii bicarb. . . . . gr. ij.
    Magnesiæ carb. (levis) . . . . gr. iij.
    Menthol . . . . gr. j.
    Cocain. hydrochlor. . . . . gr. iv.
    Sacch. lactis ; . . . . ℨjss.—M.
Sig. Use as snuff. STOWELL.

CROUP.

458—℞ Tinct. ferri chloridi . . . . ℨj-iss.
    Potassii chloratis . . . . ℨj.
    Glycerini . . . . ℨj.
    Aquæ cinnamomi . . . . ad ℥iv.—M.
Sig. A teaspoonful every two hours to a child four years old.
                        MEIGS AND PEPPER.

459—℞ Moschi . . . . gr. v.
    Syrupi acaciæ . . . . ℥ij.
    Aquæ rosæ . . . . ℥ij.—M.
Sig. Shake and give teaspoonful every two hours. (Used to
relieve laryngeal spasm.)

460—℞ Potassii chloratis . . . . ℨj.
    Ammonii chloridi . . . . ℈ij.
    Syrupi simplicis . . . . ℨj.
    Aquæ destillatæ . . . . ℥ij.—M.
Sig. A teaspoonful every three hours. HAZARD.

461—℞ Acidi lactici . . . . ℨiiss.
    Aquæ destillatæ . . . . ℥x.—M.
Sig. Apply frequently by means of a spray-producer or a
simple mop. (To dissolve false membrane.)
                      MORELL MACKENZIE.

462—℞ Apomorphinæ . . . . gr. ¼.
    Syr. simplicis,
    Aquæ . . . . āā ℨj.—M.
Sig. A teaspoonful or two every hour or two, according to
the urgency of the case. FLIESBURG.

463—℞ Hydrargyri sulphatis flavæ . . . . . . gr. iij-v.
Fiat pulvis.
Sig. As an emetic. FORDYCE BARKER.

464—℞ Pulv. aluminis . . . . ℨiss.
    Mellis albi . . . . ℥x.—M.
Sig. A half-teaspoonful every hour ; and powdered alum
blown into the throat every four hours. TROUSSEAU.

465—℞ Pulv. aluminis . . . . ℨij.
    Syr. ipecac. . . . . ℨj.—M.
Sig. One teaspoonful every twenty minutes until vomiting
is produced. A hot mustard foot-bath should be given at
the same time. J. LEWIS SMITH.

466—℞ Syr. ipecacuanhæ . . . . ℨij.
Sig. A teaspoonful every ten or fifteen minutes until vomiting is produced. Then five or ten minims every two or
three hours the next day. MEIGS AND PEPPER.

467—℞ Potassii bromidi,
    Chloral. hydratis . . . . āā ℈ij.
    Syr. acaciæ . . . . ℨij.—M.
Sig. A teaspoonful or less, according to age. ELLIS.

CROUP (Continued).

468—℞ Tinct. belladonnæ . . . . gtt. iv.
 Tinct. opii camph. . . . . gtt. l.
 Pulv. aluminis . . . . gr. vj.
 Syr. acaciæ . . . . ʒss.
 Aquæ . . . . ʒiss.—M.
Sig. A teaspoonful every two or three hours at six months of
 age.   MEIGS AND PEPPER.

469—℞ Tinct. aconiti radicis . . . . ʒss.
Sig. One drop in a teaspoonful of water every hour till
 urgent symptoms abate; then every two or three hours.
               RINGER.

CYSTITIS. (See also Catarrh.)

470—℞ Iodoformi . . . . ʒxij.
 Glycerini . . . . ʒx.
 Tragacanthæ . . . . gr. xx.
 Aquæ destillatæ . . . . ʒiiss.—M.
Ft. emulsio.
Sig. One tablespoonful in half a pint of water as an injection.
               FREY.

DEBILITY, GENERAL AND SENILE.

471—℞ Tinct. ferri chlor.,
 Syr. simplicis . . . . āā fʒj.
 Aquæ cinnamomi . . . . fʒij.—M.
Sig. A teaspoonful three times daily.   Charity Hospital, N.Y.

472—℞ Liquoris acidi arsenosi . . . . ℥Lxxx.
 Acidi hydrochlorici diluti . . . . fʒij.
 Tincturæ gentianæ compositæ . q. s. ad fʒiv.—M.
Sig.—Teaspoonful after meals.

473—℞ Quininæ sulphatis . . . . gr. xxx.
 Acidi sulphurici dil. . . . . q. s. ad ft. sol.
 Aquæ . . . . fʒij.
 Tinct. ferri chlor. . . . . fʒss.
 Spts. chloroformi . . . . fʒvj.
 Glycerini . . . . fʒiv.—M.
Sig. A teaspoonful three times daily.   LOOMIS.

474—℞ Ferri et potassii tartratis . . . . ʒss.
 Vini xerici . . . . Oj.
Solve et cola.
Sig. A tablespoonful three times a day.   BENNET.

475—℞ Infusi cocæ sacch. . . . . fʒl.
 Glycerini . . . . fʒv.
 Ext. cinchonæ fld. . . . . f℥lxxv.
 Tinct. canellæ . . . . fʒj.
 Tinct. vanillæ . . . . f℥xlv.
 Tinct. cascarillæ . . . . fʒss.—M.
Sig. A tablespoonful thrice daily.   MONIN.

476—℞ Spiritus ferri chlorati ætherei (Ph. Bo-
 russ.) . . . . fʒiij.
 Aquæ cinnamomi,
 Syrupi aurantii corticis . . . . āā fʒj.
 Infusi valerianæ . . . . fʒv.—M.
Sig. Shake well, and take a tablespoonful every two, four, or
 six hours. (In nervous debility.)
"Bestucheff's Nervine Tincture," or "Lamotte's Golden
Drops," a great favorite in Germany.   SOBERNHEIM.

477—℞ Phosphori . . . . gr. ss.
 Acidi arsenosi . . . . gr. j.
 Ferri reducti . . . . gr. xx.
 Strychninæ sulphatis . . . . gr. j.—M.
Fiant pilulæ no. lx.
Sig. One pill after meals.

D

DEBILITY, GENERAL AND SENILE (Continued).

478—℞ Pulveris aloes socotrinæ . . . . ℨj.
Pulveris zedoariæ,
Pulveris gentianæ,
Croci,
Pulveris rhei,
Agarici . . . . āā ℨj.
Spiritus vini gallici . . . . Oij.
Macera per dies septem, cola, et adde—
Syrupi simplicis . . . . f ℥ij.—M.

Sig. A tablespoonful three times a day in water. (This is the
celebrated "Baume de Vie," or " Elixir of Life.")
Hoffmann.

479—℞ Spts. chloroformi . . . . f ℥v.
Acidi hydrochlor. dil. . . . . f ℥iiss.
Inf. cinchonæ . . . . f ℥xv.—M.

Sig. Two tablespoonfuls three times daily. Fothergill.

DELIRIUM, TRAUMATIC.

480—℞ Chloral. hydratis . . . . ℨss.
Syrupi aurantii corticis,
Aquæ destillatæ . . . . āā f ℥ss.—M.

Sig. One dose, to be repeated if necessary. (In maniacal
delirium.) Liebreich.

481—℞ Potassii bromidi . . . . ℨss.
Syrupi simplicis . . . . f ℨj.
Aquæ fœniculi . . . . q. s. ad f ℥iij.—M.

Sig. A dessertspoonful every two hours. (In cases resembling
delirium tremens.) Ringer.

482—℞ Tincturæ belladonnæ . . . . f ℥iss.
Syrupi simplicis . . . . f ℥viss.
Aquæ cinnamomi . . . . f ℨj.—M.

Sig. A teaspoonful every two or three hours. (In fevers.)
S. G. Morton.

DELIRIUM TREMENS.

483—℞ Infusi digitalis . . . . f ℥iij.

Sig. A tablespoonful every four hours. (In anæmic cases with
effusion and œdema.) Bartholow.

484—℞ Sodii bromidi . . . . gr. xv.
Chloral. hydratis . . . . gr. x.
Syrupi aurantii cort.,
Aquæ . . . . āā q. s. ad ft. f ℥j. M.

Sig. As required. Also to be taken, fluid extract of coca fifteen minims, increased to tolerance. Da Costa.

485—℞ Trional . . . . ℨj.
Div. in chart. no. ii.
Sig. Give one and repeat once if necessary. H. Tucker.

486—℞ Antimonii et potassii tartratis . . . . . gr. j.
Tincturæ aconiti radicis . . . . f ℥ss.
Tincturæ opii. . . . . f ℨj.
Aquæ destillatæ. . . . . q. s. ad f ℥iv.—M.

Sig. A dessertspoonful in porter every two or three hours. (In
strong and robust patients with boisterous delirium.) Ringer.

487—℞ Potassii bromidi . . . . ℨj.
In pulv. no. viii div.
Sig. A powder dissolved in one-half tumblerful of water,
every four to six hours. (In the "horrors" preceding the delirium. Bartholow.

488—℞ Liq. morph. sulph. (U. S. P.),
Ext. valerian. fld. . . . . āā f ℨj.—M.
Sig. One or two teaspoonfuls, as required. Hartshorne.

489—℞ Hyoscyami . . . . gr. j.
Spts. vini rectif.,
Aquæ destillatæ . . . . āā f ℥j.—M.
Sig. Five to ten minims hypodermically. Bryce.

DELIRIUM TREMENS (Continued).

490—℞ Amyli hydratis . . . . ʒvj.
Syr. aurantii cort. . . . . f ʒij.
Aquæ . . . . ad f ʒviij.—M.
Sig. Two to three tablespoonfuls in a wineglassful of water.
VON MERING.

491—℞ Tinct. digitalis . . . . f ʒss.
Sig. Thirty minims, repeated in four to six hours. RINGER.

492—℞ Ammonii carbonatis . . . . ʒiss.
Extracti glycyrrhizæ fluidi . . . . . . f ʒiss.
Aquæ destillatæ . . . . f ʒivss.—M.
Sig. A tablespoonful every two or three hours. ANSTIE.

493—℞ Tincturæ lupulinæ,
Syrupi amygdalæ . . . . āā f ʒj.
Aquæ destillatæ . . . . f ʒij.—M.
Sig. A tablespoonful every two hours. HAZARD.

494—℞ Ext. cannabis indicæ . . . . gr. vj-xij.
In pil. no. xii div.
Sig. One pill every two or three hours till drowsy. PHILLIPS.

495—℞ Quininæ sulph. . . . . gr. xij.
In pil. no. xii div.
Sig. One pill two or three times daily, as a tonic. ANSTIE.

DIABETES INSIPIDUS. (See also Polyuria.)

496—℞ Ext. ergotæ fld. . . . . f ʒij.
Sig. A teaspoonful three times daily, increased to two tea-spoonfuls. DA COSTA.

497—℞ Pulv. opii . . . . gr. iv.
Acidi gallici . . . . ʒij.—M.
In chart. no. xii div.
Sig. One three or four times daily. H. C. WOOD.

498—℞ Codeinæ . . . . gr. viij.
Syrupi,
Aquæ . . . . āā ʒj.—M.
Sig. A half-teaspoonful thrice daily, gradually increased to two teaspoonfuls. PAVY.

499—℞ Auri chloridi . . . . gr. j.
Confect. rosæ . . . . gr. xx.—M.
Ft. massa et in pilulas no. xx div.
Sig. A pill after meals thrice daily. BARTHOLOW.

500—℞ Ext. glandulæ suprarenalis . . . . . . ʒij.
Pone in capsulas no. xxiv.
Sig. One three times a day.

DIABETES MELLITUS.

501—℞ Morphinæ acetatis . . . . gr. viij.
Aquæ . . . . f ʒiv.—M.
Sig. A teaspoonful four times daily, increasing rapidly, until in three months seven grains daily are taken. (To be used with restricted diet.) BRUCE.

502—℞ Ext. belladonnæ . . . . gr. xxx.
Ext. opii . . . . gr. xv.—M.
Ft. massa et in pil. no. xx div.
Sig. One three times daily, gradually increased to double the quantity. (To be used with restricted diet.) VILLEMIN.

503—℞ Iodoformi . . . . gr. ij.
In pil. no. xii div.
Sig. One pill after meals, three times daily (With restricted diet.) LEVI.

48

504—℞ Acidi arseniosi . . . . gr. iv.
Pulveris opii . . . . gr. viij.
Ammonii chloridi . . . . 3ss.
Misce et fiat massa in pilulas xxxii dividenda.
Sig. One pill after each meal. (*In thin subjects with faulty assimilation.*) MARCUS.

505—℞ Pulveris opii . . . . gr. xij.
Fellis bovini inspissati . . . . 3iiss.
Fiat massa in pilulas no. xxiv dividenda.
Sig. One pill three times a day. BETHUNE.

506—℞ Codeinæ . . . . gr. vj.
Ext. nucis vom. . . . . gr. iij.—M.
In pil. no. xxiv div.
Sig. One pill three times a day; to be increased by degrees.
J. C. WILSON.

507—℞ Pulv. jambul. sem. . . . . 3j.
Dispensa in capsulas no. xxiv.
Sig. One or two capsules thrice daily, after food. FENWICK.

508—℞ Antipyrin . . . . 3iij.
Glycerin . . . . f3j.
Aquæ . . . . q. s. ad f3vij.—M.
Sig. Teaspoonful three times daily.

509—℞ Fellis bovis purificati . . . . 3ij.
Fiant pilulæ no. xlviii.
Sig. Two pills two hours after meals. (*Used in cases with hepatic torpor.*)

510—℞ Sodii salicylat. . . . . 3iij.
Liq. potassii arsenitis . . . . f3j.
Glycerini . . . . f3j.
Aquæ cinnamomi . . . . ad f3iij.—M.
Sig. A dessertspoonful three times daily. J. C. WILSON.

511—℞ Extracti jaborandi fluidi,
Elixiris simplicis . . . . āā f3j.—M.
Sig. A teaspoonful every four hours. LAYCOCK.

512—℞ Acidi lactici . . . . f3vj.
Syrupi simplicis . . . . f3x.
Aquæ destillatæ . . . . f3ij.—M.
Sig. A dessertspoonful three times a day. FOSTER.

513—℞ Aloes capensis . . . . 3v.
Sodii bicarbonatis . . . . 3iss.
Spiritus lavandulæ compositi . . . . . f3ss.
Aquæ destillatæ . . . . Oj.—M.
Macera per dies quatuordecim et cola.
Sig. A teaspoonful after each meal. (*In obese persons, and when of hepatic origin.*) METTAUER.

514—℞ Lithii carbonat. . . . . gr. xxx.
Sodii arseniat. . . . . gr. j.
Ext. gentianæ . . . . gr. xv.—M.
Ft. massa et in pil. no. xx div.
Sig. One pill morning and evening. VIGIER.

515—℞ Potassii phosphat. . . . . gr. xvj.
Aquæ . . . . f3x.—M.
Sig. A teaspoonful in a little wine or hot tea three times daily. DUCHENNE.

516—℞ Pepsinæ cryst. . . . . 3j.
In pulv. no. xii div.
Sig. One three times daily, after meals. Gradually increased, if necessary. (*Restricted diet at first.*) GARDNER.

517—℞ Sol. cocain. mur. (4 per cent.) . . . . . f3ss.
Sig. Two drops every three hours. (*With antidiabetic diet.*) When polydipsia disappears, take with above—

518—℞ Tinct. opii . . . . f3j.
Tinct. ferri muriat. . . . . f3ix.—M.
Sig. Twenty drops three times daily. WELLER.

DIABETES MELLITUS (Continued).

519—℞ Ergotinæ . . . . ʒj.
Glycerini . . . . f ʒj.
Aquæ destillatæ . . . . f ʒvij.—M.
Sig. Five or six drops daily, hypodermically. (To diminish thirst.)
CORNILLON.

DIARRHŒA, ADULTS.

520—℞ Acidi tannici . . . . gr. xxxvj.
Pulv. opii . . . . gr. iv.—M.
In pil. no. xii div.
Sig. One pill every three or four hours.
HARTSHORNE.

521—℞ Argent. nitrat. . : . . . . gr. iv.
Ext. hyoscyami . . . . gr. xx.
Ext. opii . . . . gr. iij.
Ft. pil. xx.
Sig. One pill an hour before each meal. (Chronic diarrhœa.)
HARE.

522—℞ Creasoti . . . . gtt. v.
Pulveris opii . . . . : . . gr. iij.
Pulveris acaciæ . . . . gr. vij.
Tere simul. et divide in pilulas x.
Sig. One pill to be taken every three hours.
BLASIUS.

523—℞ Acid. sulph. aromat. . . . . f ʒss.
Olei cajuputi . . . . gtt. xl.
Ext. hæmatoxyli fl. . . . . f ʒij.
Spt. chloroformi . . . . f ʒj.
Syr. zingiberis . . . . q. s. ad f ʒiij.—M.
Sig. Teaspoonful in water every two or three hours. (Watery diarrhœa.)

524—℞ Bismuthi subnitratis . . . . ʒij.
Tinct. opii deodoratæ . . . . ℳxl.
Elixiris guaranæ . . . . q. s. ad f ʒiv.—M.
Sig. Shake the vial. A dessertspoonful every two hours.
J. C. WILSON.

525—℞ Ext. hæmatoxyli . . . . ʒss.
Tinct. opii . . . . ℳij.
Aquæ . . . . f ʒij.—M.
Sig. Three or four times daily.
PARIS.

526—℞ Tinct. opii camph.,
Spts. ætheris co.,
Ext. valerianæ fld. . . . . āā ʒss.
Olei menthæ pip. . . . . gtt. xxx.
Spts. lavandulæ co. . . . . . . q. s. ad ʒiv.—M.
Sig. A teaspoonful every two or three hours. WM. DARRACH.

527—℞ Extracti ergotæ aquosi (ergotinæ) . . . ʒj.
Extracti nucis vomicæ . . . . gr. v.
Extracti opii . . . . gr. x.
Misce et flant pilulæ no. xx.
Sig. One every four to six hours. (In chronic following acute attacks.)
DA COSTA.

528—℞ Extract. hæmatoxyli fluid. . . . . . . f ʒij.
Acid. sulphuric. aromat. . . . . f ʒss.
Spirit. chloroformi . . . . f ʒj.
Syrup. zingiberis . . . . . . q. s. ad f ʒiij.—M.
Sig. Teaspoonful in water every two or three hours. (Serous diarrhœa.)
H. A. HARE.

529—℞ Alpha-naphthol . . . . gr. xlv.
Chloroform . . . . ℳv.
Oil of peppermint . . . . ℳij.
Castor oil . . . . ʒiij.—M.
Sig. The dose of this for a child of from three to ten years is one to three teaspoonfuls. MAXIMOWITCH.

530—℞ Liquoris iodi compositi . . . . f ʒss.
Syrupi papaveris . . . . ʒviiss.
Aquæ destillatæ . . . . fʒj.—M.
Sig. A teaspoonful every two hours. (*In attacks due to atony of the mucous membrane.*) SCHMIDT.

531—℞ Alpha-naphthol . . . . gr. v.
Powdered rhubarb . . . . gr. ⅓.
Extract of belladonna . . . . gr. ¼.—M.
Sig. One or two of these tablets are taken at a dose several times a day. MAXIMOWITCH.

532—℞ Saloli . . . . ʒij.
In pulv. no. xii div.
Sig. A powder every two hours, followed by a draught of water. GOELET.

533—℞ Tincturæ krameriæ . . . . fʒj.
Aquæ calcis. . . . . fʒvj.—M.
Sig. A tablespoonful three times a day. REECE.

534—℞ Caffeinæ citratis . . . . ʒss.
Aquæ destillatæ . . . . fʒij.—M.
Sig. A teaspoonful every four hours. (*In atonic cases.*)
BARTHOLOW.

535—℞ Cupri sulphatis,
Morphinæ sulphatis . . . . āā gr. j.
Quininæ sulphatis . . . . gr. xxiv.
Misce et fiant pilulæ no. xii.
Sig. One pill three times a day. (*In chronic cases.*)
BARTHOLOW.

536—℞ Spiritus lavandulæ comp. . . . . fʒij.
Aquæ cinnamomi . . . . fʒvj.
Syrupi rubi. . . . . fʒij.
Aquæ destillatæ . . . . fʒj.—M.
Sig. A tablespoonful every two or three hours. R. P. THOMAS.

537—℞ Aquæ camphoræ . . . . fʒiij.
Spiritus lavandulæ comp. . . . . . . fʒj.
Sacchari albi . . . . ʒj..
Fiat mistura.
Sig. A tablespoonful every two hours. PARRISH.

DIARRHŒA, CHILDREN.

538—℞ Tinct. opii deodoratæ . . . . gtt. xvj.
Bismuthi subnitratis . . . . ʒij.
Syr. simplicis. . . . . fʒss.
Mist. cretæ . . . . fʒiss.—M.
Sig. Shake well and give one teaspoonful every three or four hours, to a child one year old. J. L. SMITH.

539—℞ Hydrargyri chloridi mitis . . . . gr. j.
Pulveris nucis myristicæ . . . . gr. iij.
Bismuthi subcarbonatis . . . . gr. x.
Sacchari lactis . . . . · . . ʒj.
Misce et divide in chartulas no. x.
Sig. One powder every two hours. (*For infants with green stools.*) R. A. F. PENROSE.

540—℞ Bismuthi subnitratis . . . . gr. x.
Pulveris calcii phosphatis . . . . gr. xij.
Sacchari lactis . . . . ʒss.
Misce et fiant chartulæ no. x.
Sig. One powder after each evacuation. (*In wasting diarrhœa of children.*) HAZARD.

541—℞ Argenti nitratis . . . . gr. j.
Sacchari albi . . . . ʒij.
Aquæ destillatæ . . . . fʒij.
Fiat mistura.
Sig. A teaspoonful every two hours. (*In newly-weaned infants.*) HIRSCH.

DIARRHŒA, CHILDREN (Continued).

542—℞ Bismuth salicylate . . . . gr. xxiv.
      Gum arabic . . . . ʒj.
      White sugar . . . . ʒiss.
      Water, to make . . . . f ʒvj.—M.

Sig. To be kept on ice. From one to two teaspoonfuls to be
given three to six times a day. (*For infantile diarrhœa.*)
                       MIKHREVICH.

543—℞ Creasote . . . . ʒiij.
      Alpha-naphthol . . . . gr. xlv-lx.
      Powdered iodine . . . . gr. iij.
      Cod-liver oil . . . . q. s. ad ʒvj.—M.'

Sig.—Half a teaspoonful of this may be given each day to a
child of ten years.   MAXIMOWITCH.

544—℞ Pulv. ipecac. . . . . gr. ss.
      Pulv. rhei . . . . gr. ij.
      Sodii bicarb. . . . . gr. xij.—M.

In pulv. no. xii div.
Sig. One powder every four to six hours to an infant one
year old. (*In indigestion with acidity.*)   J. LEWIS SMITH.

545—℞ Saloli . . . . gr. vj.

In pulv. no. xii div.
Sig. A powder dry on the tongue, followed by a sip of water,
every two hours, to a child of six months.   GOELET.

546—℞ Sodii bromidi . . . . ʒss.
      Mucilaginis acaciæ,
      Aquæ . . . . āā f ʒj.—M.

Sig. A teaspoonful every three hours for a child less than one
year old. (*Diarrhœa of dentition.*)   A. A. SMITH.

547—℞ Acidi nitrosi . . . . ℥x-xv.
      Sacchari albi . . . . ʒiij.
      Ext. hyoscyami . . . . gr. vj.
      Aquæ cinnamomi . . . . fʒj.—M.

Sig. A teaspoonful every three hours. (*In protracted cases.*)
                      CONDIE.

548—℞ Misturæ cretæ,
      Syrup. rhei aromat.,
      Tinct. opii camphorat.,
      Mucilag. acaciæ . . . . āā f ʒss.—M.

Sig. A teaspoonful after each stool. (*For simple diarrhœa in
young children.*)   *Western Medical Review.*

DIPHTHERIA.

549—℞ Diphtheria antitoxin.

Sig. To be used in all cases. *Dose.*—Under two years of age,
1000 units as an initial dose. Over two years of age, 1500 to
3000 units as an initial dose. To be repeated in twenty-four
hours if unimproved, and again at the same interval if
necessary. Constitutional and local treatment to be used
as adjuncts. Five hundred units is the usual prophylactic
dose.

550—℞ Menthol . . . . 10 parts.
      Tolulol . . . . 36 parts.
      Ferri sesquiox. . . . . 4 parts.
      Absolute alcohol . . . . 60 parts.—M.

Sig. Apply to affected area. (*Loefler's solution.*)

551—℞ Trypsin. . . . . gr. xxx.
      Sodii bicarb. . . . . gr. x.
      Aquæ destillatæ . . . . ʒj.—M.

Sig. Apply locally to membrane.   FERNALD.

552—℞ Pulv. pepsinæ cryst. . . . . ʒiv.
      Sacchari lactis . . . . ʒj.—M.

Sig. To be insufflated locally.   RICHMOND.

553—℞ Papayotin . . . . ʒj.
      Aquæ . . . . ʒiv.
      Glycerini . . . . ʒviij.—M.

Sig. Apply locally to membranes.   A. JACOBI.

554—℞ Acidi carbolici . . . . gtt. x.
     Liq. ferri subsulphatis . . . . ʒiij.
     Glycerini . . . . ʒj.—M.
Sig. To be applied every three to six hours with a camel's-hair brush.   J. LEWIS SMITH.

555—℞ Bromi pur.,
     Potassii bromidi . . . . āā gr. viij-xv.
     Aquæ destillatæ . . . . ʒl.—M.
Sig. Apply locally every two or three hours.   LE GENDRE.

556—℞ Liq. ferri subsulphatis . . . . ʒij.
     Glycerini. . . . . ʒij.—M.
Sig. Apply locally with brush twice daily.   DRESCHER.

557—℞ Sodii sulphitis . . . . ʒj.
     Aquæ destillatæ . . . . fʒj.—M.
Sig. Apply locally.   STILLÉ.

558—℞ Acidi lactici . . . . fʒliiss.
     Aquæ destillatæ . . . . fʒx.—M.
Sig. Apply by means of a spray-producer or a mop. (*To dissolve the exudation.*)   MORELL MACKENZIE.

559—℞ Mentholi . . . . ʒijss.
     Toluoli . . . . f ʒix.
     Liquoris ferri chloridi . . . . f ʒj.
     Alchohol absoluti . . . . fʒij.—M.
Sig. Wipe off mucous membrane with dry absorbent cotton and apply solution on cotton pledget every three hours.

560—℞ Aquæ hydrogen dioxidi (concentrated solution) . . . . fʒiv.
Sig. To be injected by a syringe into the membranes, the throat being sprayed in the intervals.

561—℞ Carbolic acid . . . . ʒss.
     Alcohol. . . . . ℳxx.
     Camphor . . . . ʒiss.
     Sweet almond oil . . . . fʒiij.—M.
Sig. Apply locally.   SOULEZ.

562—℞ Carbolic acid . . . . ʒj.
     Camphor . . . . ʒiij.
     Alcohol . . . . ʒj.
     Sweet almond oil . . . . ʒliiss.—M.
Sig. Apply locally.   SOULEZ.

563—℞ Tannic acid . . . . gr. xx.
     Mucilage . . . . fʒj.
     Alcohol . . . . fʒss.—M.
Sig. For nasal injection dilute with twice its weight of water.   COUSOT.

564—℞ Tincture of rhatany . . . . 150 grains.
     Tincture of benzoin 75   "
     Tincture of aloes. 45   " -M.
Sig. Apply with brush three times daily.   OSIECKI.

565—℞ Iodi,
     Potassii iodidi . . . . āā gr. iv.
     Alcoholis. . . . . fʒiv.
     Aquæ destillatæ . . . . fʒiv.—M.
Sig. A teaspoonful to be added to hot water, kept hot by a spirit-lamp, and the steam to be inhaled many times a day, continued from eight to twelve minutes. As the patient becomes accustomed to the iodine, the quantity of the solution may be increased to half an ounce.
     WARING-CURRAN.

566—℞ Olei eucalypti . . . . ʒij.
     Olei terebinthinæ . . . . ʒviij.—M.
Sig. Place in shallow vessels and keep boiling, or at least simmering, over the stove.   J. LEWIS SMITH.

567—℞ Coal tar. . . . . ʒvij.
     Oil of turpentine . . . . ʒij ʒvj.—M.
Sig. Light and keep burning in the sick-room.   DELTHIL.

568—℞ Olei terebinthinæ . . . . ʒiv.

Sig. Put in a cup and set it in a basin of water on the top of
the stove, so that the vapor fills the room. Renew when
necessary.   ELLIOTT.

569—℞ Tinct. ferri chloridi . . . . ʒss.

Sig. One drop every quarter of an hour.   (*In the phlegmonous
form.*)   LUNIN.

570—℞ Olei terebinthinæ . . . . ʒij.

Sig. Ten minims to one teaspoonful, one to three times daily,
in milk, sugar-water, or gruel, with alcoholic stimulants.
                                                         SCHENKER.

571—℞ Tinct. ferri chloridi . . . . ʒj.
       Syr. simplicis . . . . ʒiij.—M.

Sig. A teaspoonful every hour to a child ten years old, or
half a teaspoonful every half-hour.   FERGUSON.

572—℞ Tinct. ferri chlor. . . . . ʒj.
       Glycerini,
       Aquæ . . . . āā ʒj.—M.

Sig. A teaspoonful every hour.   BILLINGTON.

573—℞ Sodii phosphatis . . . . ʒiss.
       Aquæ ferventis . . . . f ʒiij.
Solve, et adde—
       Acidi salicylici . . . . ʒiss.—M.

Sig. One to two teaspoonfuls every hour or two. LETZERICH.

574—℞ Potassii chloratis . . . . ʒj.
       Acidi hydrochlorici dil. . . . . f ʒiss.
Misce, et adde—
       Tincturæ ferri chloridi . . . . f ʒij.
       Aquæ destillatæ . . . . q. s. ad f ʒiv.—M.

Sig. A teaspoonful every two hours.   WAUGH.

575—℞ Potassii permanganatis . . . . gr. ij.
       Aquæ destillatæ . . . . f ʒij.
Solve.
Sig. A teaspoonful every three hours for a child eight or ten
years old. (Keep in a glass-stoppered bottle.) BARTHOLOW.

576—℞ Pilocarpinæ muriatis . . . . gr. ½-⅔.
       Pepsinæ cryst. . . . . gr. x-xij.
       Acidi hydrochlorici . . . . gtt. ij.
       Aquæ destillatæ . . . . ʒij ʒiss.—M.

Sig. A teaspoonful every hour, with a small amount of wine
following it.   LAX.

577—℞ Tinct. iodi . . . . gtt. viij.
       Potassii iodidi . . . . , ... gr. iss.
       Syr. simplicis,
       Aquæ . . . . āā ʒij.—M.

Sig. To be taken in one dose. (*Prevention for exposed children.*)
                                                         DUMAS.

578—℞ Salinaphthol. . . . . gr. xx-xxv.
       Spts. vini rectif. . . . . ʒj.—M.

Sig. A dessertspoonful in two-thirds of a tumbler of water as
a gargle. Salinaphthol may also be used internally in doses
of one or two drachms daily in children.   GEORGI.

579—℞ Pilocarpinæ muriatis . . . . gr. iss.
       Pepsinæ cryst. . . . . gr. xxx.
       Acidi hydrochlorici . . . . gtt. iij.
       Aquæ destillatæ . . . . ʒviij.—M.

Sig. A tablespoonful every half-hour, in wine. (*For adults.*)
                                                         GUTTMANN.

580—℞ Hydrarg. cyanidi . . . . gr. ⅟₁₆.
       Tinct. aconiti radicis . . . . ♏xv.
       Aquæ destillatæ . . . . ʒxv.—M.

Sig. One teaspoonful hourly.   LE GENDRE.

581—℞ Tinct. ferri chloridi . . . . ʒii-iij.
       Potassii chloratis . . . . ʒj.
       Acidi muriatici dil. . . . . gtt. x.
       Syr. simplicis . . . . ʒiv.—M.

Sig. A teaspoonful every hour or two.   J. LEWIS SMITH.

DIPHTHERIA (Continued).

582—℞ Hydrarg. bichloridi . . . . gr. ss.
    Spts. frumenti . . . . ℨj.
    Syr. simplicis. . . . . ℨj.—M.
Sig. A teaspoonful every three hours, night and day.
                                  DRESCHER.

583—℞ Hydrarg. chlor. cor. . . . . gr. j.
    Spts. vini rectif. . . . . ℨij.
    Elix. bismuthi et pepsinæ . . . . . ad ℨiv.—M.
Sig. A teaspoonful every two hours for a child six years old.
                                J. LEWIS SMITH.

584—℞ Hydrarg. chlorid. mit. . . . . ℨj.
In pulv. no. xxiv div.
Sig. One or two powders every one, two, or three hours until
free catharsis follows, and then at longer intervals, so that
three or four evacuations are produced daily. W. C. RESTER.

585—℞ Acidi carbolici . . . . ℨx.
    Acidi salicylici . . . . ℨij.
    Acidi benzoici . . . . ℨiv.
    Spts. vini rectif. . . . . . . q. s. ut ft. sol.—M.
Sig. To water constantly boiling add a spoonful of above
solution, using the whole quantity above in twenty-four
hours. The quantity may be increased if the size of the
room, age of the patient, or severity of the disease require
it.   RENOU.

586—℞ Olei terebinthinæ . . . . ℨiv.
Sig. A tablespoonful twice daily, or, in addition, ten drops
every hour. (*In fibrinous forms.*)   LUNIN.

DIPSOMANIA. (See Alcoholism.)

DROPSY.

587—℞ Infusi digitalis . . . . f℥iv.
Sig. A tablespoonful two or three times daily. BARTHOLOW.

588—℞ Spts. chloroformi . . . . ♏xx.
    Tinct. digitalis . . . . ♏x.
    Infusi buchu . . . . f℥j.—M.
Sig. To be taken three or four times daily, and followed by a
good drink of water. (*In renal dropsy.*) FOTHERGILL.

589—℞ Potassii acetatis . . . . ℨij.
    Spiritus ætheris nitrosi . . . . f℥ij.
    Aquæ cinnamomi . . . . f℥iss.
    Infusi digitalis . . . . f℥iv.—M.
Sig. A tablespoonful every four hours. (*In dropsy due to heart-
disease.*)   KILGOUR.

590—℞ Scillæ pulv.,
    Digitalis pulv.,
    Caffeina citrata . . . . āā gr. xxx.
    Hydrarg. chloridi mitis . . . . gr. v.—M.
Divid. in pil. xxx.
Sig. One three times a day, after meals. (*Cardiac dropsy.*)

591—℞ Potassii bicarb. . . . . gr. x.
    Ferri et ammonii citratis . . . . gr. v.
    Tinct. digitalis . . . . ♏x.
    Infusi buchu . . . . f℥j.—M.
Sig. To be taken three times daily. (*In cardiac dropsy with
gouty tendency or debility.*) FOTHERGILL.

592—℞ Magnes. sulph. . . . . ℨj.
    Aquæ. . . . . f℥iiss.
    Syr. zingiberis . . . . f℥ss.—M.
Sig. Two teaspoonfuls daily on waking.   SMITH.

593—℞ Antimonii et potassii tartratis . . . . . gr. ij.
    Pulveris scillæ . . . . ℨj.
    Potassii sulphatis . . . . ℨss.
    Potassii bitartratis . . . . ℨiss.—M.
Fiat pulvis et divide in partes æquales no. xx.
Sig. One powder four times daily. (*In general dropsy.*)
                                    EBERLE.

DROPSY (Continued).

594—℞ Potassii bicarbonatis . . . . ℨj.
    Potassii acetatis . . . . ℨv.
    Tincturæ scillæ . . . . fℨj.
    Spiritus juniperi compositi . . . . fℨj.
    Aquæ destillatæ . . . . f℥xij.
Fiat mistura.
Sig. Two tablespoonfuls three times a day. (*In local and general dropsy.*) BROWN.

595—℞ Pil. scillæ co.,
    Pil. colocynth. co. . . . . ää ℈ij.
    Olei tiglii . . . . ℳvj.—M.
Ft. massa et in pil. no. xviii div.
Sig. Three pills twice a week. SELWYN.

596—℞ Triturationis elaterini . . . . ◄ . gr. iij.
Fiant chartulæ no. vi.
Sig. One powder on tongue every hour until profuse watery discharge.

597—℞ Pulveris jalapæ . . . . ℨj.
    Potassii bitartratis . . . . ℨvj.
Misce et divide in chartulas vi.
Sig. One powder every three hours, in molasses. (*In general dropsy due to kidney-disease.*) N. CHAPMAN.

598—℞ Pulveris opii . . . . gr. iv.
    Hydrargyri chloridi mitis . . . . gr. vj.
    Pulveris digitalis . . . . gr. xij.
    Confectionis rosæ . . . . q. s.
Misce et fiant pilulæ no. xii.
Sig. One to be taken every eight hours. (*In hydrothorax and ascites.*) ELLIS.

599—℞ Pûlv. jalapæ . . . . gr. xv-xx.
    Potass. bitart. . . . . ℨij.
    Pulv. zingiberis . . . . gr. v.—M.
Sig. To be taken before breakfast, two or three times a week. WARING.

600—℞ Potassii bitartratis . . . . ℨij.
    Mucilaginis acaciæ . . . . fℨj.
    Spiritus ætheris nitrosi,
    Extracti taraxaci fluidi . . . . . . ää f℥ss.
    Aquæ destillatæ . . . . f℥ij.—M.
Sig. A dessertspoonful every four hours. (*In cases associated with disease of the liver and portal system.*) HILDENBRAND.

601—℞ Resinæ podophylli . . . . gr. iv.
    Potassii bitartratis . . . . ℨij.
Misce et divide in pulveres viii.
Sig. One powder every two hours. (*In anasarca.*) V. C. HOWE.

602—℞ Pilocarpinæ hydrochloratis . . . . . . gr. j.
    Sacchari lactis . . . . gr. xx.
    Alcohol . . . . q. s.
Misce et fiant tabellæ triturationes no. xii.
Sig. One or more tablets twice daily to induce free sweating. (*Used in renal dropsy.*)

603—℞ Acidi arseniosi . . . . gr. j.
    Sacchari albi . . . . gr. j.
Tere simul in pulverem subtilem, dein adde—
    Micæ panis . . . . q. s.
Misce bene et divide in pilulas xx.
Sig. One pill twice daily. (*In swelling of the feet of old people.*) WOOD.

604—℞ Vini colchici sem. . . . . f℥ss.
    Liq. ammonii acetat. . . . . f℥iss.
    Infusi petroselini . . . . f℥v.—M.
Sig. A teaspoonful every four hours. (*Especially adapted to scarlatinal dropsy.*) BARTHOLOW.

605—℞ Mist. ferri et ammon. acetat. (U.S.P.) . . f℥vj.
Sig. One or two teaspoonfuls three or four times daily. BASHAM.

DROPSY (Continued).

606—℞ Extracti jaborandi fluidi,
Elixiris simplicis . . . . āā f℥j.
Aquæ destillatæ . . . . f℥j.—M.
Sig. A tablespoonful every four hours. (*In hydrothorax and ascites.*)   GUBLER.

607—℞ Juniperi contusi,
Sinapis,
Zingiberis . . . . āā ℥ss.
Armoraciæ contusæ,
Petroselini . . . . āā ℥j.
Succi fermenti pomorum . . . . Oij.
Macera per diem unam et cola.
Sig. A wineglassful three or four times a day. (*In cases of general dropsy which admit of stimulation.*) The cider should be old and sound.   JOSEPH PARRISH.

608—℞ Juniperi contusi . . . . ℥iv.
Aquæ bullientis . . . . f℥xij,
Macera per horas duodecim et exprime, dein adde—
Spiritus juniperi compositi . . . . . . f℥iv.—M.
Sig. A wineglassful mixed with a teaspoonful of cream of tartar three times a day.   W. PROCTOR, JR.

609—℞ Potassii iodidi . . . . ℥ss-℥j.
Aquæ destillatæ . . . . f℥vj.—M.
Sig. A tablespoonful three times a day. (*In anasarca with scanty urine.*)   RINGER.

DYSENTERY.

610—℞ Hydrarg. chlorid mit. . . . . ℥j.
In pulv. no. viii div.
Sig. A powder two or three times daily. (*In the epidemic form.*)   HULL.

611—℞ Hydrargyri chloridi corrosivi . . . . . gr. j.
Syrupi simplicis . . . . f℥j.
Aquæ destillatæ . . . . f℥viij.—M.
Sig. A teaspoonful every hour or two. (*Where there is much mucus.*)   RINGER.

612—℞ Plumbi acetat. . . . . gr. xxiv.
Pulv. ipecac. . . . . gr. iij.
Pulv. opii. . . . . gr. iij.—M.
Ft. massa et in pil. no. xii div.
Sig. One pill every two hours until blood ceases; then at longer intervals.   DA COSTA.

613—℞ Tinct. opii . . . . ℥ss.
Sig. Twenty drops to be given after a mustard plaster has been put over the stomach, and one hour later give the following:

℞ Pulv. ipecac. . . . . ℥ii-iiss.
In pulv. no. vi div.
Sig. One powder, stirred in a little water, to be taken every evening at bedtime.   MCDOWELL.

614—℞ Neutral aluminum and potassium sul-
phate . . . . gr. ¾.
Lead acetate . . . . gr. 1½.
Cocoa butter . . . . ℥v.
Beeswax . . . . gtt. xx.—M.
Sig. Divide into ten suppositories. One is to be introduced every three or four hours.   M. T. GUIDA.

615—℞ Argenti nitratis . . . . ℥j.
Aquæ destillatæ . . . . ℥j.—M.
Sig. One drachm of solution to three pints of water, to be introduced by a colon tube attached to a fountain syringe daily. (*Tubercular and chronic colitis.*)   H. TUCKER.

616—℞ Sol. hydrarg. bichlorid. (1-10,000) . . . . Oij.
Sig. The whole quantity to be used as an irrigating enema, after the rectum has been washed out with water as hot as can be borne. To be repeated every twelve hours, and each time followed by—

617—℞ Suppositorium opii . . . . no. j.
Sig. Introduce into the rectum.   FORDYCE.

618—℞ Thymoli . . . . ʒj.
Ft. massa et in pil. no. xxiv. div.
Sig. Two pills every six hours.   MARTINI.

619—℞ Tinct. opii deodoratæ . . . . ʒss.
Bismuthi subnitratis . . . . ʒij.
Aquæ menthæ pip.,
Syr. zingiberis . . . . āā fʒj.—M.
Sig. Shake bottle. Give one teaspoonful every two to four
hours, to a child five years of age. Half dose for child one
year of age.   J. LEWIS SMITH.

620—℞ Vini ipecac.. . . . . fʒss.
Sig. One drop every hour. (*In the acute or chronic form of
children, with slimy stools.*)   RINGER.

621—℞ Iodoformi . . . . ʒj.
Olei olivæ . . . . fʒiij.—M.
Sig. Keep on ice. Tablespoonful injected into rectum every
four to six hours.

622—℞ Pure creasote . . . . ℥xv.
Laudanum . . . . ℥v.
Milk or bouillon . . . . ʒv.
Sig. To be added to six ounces of boiled water and given as
one injection. (*Acute dysentery.*)   TESTEVIN.

623—℞ Cupri sulphatis . . . . gr. ss.
Magnesii sulphatis . . . . ʒj.
Acidi sulphurici diluti . . . . fʒj.
Aquæ destillatæ . . . . fʒiv.—M.
Sig. A tablespoonful every four hours. (*In acute dysentery.*)
BARTHOLOW.

624—℞ Naphthalini . . . . ʒiss.
Dispensa in capsulas no. xviiL
Sig. Two capsules every three hours. At least twelve to be
taken during the twenty-four hours.   HOLT.

625—℞ Ext. quebracho alc. . . . . ʒss.
Sig. Twenty to thirty drops every two or four hours. (*In
asthenic cases.*)   BOURDEAUX.

DYSMENORRHŒA.

626—℞ Chloroform. (pur.),
Spts. camphoræ . . . . āā fʒss.
Spts. æther. nitrosi,
Spts. æther. comp. . . . . āā fʒiss.—M.
Sig. fʒss-j in ʒj of water containing ʒj of spiritus frumenti
every half-hour for three doses.   J. C. DA COSTA.

627—℞ Alcohol of melissa,
Tincture of saffron,
Tincture of iodine, ... of each fʒj.—M.
Sig. Twelve drops daily, before each of the two principal
meals.   MONIN.

628—℞ Fluid extract of cimicifuga . . . . ʒij.
Fluid extract of gelseminum semper-
virens (green root) . . . . ʒj.—M.
Sig. Ten drops every two or three hours. Begin treatment
one day prior to expected menstruation.   HOUSMAN

629—℞ Antipyrin. . . . . gr. ix.
Ext. cannabis indicæ,
Ext. digitalis,
Camphoræ . . . . āā gr. ⅒.
Sig. For one cachet. To be taken every two hours until the
pain ceases, but not more than six to be taken. P. MÉNIÈRE.

DYSMENORRHŒA (Continued).

630—℞ Antipyrin. . . . . ʒij.
Syr. tolutani . . . . fʒij.—M.

Sig. Two teaspoonfuls at first; one teaspoonful every hour or two afterwards until pain is relieved. DELLENBAUGH.

631—℞ Antipyrin. . . . . gr. xxviiiss.
Cocain. muriatis . . . . gr. iss.
Aquæ bullientis . . . . fʒij.—M.

Sig. Ten to twenty minims hypodermically. (*In neuralgic and congestive forms.*) May also be taken by mouth.
P. MÉNIÈRE.

632—℞ Phenacetin. . . . . ʒj.

In pil. (compressas) no. xx div.
Sig. One pill every half-hour till relieved: no more than six in one series. J. C. WILSON.

633—℞ Liq. ammonii acetat. . . . . : . fʒiv.

Sig. A tablespoonful every two or three hours, with the following:

634—℞ Pulv. ipecac. . . . . gr. iv.

In pil. no. xii div.
Sig. One every two or three hours. EMMET.

635—℞ Extracti cannabis indicæ. . . . . gr. iij.
Sacchari lactis . . . . ʒss.

Misce et fiant chartulæ no. vi.
Sig. One powder every two or three hours. H. C. WOOD.

636—℞ Crotonis chloralis. . . . . gr. xxiv.
Pulveris tragacanthæ,
Glycerini . . . . āā q. s.

Misce et fiant pilulæ no. xii.
Sig. Two pills every two hours. (*In neuralgic dysmenorrhœa.*)
LOUIS LEWIS.

637—℞ Tinct. pulsatillæ radicis . . . . fʒss.

Sig. Two or three drops every two hours for ten days preceding the period. BROWN.

638—℞ Tincturæ opii deodoratæ . . . . fʒij.
Extracti cimicifugæ . . . . . . ⸱. . . . fʒss.
Syrupi simplicis . . . . fʒx.—M.

Sig. A teaspoonful every three or four hours. (*To restore the menstrual flow after it has been suddenly checked.*) RINGER.

639—℞ Cupri arseniatis . . . . gr. ¹⁄₈.
Tinct. pulsatillæ . . . . ℳxv.
Tinct. nucis vom. . . . . ℳviij.
Aq. dest. . . . . fʒiiiss.—M.

Sig. One teaspoonful every hour, or half-hour, until the pain is relieved. Lancet.

640—℞ Potassii bromidi,
Chloral. hydratis . . . . āā ʒiv.
Syrupi simplicis,
Aquæ. . . . . āā fʒij.—M.

Sig. Two tablespoonfuls to be used as an enema, as required for pain. MÉNIÈRE.

641—℞ Tinct. guaiaci ammoniatæ . . . . fʒij.

Sig. One-half to one teaspoonful in milk every two or three hours until pain is relieved. SIR JAMES SAWYER.

642—℞ Apiolis . . . . fʒj.
Alcoholis . . . . fʒij.
Syrupi simplicis . . . . fʒss.
Aquæ destillatæ . . . . fʒij.—M.

Sig. A teaspoonful every two hours. (*In anæmic cases.*)
JORET ET HOMOLLE.

643—℞ Extracti gelsemii fluidi . . . . fʒiiss.
Elixiris simplicis. . . . . fʒvss.
Syrupi aurantii corticis . . . . fʒj.—M.

Sig. A teaspoonful every two hours. PORCHER.

59

DYSMENORRHŒA (Continued).

644—℞ Gossypii radicis contusi . . . . ℨii.
Aquæ bullientis . . . . Oij.
Misce, coque ad Oj, et cola.
Sig. A wineglassful every hour.   T. J. SHAW.

645—℞ Amyli nitritis . . . . f ℨj.
Sig. Five drops upon handkerchief by inhalation to relieve
severe pain. (*Used in spasmodic dismenorrhœa to relieve
pain.*)

646—℞ Camphoræ . . . . ℈j.
Alcoholis . . . . q. s. ut fiat pulvis.
Dein adde—
Pulveris acaciæ,
Sacchari albi . . . . āā ℨj.
Aquæ cinnamomi . . . . f ℨj.
Fiat mistura.
Sig. The one-half the instant pain is felt; if not relieved in
an hour or two, give the remainder.   DEWEES.

DYSPEPSIA.

647—℞ Tinct. nucis vomicæ . . . . f ℨiss.
Resorcin. . . . . gr. vij.—M.
Sig. Dose, five to ten drops three times daily.
     Therapeutic Gazette.

648—℞ Salicylate of bismuth,
Naphthol,
Magnesia . . . . āā gr. x.
Divide into thirty powders.
Sig. One powder after each meal.   SONNEBERG.

649—℞ Acidi hydrochlorici diluti . . . . f ℨvj.
Tincturæ capsici . . . . f ℨiv.
Tincturæ nucis vomicæ . . . . f ℨij.
Tincturæ quassiæ. . . . . q. s. ad f ℨiv.—M.
Sig. Teaspoonful in water after meals.

650—℞ Creasote (beechwood) . . . . gtt. iij.
Alcohol . . . . ℳ xv.
Powdered acacia . . . . ℨiss.
Syrup. . . . . f ℨj.
Orange-flower water . . . . f ℨiss.
Water . . . . q. s. ad f ℨiij.
Sig. A teaspoonful for children, a tablespoonful for adults,
three times daily, before meals.   ZANGGER.

651—℞ Tinct. opii deodoratæ . . . . gtt. xij.
Magnesii calcinati . . . . gr. xij-xxiv.
Sacchari albi . . . . ℨj.
Aquæ anisi . . . . f ℨiss.—M.
Sig. Shake bottle. One teaspoonful every two hours to a
child one year old, until relieved. If much pain, add a
little chloroform or Hoffmann's Anodine to the mixture.
     J. LEWIS SMITH.

652—℞ Pepsini (scale) . . . . ℨiv.
Peptonoidi liquidi (Arlington) . . . . . f ℨvj.—M.
Sig. Shake. Wineglassful every half-hour.

653—℞ Bismuthi subnitratis,
Sodii bicarbonatis,
Pulv. cubebæ . . . . āā ℨj.
Pulv. zingiberis . . . . ℈j.—M.
In pulv. no. xii div.
Sig. A powder in a wineglassful of water before each meal.
     ALONZO CLARK.

DYSPEPSIA (Continued).

654—℞ Extracti pancreati . . . . ℨiv.

Fiant chartulæ no. xii.
Sig. One powder with about half its bulk of bicarbonate of
soda two hours after meals.

655—℞ Naphthalini . . . . ℨiss.

Dispensa in capsulas no. xviii.
Sig. One or two capsules every three to six hours. (*In flatulent dyspepsia and intestinal indigestion.*)   HOLT.

656—℞ Ammonii salicylatis . . . . ℨij.
    Syr. aurantii cort. . . . . f℥j.
    Aquæ menthæ pip. . . . . ad f℥iv.—M.

Sig. A tablespoonful half an hour before meals. (*In fermenta-
tive dyspepsia.*)   SULLIVAN.

657—℞ Sodii sulpho-carbolat. . . . . ℨiv.
    Glycerini . . . . ℨij.
    Infusi quassiæ . . . . f℥vj.—M.

Sig. A tablespoonful before meals. (*In flatulent dyspepsia.*)
          DELAFIELD.

658—℞ Carbonis ligni . . . . ℨj.
    Bismuthi subnitratis . . . . ℈ij.

Misce et fiant chartulæ iv.
Sig. One powder three times a day. (*With flatulence.*)
          RINGER.

659—℞ Pulveris zingiberis . . . . ℈j.
    Magnesii carbonatis . . . . ℈ij.
    Carbonis ligni . . . . ℨj.

Misce et divide in chartulas iv.
Sig. One powder three times a day. (*With acidity.*)
          DUNGLISON.

660—℞ Potassii iodidi,
    Manganesii sulphatis exsiccati . . . āā ℨj.   .
    Mellis despumati . . . . q. s.

Fiat massa, in pilulas no. xxx dividenda.
Sig. One pill morning and night. (Keep in well-stoppered
bottle.)   HANNON.

661—℞ Sol. iodi trichlor. (1–1500) . . . . f℥iv.—M.

Sig. A teaspoonful every two hours. (*When due to presence of
bacteria.*)   LANGENBUCH.

662—℞ Tinct. capsici . . . . ℳxvj.
    Tinct. nucis vomicæ . . . . f℥ij.
    Tinct. gentianæ co. . . . . ad f℥ij.—M.

Sig. A teaspoonful in water three times daily, with gr. ¼ aloin
at bedtime, avoiding starchy diet.   DA COSTA.

EARACHE. (See Otitis.)

ECTHYMA. (See Skin Diseases.)

ECZEMA. (See Skin Diseases.)

EMISSIONS. (See Spermatorrhœa.)

EMPHYSEMA. (See Asthma and Bronchitis.)

EMPYEMA.

663—℞ Mist. ferri et ammonii acetatis . . . . . f℥iv.

Sig. One to two teaspoonfuls three or four times daily, with
quinine and stimulants. (*In chronic cases.*)   DA COSTA.

664—℞ Aquæ chlori . . . . f℥j.
    Aquæ destillatæ . . . . f℥ix.—M.

Sig. To wash out the pleural cavity after the evacuation of
the pus.   RINGER.

61

EMPYEMA (Continued).

665—℞ Quininæ sulphatis . . . . ʒij.
Aquæ . . . . f ʒxij.—M.
Sig. Inject after evacuating the pus.   RINGER.

666—℞ Liquor iodi co. . . . . f ʒj.
Aquæ destillatæ . . . . f ʒxv.—M.
Sig. Inject after aspirating the pus.   BARTHOLOW.

667—℞ Ext. belladonnæ . . . . gr. ij.
Strychninæ sulph. . . . . gr. j.—M.
In pil. no. xxx div.
Sig. One pill four times daily, as a respiratory stimulant.
                                              J. C. WILSON.

ENDOCARDITIS.

668—℞ Tinct. veratri viridis . . . . f ʒj.
Sig. Two drops every two or three hours.   J. C. WILSON.

669—℞ Tinct. digitalis . . . . f ʒj.
Sig. Ten or fifteen drops every four hours. (*When heart's
action is irregular.*)   DA COSTA.

670—℞ Tinct. aconiti radicis . . . . f ʒss.
Sig. One drop every hour or two.   RINGER.

671—℞ Tincturæ aconiti . . . . ♏xij.
Aquæ . . . . f ʒiij.—M.
Sig. One teaspoonful every hour until heart is calmed, then
reduce dose or discontinue. Ice-bags to præcordium. (*Used
in acute sthenic cases with bounding pulse of high tension.*)
                                              H. A. HARE.

672—℞ Emplastri cantharidis . . . . 3 in. ✕ 3 in.
Sig. Apply over heart. When drawn, poultice blister till
full, then cut and dress with simple cerate. (*To promote
absorption of effusion.*)   WARING.

ENTERITIS.

673—℞ Pulv. opii . . . . gr. v.
Bismuthi subnitratis . . . . ʒij.—M.
Divide in pulveres no. xx.
Sig. A powder every two to four hours, for a child of five
years.   J. LEWIS SMITH.

674—℞ Hydrargyri chloridi mitis . . . . gr. vj.
Pulveris opii . . . . gr. iij.
Quininæ sulphatis . . . . gr. xij.
Syrupi simplicis . . . . q. s.
Fiat massa, in pilulas xii dividenda.
Sig. One pill night and morning.   CHANNING.

675—℞ Olei ricini . . . . ʒj.
Pulv. acaciæ,
Sacch. albi . . . . āā ℈iss.
Tinct. opii . . . . ♏lij.
Aquæ cinnamomi . . . . f ʒxj.—M.
Sig. A teaspoonful every four hours, for a child of one year.
                                              TANNER.

676—℞ Liq. potassii arsenitis . . . . gtt. l.
Tinct. opii . . . . gtt. cxx.
Aquæ . . . . ad f ʒiij.—M.
Sig. A teaspoonful before meals thrice daily. (*In the chronic
form.*)   BARTHOLOW.

677—℞ Tinct. opii deodoratæ . . . . f ʒj.
Sig. Ten drops every second or third hour, according to age,
to the point of tolerance.   DA COSTA.

678—℞ Salol . . . . gr. ¼-j.
Bismuth. subnit. . . . . gr. x.
Mucilag. acaciæ . . . . ʒij.
Sig. Repeat every two hours. (*Gastro-enteritis of children.*)
                                              GRAHAM.

ENTERITIS (Continued).

679—℞ Hydrargyri chloridi corrosivi . . . . . gr. j.
Tincturæ rhei,
Tincturæ cinchonæ . . . . āā f3j.—M.

Sig. A teaspoonful twice a day. (*In chronic cases.*)
ASTLEY COOPER.

680—℞ Extracti chrysophylli . . . . 3ss.
Aquæ destillatæ . . . . f3ij.
Tere simul, cola, et adde—
Syrupi acaciæ . . . . f3j.—M.

Sig. A teaspoonful every four hours. TROUSSEAU.

681—℞ Hydrarg. chlor. mit.,
Pulv. ipecac. . . . . āā gr. ij.
Ext. hyoscyami . . . . gr. iv-vj.
Plumbi acetatis . . . . gr. viij-xij.—M.

Ft. massa et in pil. no. xii div.
Sig. One pill every three hours. For children. CONDIE.

682—℞ Pulv. ipecac. co. . . . . 3j.
Bismuthi subnitratis . . . . 3ij.—M.

In pulv. no. xxiv div.
Sig. A powder every two to four hours, for a child five years
old. J. LEWIS SMITH.

683—℞ Iodoformi . . . . 3j.
Saloli . . . . 3j.
Acidi tannici . . . . 3ij.

Pone in cachetas no. xxiv.
Sig. One cachet three times a day. (*Used in tubercular enteritis.*)

EPILEPSY.

684—℞ Nickel. bromidi . . . . gr. xvj.
Aquæ destillatæ . . . . 3ij.—M.

Sig. A teaspoonful several times daily, according to tolerance.
DA COSTA.

685—℞ Ammonii bromidi,
Potassii iodidi . . . . āā ɔviij.
Potassii bromidi . . . . 3vj.
Sodii bicarbonatis . . . . 3ij.
Tincturæ calumbæ . . . . f3ij.
Aquæ destillatæ . . . . f3vj.—M.

Sig. A dessertspoonful after each meal, and a tablespoonful
at bedtime. BROWN-SÉQUARD.

686—℞ Ferri bromidi . . . . gr. iv.
Potassii bromidi . . . . 3j.
Aquæ destillatæ . . . . f3ij.
Syrupi simplicis . . . . f3vj.—M.

Sig. A tablespoonful twice daily. (*In anæmic subjects.*)
BARTHOLOW.

687—℞ Extracti solani carolinensis fluidi . . . f3j.

Sig. Ten to thirty drops in water three times a day. (*Used in
epileptics with arterial relaxation.*)

688—℞ Acetanilid. (antifebrin.) . . . . 3j.
Spts. vini gallici . . . . 3j.
Syr. simplicis . . . . ad 3iss.—M.

Sig. A teaspoonful two or three times daily. LEIDY, JR.

689—℞ Chloralis hydratis . . . . 3ss.
Syrupi simplicis,
Aquæ destillatæ . . . . āā f3ij.

Misce et fiat haustus.
Sig. At bedtime. (*To prevent nocturnal fits.*) DA COSTA.

690—℞ Iodi . . . . gr. ij.
Potassii iodidi . . . . 3iv.
Aquæ menthæ piperitæ . . . . f3vj.

Fiat solutio.
Sig. A teaspoonful thrice daily. MAGENDIE.

63

EPILEPSY (Continued).

691—℞ Tab. duboisinc sulphat . . . . . . āā gr. 〱.
No. xii.
Sig. One given hypodermically as indicated.   CIVIDALI.

692—℞ Extracti glandulœ suprarenalis . . . . ʒij.
Ponc in capsulas no. xxiv.
Sig. One capsule three times a day. (*Used along with bromides
in epileptics with lowered arterial tension.*)

693—℞ Ext. conii fld. (Squibb) . . . . ʒij.
Sig. Fifteen to sixty minims, not over three times daily.
SPITZKA.

EPISTAXIS.

694—℞ Ext. hamamelidis ud. . . . . fʒij.
Sig. A teaspoonful every one to three hours. If pulse is
rapid and bounding, add veratrum viride and morphine.
J. V. SHOEMAKER.

695—℞ Ext. geranii mac. fld. . . . . fʒj.
Aquæ . . . . fʒiij.—M.
Sig. Syringe the nostrils, or plug with cotton saturated with
the fluid.   J. V. SHOEMAKER.

696—℞ Olei erigerontis (canad.) . . . . fʒj.
Sig. Five to fifteen drops on sugar every hour, or repeated as
required.   ELLWOOD WILSON.

697—℞ Tincturæ aconiti radicis . . . . ℳviij.
Liquoris ammonii acetatis . . . . . . fʒj.—M.
Sig. A teaspoonful every half-hour. (*In plethoric cases.*)
THOMAS.

698—℞ Pulv. ipecac. . . . . gr. xx.
Olei theobromæ . . . . ʒss.—M.
Ft. suppositor. no. i.
Sig. Introduce into the rectum, and when vomiting ceases
give—

699—℞ Pulv. ipecac.,
Ext. glycyrrhizæ . . . . āā ʒss.—M.
Sig. A powder every three hours.   PEPPER.

700—℞ Pulv. aluminis,
Pulv. acidi tannici . . . . . āā partes æquales.—M.
Sig. To be insufflated into the nares anteriorly and poste-
riorly.   SAJOUS.

701—℞ Corrosive sublimate . . . . gr. j.
Dilute hydrochloric acid,
Tincture of cannabis indica . . . . āā ʒij.
Ergotin . . . . gr. xxx.
Simple syrup . . . . ʒj.
Infusion of quassia . . . . ʒviij.—M.
Sig. Three large teaspoonfuls of this solution may be taken
each day in a glass of water.

702—℞ Liquoris ferri persulphatis . . . . fʒj.
Aquæ destillatæ . . . . fʒij.—M.
Sig. Inject into the nostril.   R. J. LEVIS.

703—℞ Antipyrin. . . . . ʒij.
In capsulas no. xxiv div.
Sig. One, two, or three to be taken as required. To be used
with local treatment.   BEVERLEY ROBINSON.

704—℞ Pulveris aluminis,
Pulveris acaciæ . . . . . . āā partes æquales.—M.
Sig. To be blown into the nostrils.   LECLUYSE.

705—℞ Pulv. acidi tannici . . . . ʒij.
Sig. To be insufflated after a small quantity of cocaine has
been applied.   FLETCHER INGALS.

706—℞ Tannic acid,
 Camphor . . . . āā ℥iij.
 Spirit of ether . . . . f℥iij.
Sig. To be applied hourly for four or five times. REHBINDER.

707—℞ Ichthyol . . . . ℈ss.
 Ætheris,
 Glycerini . . . . āā ℥ij.—M.
Sig. Apply locally.   LORENZ.

708—℞ Aristol. . . . . gr. xx.
 Collodii . . . . ℥j.—M.
Sig. Apply with camel's-hair brush over and slightly beyond inflamed area, and renew when it scales off.
            West. Med. Rev.

709—℞ Creolin . . . . 1 part.
 Iodoform . . . . 4 parts.
 Lanolin . . . . 10 "
Sig. Paint on.   KOCH.

710—℞ Acidi carbolici puri,
 Alcoholis absoluti . . . . āā ℳxlv.
 Aquæ destillatæ . . . . f℥iij.—M.
Sig. For hypodermic injection,   HUNTER.

711—℞ Acetanilid. (antifebrin.) . . . . ℈j.
Dispensa in capsulas no. xv.
Sig. Two capsules as required. (To reduce the temperature.)
             OSLER.

712—℞ Acidi sulphurosi,
 Glycerini . . . . āā f℥iss.—M.
Sig. Apply locally to inflamed part.   DEWAR.

713—℞ Sodii salicylat. . . . . ℈ss.
 Ungt. aquæ rosæ . . . . ℥ij.—M.
Sig. Apply locally.   H. TUCKER.

714—℞ Sol. hydrarg. bichlor. (3–1000) . . . . . q. s.
Sig. Bathe the parts and irrigate the wounds, and cover with iodoform gauze wet with the solution. Apply tar to the red portions of the skin and a little beyond. Then cover with a wet dressing made with "Burow's Fluid" (No. 717, infra).

715—℞ Plumbi acetatis . . . . ℈j.
 Tinct. opii . . . . ℥j.
 Aquæ . . . . ad Oj.—M.
Sig. Shake the bottle well, and wet cloths or lint thoroughly with the lotion and apply to affected parts.
          Charity Hospital, N.Y.

716—℞ Cretæ præparatæ,
 Adipis . . . . āā ℈j.
 Acidi carbolici . . . . ℈j.—M.
Ft. unguentum.
Sig. Apply externally and cover with lint.
       SIR DYCE DUCKWORTH.

717—℞ Aluminis crudi . . . . ℈j.
 Plumbi acetatis cryst. . . . . ℈v.
 Aquæ destillatæ . . . . ℥xiiss.—M.
Sig. "Burow's Fluid."   FRAIPONT.

718—℞ Pilocarpinæ hydrochloratis . . . . . . gr. j.
 Aquæ . . . . f℥iss.—M.
Sig. Ten drops hypodermically every half-hour until free perspiration. (Used only in sthenic subjects.)

719—℞ Tincturæ ferri chloridi . . . . f℥vj-f℥iss.
 Syrupi simplicis . . . . f℥ij.
 Aquæ destillatæ . . . . q. s. ad f℥vj.—M.
Sig. A tablespoonful every two hours. GOLDBERG.

720—℞ Potassii permanganatis . . . . gr. vj.
 Aquæ destillatæ . . . . f℥vj.—M.
Sig. A tablespoonful three times a day. (Keep in glass-stoppered bottle.)   BARTHOLOW.

ERYSIPELAS (Continued).

721—℞ Ammonii carbonatis . . . . ℨij.
        Extracti glycyrrhizæ fluidi . . . . . . f℥j.
        Liquoris ammonii acetatis . . . . f℥iij.—M.
   Sig. A dessertspoonful every three hours,   BRANDE.

ERYTHEMA. (See Skin Diseases.)

FAVUS. (See Skin Diseases.)

FETOR OF AXILLÆ, BREATH, AND FEET.

722—℞ Sodii bicarbonatis . . . . ℨij.
        Aquæ . . . . f℥viij.—M.
   Sig. Apply as a lotion frequently.   BARTHOLOW.

723—℞ Potassii permanganatis . . . . gr. x-xxx.
        Aquæ . . . . f℥viij.—M.
   Sig. Apply locally frequently.   BARTHOLOW.

724—℞ Atropinæ sulphatis . . . . gr. iv-vij.
        Aquæ rosæ . . . . f℥ij.—M.
   Sig. Apply to the part with a brush.   BARTHOLOW.

725—℞ Aluminii chloridi . . . . ℨss.
        Aquæ . . . . Oj.—M.
   Sig. Apply locally.   GOLDBERG.

726—℞ Sodii bicarbonatis . . . . ℨss.
        Aquæ . . . . Oj.—M.
   Sig. Apply locally.   GOLDBERG.

727—℞ Sodii biboratis . . . . gr. xv.
        Thymoli . . . . gr. viiss.
        Aquæ destillatæ . . . . f℥lxxv.—M.
   Ft. sol.
   Sig. Mouth-wash. (For fetor of breath due to carious teeth.)
                                           MAGITOT.

728—℞ Pepsini (scale) . . . . ℨiv.
        Acidi hydrochlorici diluti . . . . . . f℥iv.
        Strychninæ sulphatis . . . . gr. ¼.
        Aquæ . . . . q s. ad f℥viij.—M.
   Sig. Tablespoonful in water after meals.

729—℞ Acidi salicylici . . . . gr. xxx.
        Pulv. amyli . . . . ℥v.
        Pulv. talci . . . . ℨxxij.—M.
   Sig. Dust in socks.   J. C. WILSON.

FEVERS, ERUPTIVE AND SIMPLE.

730—℞ Antipyrin . . . . ℨj.
        Syr. simplicis . . . . f℥ss.
        Aquæ cinnamomi . . . . ad f℥ij.—M.
   Sig. One-half to one teaspoonful every hour or two for children.   PENZOLDT.

731—℞ Antifebrin . . . . ℨj-ij.
        Spts. vini gallici . . . . f℥ss.
        Syr. simplicis . . . . ad f℥ij.—M.
   Sig. A teaspoonful every four hours, or as required. (To
   reduce the temperature.)   HEINZELMANN.

732—℞ Amyli hydratis . . . . ℨij.
        Syr. simplicis . . . . f℥j.
        Aquæ . . . . ad f℥iv.—M.
   Sig. Two tablespoonfuls at bedtime, in water, for adult. (For
   insomnia of fevers.)   VON MERING.

733—℞ Ammonii salicylatis . . . . ℨj.
        Syr. simplicis . . . . f℥ss.
        Aquæ menthæ pip. . . . . ad f℥iiss.—M.
   Sig. A teaspoonful every four hours to a child three years
   old. To adults, two or three teaspoonfuls may be given
   every four hours.   SULLIVAN.

F

FEVERS, ERUPTIVE AND SIMPLE (Continued).

734—R, Tincturæ aconiti folii . . . . f3v.
    Extracti veratri viridis fluidi . . . . . f3j.—M.
Sig. Twelve drops every two hours, watching effects.
    WEBER.

735—R, Tincturæ aconiti radicis . . . . ℔xxx.
    Syrupi limonis . . . . f3ss.
    Liquoris ammonii acetatis . . . . . . f3ij.—M.
Sig. A dessertspoonful every three hours. R. P. THOMAS.

736—R, Sodii bromidi . . . . gr. x-xx.
    Syr. aurantii cort.. . . . . f3ss.
    Aquæ . . . . ad f3iiss.—M.
Sig. A teaspoonful every quarter of an hour for children.
    A. A. SMITH.

737—R, Liq. ammonii acetatis . . . . f3iiss.
    Spts. ætheris nitrosi . . . . ad f3iv.—M.
Sig. A teaspoonful to a tablespoonful, according to age.
    HARTSHORNE.

738—R, Antimonii et potassii tartratis . . . . . gr. viij.
    Aquæ destillatæ . . . . f3viij.—M.
Sig. Sponge the scalp frequently. (*For loss of hair after fever.*)
    POULAIN.

739—R, Antimonii et potassi. tartratis,
    Morphinæ sulphatis . . . . āā gr. j.
    Hydrargyri chloridi mitis . . . . . . gr. iij.
    Potassii nitratis . . . . 5j.
Misce et fiant chartulæ no. xii.
Sig. One powder every two or three hours. PENDLETON TUTT.

740—R, Vini antimonii . . . . . . ; . . . . f5j.
    Potassii vel sodii nitratis . . . . 5j.
    Spiritus ætheris nitrosi . . . . f3iij.
    Liquoris morphinæ sulphatis . . . . f3j.
    Syrupi acidi citrici . . . . f3ss.
    Liquoris potassii citratis . . . . f3iv.—M.
Sig. A tablespoonful every two hours. CARSON.

741—R, Cocain. hydrochloratis . . . . gr. iv.
    Aquæ destillatæ . . . . f3ij.
Sig. Seven to fifteen minims hypodermically every two hours.
(*In low fevers with weak circulation.*) DA COSTA.

742—R, Tincturæ opii deodoratæ . . . . gtt. xlv.
    Vini antimonii . . . . f3iss.
    Spiritus ætheris nitrosi . . . . f3ij.
    Syrupi limonis . . . . f3ij.
    Liquoris ammonii acetatis . . . . . . f3vj.
Fiat mistura.
Sig. A tablespoonful every two hours. EBERLE.

743—R, Glycerini . . . . f3viiss.
    Acidi citrici vel tartarici . . . . 5ss.
    Aquæ . . . . f3xix.—M.
Sig. One to two tablespoonfuls every hour as a beverage.
(*When used freely, the excretion of urea is diminished.*)
    SEMMOLA.

FEVER, HECTIC.

744—R, Antipyrin. . . . . 3ij.
    Aquæ . . . . f3viij.—M.
Sig. Two tablespoonfuls, followed by one tablespoonful
every hour till temperature is normal. PRIBRAM.

745—R, Quininæ sulphatis . . . . 5j.
In pulv. no. xii div.
Sig. A powder, in water, three or four times daily. PHILLIPS.

746—R, Quininæ hydrochloratis . . . . gr. xxxij.
    Acidi hydrochlorici diluti . . . . f3j.
    Syrupi aurantii rubri . . . . f3vij.
    Aquæ . . . . f3iij.—M.
Sig. A dessertspoonful every four hours. ELLWOOD WILSON.

FEVER, HECTIC (Continued).

747—℞ Syr. calcis lactophosphatis . . . . . . f ʒiv.
Sig. A teaspoonful three or four times daily. BENEKÉ.

748—℞ Syrupi phosphatum compositi . . . . . f ʒiij.
Sig. A teaspoonful every four hours. PARRISH.

749—℞ Tinct. digitalis . . . . f ʒiij.
Tinct. ferri chlor. . . . . f ʒv.—M.
Sig. Fifteen drops three or four times daily, well diluted.
BARTHOLOW.

FEVER, INTERMITTENT AND REMITTENT.

750—℞ Quininæ sulphatis . . . . ℈ij.
Acidi sulphurici diluti . . . . f ʒj.
Syrupi zingiberis . . . . f ʒj.
Aquæ destillatæ . . . . q. s. ad f ʒiv.—M.
Sig. A dessertspoonful every two hours during the intermission.
DA COSTA.

751—℞ Quininæ sulphatis . . . . gr. vj.
Acidi tartarici . . . . gr. iij.
Syrupi simplicis . . . . f ʒj.—M.
Sig. A teaspoonful. CASOVATI.

752—℞ Quininæ ferrocyanatis . . . . gr. iv.
Alcoholis . . . . f ʒj.
Solve, et adde—
Aquæ camphoræ . . . . f ʒvij.—M.
Sig. A teaspoonful every hour or two. ELLIS.

753—℞ Quininæ sulphatis . . . . ℈ij.
Acidi salicylici . . . . ʒiiss.
Misce et divide in chartulas xvi.
Sig. One powder every three hours. SARZANCE.

754—℞ Extracti nucis vomicæ . . . . gr. iv.
Quininæ sulphatis . . . . ʒss.
Glycerini . . . . q. s. ut fiat massa in
pilulas xvi dividenda.
Sig. One pill three times a day. DA COSTA.

755—℞ Quininæ sulphatis . . . . gr. xlv.
Ferri et potassii tartratis . . . . gr. cv.
Aquæ destillatæ . . . . f ʒx.
Liquoris potassii arsenitis . . . . gtt. xxv.-M.
Sig. One to three tablespoonfuls daily. BACCELLI.

756—℞ Quininæ hydrochloratis . . . . gr. xv.
Sodii chloridi . . . . gr. xij.
Aquæ destillatæ . . . . ʒiij ʒj.—M.
Sig. For hypodermic injection. BACCELLI

757—℞ Cinchoninæ sulphatis . . . . ʒss.
Liquoris potassii arsenitis . . . . f ʒiss.
Tincturæ ferri chloridi . . . . f ʒss.
Syrupi zingiberis . . . . f ʒiss.
Aquæ destillatæ . . . . q. s. ad f ʒiv.—M.
Sig.—A dessertspoonful after meals. (*In chronic cases.*)
PENDLETON TUTT.

758—℞ Antimonii et potassii tartratis . . . . . gr. iij.
Quininæ sulphatis . . . . gr. x.
Misce et divide in partes æquales vi.
Sig. One powder every two hours during intermission. GOLA.

759—℞ Salicini . . . . gr. xxiv
Sacchari albi. . . . . ℈iv.
Misce et divide in partes æquales viii.
Sig. One powder three times a day. KROMBHOLZ.

760—℞ Ferri ferrocyanidi,
Pulveris guaiaci resinæ . . . . . . āā ʒj.
Misce et divide in chartulas xii.
Sig. One powder three times a day. (*In obstinate intermittens.*)
ELLIS.

761—℞ Cupri sulphatis . . . . gr. iv.
Extracti cinchonæ . . . . gr. xxxij.
Syrupi simplicis . . . . q. s. ut fiat massa in
pilulas xvi dividenda.
Sig. One to be taken three times a day. (*In obstinate cases.*)
CHAPMAN.

762—℞ Ferri redact.,
Quin. sulphat. . . . . āā gr. xlviij.
Acid. arseniosi . . . . gr. ss.
Ol. capsici . . . . ℥j.—M.
Fiant in pil. no. xxiv.
Sig. One after meals. C. J. MANLY.

763—℞ Extracti hydrastis fluidi,
Tincturæ eucalypti . . . . āā f℥iss.
Elixiris simplicis . . . . f℥j.
Vini xerensis . . . . f℥ij.—M.
Sig. A tablespoonful three times a day. (*In convalescents with hepatic and splenic enlargement.*) BARTHOLOW.

764—℞ Quininæ muriatis . . . . gr. vj.
Aquæ bullientis . . . . ℥lxij.—M.
Sig. Inject deeply into the tissues four to six minims of the hot solution. PULAWSKI.

765—℞ Quininæ sulphatis . . . . ℈iv.
Acidi sulphurici diluti . . . . q. s. ut ft. sol.
Spts. ætheris nitrosi . . . . f℥ss.
Syr. tolutani,
Aquæ . . . . āā q. s. ad f℥ij.—M.
Sig. A teaspoonful three or four times daily. DA COSTA.

766—℞ Quin. sulphat. . . . . gr. xv.
Syr. yerba santa co. . . . . f℥ij.—M.
Sig. Teaspoonful three times daily. (*For child of one year.*) C. J. MANLY.

767—℞ Chinoidini . . . . ℈ij.
Resinæ podophylli . . . . gr. iv.
Ferri sulph. exsic. . . . . ℈j.—M.
Ft. massa et in pil. no. xx div.
Sig. One three times daily. BARTHOLOW.

768—℞ Tetramethyli thionin-chloridi (methylene blue) . . . . ℈j.
Pone in capsulas no. xxiv.
Sig. One capsule every four hours.

769—℞ Tincturæ Warburgi . . . . f℥iv.
Sig. Tablespoonful and repeat in four hours to prevent attack. One to two teaspoonfuls after meals as prophylactic.

770—℞ Acidi carbolici . . . . gr. xlviij.
Syrupi acaciæ . . . . f℥iss.
Aquæ cinnamomi . . . . ad f℥iv.—M.
Sig. A teaspoonful every three hours until five doses are taken daily. LUZZATO.

771—℞ Acidi arseniosi . . . . gr. j.
Extracti taraxaci . . . . ℈j.—M.
Ft. massa et in pil. no. xl div.
Sig. One to four pills every three or four hours until twenty or thirty pills are taken. (*In hemorrhagic malarial fever.*) RIGGS.

772—℞ Pulv. opii . . . . gr. xij.
Pulv. capsici . . . . gr. xxxvj.
Quininæ sulph. . . . . ℈j.—M.
In pulveres no. xii div.
Sig. One powder three times daily. (*In inveterate forms.*) ALONZO CLARK.

773—℞ Ext. ergotæ aquosi (Bonjean) . . . . . gr. xxx.
Aquæ destillatæ,
Glycerini . . . . āā f℥iss.—M.
Sig. Inject a hypodermic syringeful into the spleen once or twice, at intervals of a few days. ROUQUETTE.

774—℞ Olei phosphorati . . . . f̃ss.
Sig. Five drops, well diluted, three times daily.   SOZINSKY.

775—℞ Potassii permanganatis . . . . gr. xij.
Aquæ destillatæ . . . . f̃iij.—M.
Sig. One or two teaspoonfuls three times daily. (*In chronic malarial cases.*)   JOS. LEVI.

776—℞ Antipyrin. . . . . ʒiv.
Syr. tolutani . . . . f̃iss.
Aquæ. . . . . ad f̃iij.—M.
Sig. One or two teaspoonfuls thrice daily.   ANTONY.

777—℞ Tinct. Iodi . . . . f̃vj.
Potassii Iodidi . . . . ʒij.
Aquæ cinnamomi . . . . ad f̃iij.—M.
Sig. A teaspoonful three times daily.   *Charity Hospital, N.Y.*

778—℞ Hydrochlorate of quinine . . . . gr. iv.
Warm infusion of chamomile . . . . . f̃ij.
Sydenham's laudanum . . . . gtt. ss.—M.
Sig. Give per rectum. (*Malaria in children.*)

779—℞ Ammonii picratis . . . . ʒj.
Ft. massa et in pilulas no. xl div.
Sig. One to three pills four or five times daily.   H. M. CLARK.

FEVER, TYPHOID.

780—℞ Acidi carbolici . . . . ℳxxiv.
Glycerini . . . . f̃ij.
Liquid. pepsin. aromat. . . . . f̃j.
Aquæ menthæ pip. . . . . f̃ij.—M.
Sig. A teaspoonful one hour after food.   McCOCKLE.

781—℞ Hydrarg. chlorid. mit. . . . . gr. xxij.
In pulv. no. iii div.
Sig. One powder every half-hour till three are taken. (*Only during the first week.*)   VON ZIEMSSEN.

782—℞ Hydrargyri chloridi mitis . . . . . . gr. vj.
Sacchari albi . . . . ʒij.
Misce et fiant chartulæ xii.
Sig. One every three hours. (*During first nine days, carefully avoiding ptyalism.*)   PARKES.

783—℞ Hydrarg. chlorid. mit. . . . . gr. x.
Sodii bicarb. . . . . gr. xv.—M.
In chartulas no. ii div.
Sig. One at night. To be given the first and third night of treatment, if before the tenth day.   J. C. WILSON.

784—℞ Antipyrin. . . . . ʒviij.
Syr. tolutani . . . . f̃j.
Aquæ . . . . ad f̃ij.—M.
Sig. Two or three teaspoonfuls at first, and one teaspoonful hourly thereafter, until temperature is reduced.   MINOT.

785—℞ Thallin. sulphat. . . . . gr. xxxij.
Aquæ menthæ pip. . . . . f̃j.—M.
Sig. A teaspoonful when required. (*For pyrexia of typhoid.*)   MINOT.

786 ℞ Antifebrin. . . . . ʒss-j.
Elixiris simplicis . . . . f̃j.—M.
Sig. A teaspoonful when required. (*For pyrexia.*)   BEREZOVSKY.

787—℞ Sodii salicylatis . . . . ʒss.
Syrupi simplicis . . . . f̃ss.
Aquæ destillatæ . . . . q. s. ad f̃ij.—M.
Sig. A tablespoonful every other night. (*To lower temperature.*)   MOELI.

788—℞ Acidi hydrochlorici diluti . . . . f℥j.
Syrupi . . . . f℥vij.
Aquæ destillatæ . . . . f℥ij.—M.
Sig. A dessertspoonful every two or three hours. (*In uncomplicated cases.*) DA COSTA.

789—℞ Olei terebinthinæ . . . . f℥iss.
Pulv. acaciæ,
Syrupi simplicis,
Aquæ destillatæ . . . . āā q. s.
Fiat emulsio, secundum artem, ad f℥ij.
Sig. A teaspoonful every two or three hours. (*With diarrhœa and tympanitis.*) G. B. WOOD.

790—℞ Pulveris ipecacuanhæ compositi . . . . gr. x.
Divide in chartulas iv.
Sig. One every hour or two. (*Used at night in wakeful delirium.*) RINGER.

791—℞ Strychniæ . . . . gr. ¹⁄₂₀,
Aquæ . . . . q. s.—M.
Sig. Use hypodermically in cardiac asthenia. J. C. WILSON.

792—℞ Guaiacoli carbonatis . . . . gr. xx.
Saloli . . . . gr. xl.—M.
Pone in capsulas no. xx.
Sig. One every eight hours.

793—℞ Thymoli . . . . ℈j.
Ext. gentianæ . . . . q. s.
Ft. massa et in pil. no. xxiv div.
Sig. Two pills every six hours. (*For diarrhœa and dry tongue of typhoid.*) HENRY.

794—℞ Benzonaphthol,
Salol,
Sodii bicarbonat.,
Magnesiæ . . . . āā gr. iij.
For one capsule.
Sig. One every four hours for intestinal antisepsis. (*Typhoid fever.*) J. D. RIBEIRO.

795—℞ Tinct. strophanth. hisp. (1-20) . . . . . f℥ss.
Sig. Four to eight minims three or four times daily. (*For weak heart of typhoid.*) QUINLAN.

796—℞ Acidi sclerotici . . . . ℈j.
Aquæ destillatæ . . . . f℥v.—M.
Sig. A hypodermic syringeful every half-hour as a styptic. (*In typhoid intestinal hemorrhage.*) VON ZIEMSSEN.

797—℞ Extracti ergotæ aquosi (ergotinæ) . . . gr. xv.
Syrupi aurantii corticis . . . . f℥j.
Aquæ destillatæ . . . . f℥iij.—M.
Sig. A tablespoonful every hour or two. (*In alarming intestinal hemorrhage.*) BONJEAN.

798—℞ Caffeine . . . . 6 gr.
Salicylate of sodium . . . . 4½ gr.
Distilled water . . . . up to 16 minims.—M.
Dissolve with the aid of heat. Sixteen minims of the solution contain six grains of caffeine. (*For hypodermic injections for heart-failure in enteric fever.*) TANRET.

FEVER, TYPHUS.

799—℞ Ext. opii . . . . gr. vj.
In pil. no. xii div.
Sig. One pill every three hours, until quiet. (*For restlessness, when there is no lung-complication present.*) TANNER.

800—℞ Tinct. digitalis,
Spts. chloroformi . . . . āā f℥ss.
Syr. aurantii cort. . . . . f℥ij.—M.
Sig. A teaspoonful every two hours. (*In cardiac asthenia.*) J. C. WILSON.

801—℞ Guaiacoli . . . . f ʒiv.

Sig. Ten to twenty drops in teaspoonful of sweet oil applied over abdomen. (*To reduce fever.*)

802—℞ Antimonii et potassii tartratis . . . . . gr. iv.
Tincturæ opii . . . . ƒʒj.
Aquæ camphoræ . . . . f ʒviij.—M.

Sig. A tablespoonful every two hours. (*With sleeplessness and extreme nervous excitement.*) GRAVES.

803—℞ Moschi optimi . . . . gr. x-ɔj.
Tincturæ castorei . . . . fʒij.
Syrupi zingiberis . . . . fʒij.
Aquæ destillatæ . . . . fʒj.

Misce et fiat haustus.
Sig. One dose, given in coma and last stage of typhus.
E. J. CLARK.

804—℞ Quininæ sulphatis . . . . ɔiv.
Acidi sulphurici dil. . . . . . . q. s. ut ft. sol.
Syr. simplicis. . . . . fʒss.
Aquæ. . . . . ad f ʒj.—M.

Sig. A teaspoonful every two hours until fever is lessened.
GOOLDEN.

805—℞ Acidi phosphorici dil. . . . . fʒj.

Sig. Twenty to thirty minims, well diluted, every four or six hours. TANNER.

806—℞ Tinct. belladonnæ . . . . ʒss.
Tinct. aconiti radicis . . . . ʒss.—M.

Sig. Ten drops every two hours. HARLEY.

FEVER, YELLOW.

807—℞ Hydrargyri chloridi mitis . . . . gr. xx.
Quininæ sulphatis . . . . gr. xxiv.

Misce et fiat chartula.
Sig. One dose, given in simple syrup, to be repeated every four to six hours until four doses are taken. (*Given at the very onset to abort the disease.*) BLAIR.

808—℞ Morphinæ sulphatis . . . . gr. j-ij.(!!)

Fiat chartula.
Sig. One dose. (To be given at the *very commencement after* a free mercurial purge followed by a saline cathartic.)
EDWARD FOWLER.

809—℞ Hydrarg. chloridi mitis,
Pulv. jalapæ . . . . ãã gr. x.—M.

Ft. pulv. no. i.
Sig. To be given early in the disease. RUSH.

810—℞ Tinct. iodidi . . . . ℳ viij.
Liq. ferri perchloridi . . . . ʒss.
Syr. piper. menth. . . . . fʒj.
Aquæ . . . . q. s. ad f ʒvj.—M.

Sig. Two teaspoonfuls every hour or two. (*For children.*)
TEIXERIA.

811—℞ Tincturæ aconiti foliorum . . . . gtt. x.
Spiritus ætheris nitrosi . . . . fʒj.—M.

In water every three or four hours. In forty or fifty hours the fever subsides and the stage of calm comes on. When much exhaustion during this stage, stimulants: when much restlessness, valerianate of zinc, gr. v-x, or morphine, gr. ¼, repeated as necessary. When retching and vomiting supervene, give—

812—℞ Morphinæ sulphatis . . . . gr. iv.
Creasoti . . . . ʒj.
Spiritus vini gallici . . . . f ʒiv.—M.

Sig. A tablespoonful every three hours as needed.
DOWELL.

813—℞ Chloroformi . . . . f 3j.
Syr. acaciæ . . . . f 3ij.—M.
Sig. A teaspoonful before nourishment. MacDonald.

814—℞ Sodii chloridi . . . . 3ss.
Olei olivæ . . . . f 3ss.
Olei terebinthinæ . . . . f 3j.
Aquæ ferventis . . . . Oiss.—M.
Sig. Use as an enema. Lawson.

815—℞ Ergotin . . . . 3j.
Acid. tannic. . . . . 3j.
Syr. krameriæ . . . . q. s. ad f 3iij.—M.
Sig. Teaspoonful diluted every third hour. (*For black vomit.*)
Teixeira.

816—℞ Olei terebinthinæ . . . . f 3iss.
Mucilaginis acaciæ . . . . f 3xivss.—M.
Sig. A teaspoonful every hour or two. (*To allay retching and vomiting.*) La Roche.

817—℞ Cocainæ . . . . gr. xxiv.
Aquæ . . . . f 3iij.—M.
Sig. Teaspoonful every two hours. (*For vomiting.*)

818—℞ Pilocarpinæ muriatis . . . . gr. iij.
Aquæ destillatæ . . . . f 3iij.—M.
Sig. Ten minims hypodermically. (*To favor diaphoresis.*)
Hebersmith.

819—℞ Potassii iodidi . . . . gr. ij.
Liquoris potassii arsenitis . . . . gtt. ij.—M.
Sig. One dose every two or three hours. (This should be given throughout the entire course of the disease, beginning with the second day.) Edward Fowler.

820—℞ Tincturæ ferri chloridi . . . . f 3iij.
Syrupi acidi citrici . . . . f 3xiij.—M.
Sig. A teaspoonful in ice-water every three or four hours.
Bailey.

821—℞ Creasoti . . . . 3j-iss.
Alcoholis . . . . q. s. ut fl. sol.
Liq. ammonii acetatis . . . . . . ad f 3iv.—M.
Sig. A teaspoonful every three or four hours. Lewis.

FISSURE OF ANUS AND NIPPLES.

822—℞ Extracti hydrastis fluidi . . . . f 3ss.
Sig. Apply to the affected part. Bartholow.

823—℞ Bismuthi subnit. . . . . gr. x.
Aristol . . . . gr. ij.
Pulv. opii . . . . gr. ss.
Ol. theobrom. . . . . q. s. ad sup. 1.—M.
Sig. Introduce an hour before the bowels move. W. J. Hearn.

824—℞ Liquoris ferri subsulphatis . . . . f 3ij.
Glycerini . . . . f 3vj.—M.
Sig. Apply with camel's-hair brush to affected parts. (*For nipple.*) Bartholow.

825—℞ Plumbi nitratis . . . . gr. x.
Glycerini . . . . f 3j.—M.
Sig. Apply after each nursing, carefully washing before next nursing. (*For excoriated and fissured nipple.*) Bartholow.

826—℞ Acidi carbolici . . . . gr. xxiv.
Aquæ . . . . f 3j.—M.
Ft. lotio.
Sig. Apply several times daily to the nipples. Parvin.

827—℞ Cocoa butter . . . . 3v.
Oil of almond . . . . ℳxv.
Extract of krameria . . . . gr. xv.—M.
Sig. Make into an ointment. Apply to the nipples.
Gazette hebdom.

828—℞ Acidi boracici . . . . gr. xx.
Mucilag. acaciæ . . . . ȝj.—M.
Sig. Use a nipple-shield, and, after nursing, dry the nipple
well with absorbent cotton and apply the lotion with a
camel's-hair brush. Should this fail, touch the fissure with
a point of argenti nitras every other day. STARR.

829—℞ Boric acid (powdered) . . . . gr. x.
Lanolin,
Cosmolin . . . . āā ȝss.—M.
Sig. Apply after each nursing. E. P. DAVIS.

830—℞ Acidi tannici . . . . ȝj.
Glycerini . . . . f ȝij.—M.
Sig. Introduce into the rectum night and morning on a tent.
(For fissure of anus.) WARING.

831—℞ Potassii bromidi . . . . ȝj.
Glycerini . . . . f ȝv.—M.
Sig. Apply locally. (For anus.) RINGER.

FISTULÆ.

832—℞ Camphor . . . . ȝj.
Salol . . . . ȝss.
Ether . . . . f ȝj.—M.
Sig. Use as an injection. St. Louis Hospital, Paris.

833—℞ Argenti nitratis . . . . gr. xij.
Aquæ destillatæ . . . . f ȝviij.
Solve.
Sig. Inject once daily. (Fistula in ano.) DRUITT.

834—℞ Acidi carbolici (pur.) . . . . gr. viij.
Ol. olivæ (boiled) . . . . f ȝj.
Sig. Apply on absorbent cotton. HEARN.

835—℞ Ext. sanguinariæ fld. . . . . f ȝij.
Sig. Inject a quantity sufficient to fill and distend the fistula.
PHILLIPS.

836—℞ Hydrargyri chloridi corrosivi . . . . . gr. ij.
Aquæ destillatæ . . . . f ȝviij.
Misce et fiat collyrium.
Sig. Apply to inner canthus of the eye twice daily. (In lach-
rymal fistula.) DRUITT.

837—℞ Formaldehydi (40 per cent. sol.) . . . . f ȝj.
Sig. Five to ten drops in half-pint of water, and inject into
fistula once daily.

838—℞ Methyl violet (blue pyoktanin) . . . . . ȝj.
Water . . . . f ȝiij.—M.
Sig. Inject every two or three days. (Sinus communicating
with carious cartilage after enteric fever.) J. C. WILSON.

FLATULENCE. (See also Acidity, Colic, and Dys-
pepsia.)

839—℞ Pulv. carbonis ligni . . . . ȝi-ij.
In pulv. no. xii div.
Sig. A powder at the time the flatulence usually appears.
RINGER.

840—℞ Tinct. asafœtidæ . . . . f ȝj.
Aquæ . . . . f ȝviij.—M.
Sig.—A teaspoonful three or four times daily. (For children.)
RINGER.

841—℞ Spiritus armoraciæ,
Elixiris simplicis . . . . āā f ȝss.—M.
Sig. A teaspoonful. RINGER.

842—℞ Olei caryophylli . . . . gtt. iij.
Camphoræ monobromatis . . . . gr. xij.—M.
In pil. no. xii div.
Sig. One pill an hour after meals. J. C. WILSON.

843—℞ Tinct. nucis vomicæ,
Tinct. physostigmatis,
Tinct. belladonnæ . . . . āā f3j.—M.
Sig. Fifteen drops, in a little water, two or three times daily.
BARTHOLOW.

844—℞ Pulv. calumbæ,
Pulv. zingiberis . . . . āā 3ss.
Sennæ fol. . . . . 3j.
Aquæ bullientis . . . . Oj.—M.
Ft. infusum.
Sig. A wineglassful three times daily. BARTHOLOW.

845—℞ Olei terebinthinæ . . . . f3j.
Sig. Three to five drops on sugar. BARTHOLOW.

846—℞ Magnesiæ . . . . 3j.
Spiritus ammoniæ aromatici . . . . . f3j.
Spiritus cinnamomi . . . . f3iij.
Aquæ destillatæ . . . . f3vj.—M.
Sig. A tablespoonful every two hours. (*In sour eructations.*)
ELLIS.

847—℞ Aloes . . . . gr. xxiv.
Asafœtidæ . . . . gr. xlviij.—M.
Fiant pilulæ no. xxiv.
Sig. One after meals. (*Used in flatulency and constipation of old people.*)

848—℞ Olei cajuputi . . . . : . . . . f3j.
Mucilaginis acaciæ . . . . f3ss.
Syrupi simplicis . . . . f3j.
Aquæ destillatæ . . . . q. s. ad f3vj.—M.
Sig. A tablespoonful. SWEDIAUR.

849—℞ Acidi sulphurosi . . . . f3iss.
Syrupi zingiberis . . . . f3viss.
Aquæ destillatæ. . . . . f3j.—M.
Sig. A teaspoonful. POLLI.

850—℞ Olei cajuputi . . . . 3ss.
Spts. lavandulæ co. . . . . f3ss.
Syr. zingiberis . . . . f3ij.
Mucil. acaciæ . . . . ad f3ij.—M.
Sig. A dessertspoonful, as required. HARTSHORNE.

851—℞ Aquæ anisi,
Liq. calcis . . . . āā f3ss.
Syr. acaciæ . . . . f3j.—M.
Sig. Add from ten to thirty drops of chloroform, according to age of child, and give a teaspoonful every two hours.
CONDIE.

FRECKLES, SUNBURN, AND TAN. (See Skin Diseases.)

FROST-BITE. (See also Chilblains.)

852—℞ Acidi carbolici . . . . 3j.
Tinct. iodi . . . . 3ij.
Acidi tannici . . . . 3ij.
Cerati simplicis . . . . 3iv.—M.
Ft. ungt.
Sig. Apply locally. BARTHOLOW.

853—℞ Acidi sulphurosi . . . . f3iij.
Glycerini,
Aquæ. . . . . āā f3j.—M.
Sig. Apply to affected part. BARTHOLOW.

854—℞ Fellis bovini recentis . . . . Oss.
Sig. Warm and rub in well daily. HUGH SMITH.

855—℞ Fellis bovini recentis . . . . f3ij.
Balsami peruviani . . . . f3j.—M.
Sig. Apply two or three times a day. (*With broken or unbroken skin.*)
HUGH SMITH.

FROST-BITE (Continued).

856—℞ Olei caryophylli,
Olei succini rectificati . . . . āā f℥ss.
Olei olivarum . . . . f℥j.—M.
Sig. Apply twice daily. ROCHE.

857—℞ Tinct. capsici . . . . f℥ss.
Sig. Paint over the unbroken surfaces. RINGER.

858—℞ Tinct. benzoini . . . . ℥ij.
Olei lini . . . . ℥iv.
Ceræ flavæ . . . . ℥j.
Glycerini . . . . q. s.—M.
Ft. ungt.
Sig. Apply locally. REVEIL.

859—℞ Iodi . . . . ℈j.
Potassii iodidi . . . . gr. iv.
Aquæ destillatæ . . . . ℳvj.
Adipis . . . . ℥j.—M.
Sig. Apply once daily. (*With unbroken skin.*) HEBRA.

860—℞ Olei cajuputi . . . . f℥vij.
Olei amygdalæ dulcis . . . . f℥xvij.—M.
Sig. Apply three times a day on lint. (*With broken skin.*)
RADIUS.

861—℞ Camphoræ . . . . ℥j.
Olei cajuputi . . . . f℥ij.
Ætheris . . . . f℥j.—M.
Ft. linimentum.
Sig. Apply locally to the unbroken skin. TORTUAL.

862—℞ Linimenti camphoræ,
Linimenti saponis comp.,
Olei cajuputi . . . . āā f℥j.—M.
Ft. linimentum.
Sig. Apply locally to the unbroken skin. BRANDE.

FURUNCLE. (See Carbuncle.)

GALACTORRHŒA.

863—℞ Atropinæ sulph. . . . . gr. iv.
Aquæ rosæ . . . . f℥j.—M.
Sig. Apply on lint around the breast, and remove when the
throat becomes dry. BARTHOLOW.

864—℞ Cocaine hydrochlor. . . . . ℥j.
Aquæ,
Glycerini . . . . āā f℥ss.—M.
Sig. Apply by means of gauze. JOHIE.

865—℞ Potassii iodidi . . . . ℥j.
Aquæ . . . . f℥j.—M.
Sig. Twenty-five to thirty drops in water once or twice daily.
ROUSSEL.

GALL-STONES. (See Calculi.)

GANGRENE.

866—℞ Creasoti . . . . f℥ss.
Tincturæ gentianæ . . . . f℥j.
Spiritus vini (95°) . . . . f℥ij.
Vini xerici . . . . f℥vj.—M.
Sig. From three to five tablespoonfuls a day, with milk.
ROMANOVSKY.

867—℞ Pulveris ligni carbonis,
Micæ panis,
Lactis . . . . āā q. s.
Fiat cataplasma.
Sig. Apply to correct fetor. GROSS.

868—℞ Acidi chromici . . . . ℥v.
Aquæ . . . . f℥iij.—M.
Sig. Apply to slough. BARTHOLOW.

76

GANGRENE (Continued).

869—℞ Pulv. acidi salicylici . . . . ᴣj.
Ft. chart. no. i.
Sig. Use locally as a dusting powder. (*To destroy fetor and change morbid action.*) BARTHOLOW.

870—℞ Acidi carbolici . . . . ᴣij.
Glycerini . . . . fᴣviij.—M.
Sig. Apply on lint. LISTER.

871—℞ Potassii bromidi . . . . ᴣij ᴣij.
Aquæ destillatæ . . . . fᴣij.
Solve. Dein adjice—
Bromi . . . . ᴣj (by weight).
Aquæ destillatæ . . . . . . q. s. ad fᴣiv.—M.
Sig. Apply to slough. (*In hospital gangrene.*)
J. LAWRENCE SMITH.

872—℞ Sodii sulphitis . . . . ᴣj-ij.
Aquæ . . . . fᴣx.—M.
Ft. lotio.
Sig. Use as a lotion, or apply on compresses. WARING.

873—℞ Liquor. hydrogenii peroxidi (10 vol.) . fᴣiv.
Sig. Apply locally, pure or diluted.

874—℞ Acidi nitrici . . . . fᴣj.
Sig. Apply to the ulcer with a glass rod until it is converted into a firm, dry mass. WARING.

875—℞ Brominii . . . . ᴣj.
Sig. Apply to the slough with a glass rod. (*Hospital gangrene.*)
BARTHOLOW.

GASTRALGIA. (See Neuralgia, Catarrh, Colic, and Dyspepsia.)

GASTRIC ULCER. (See Ulcer.)

GLANDS, ENLARGED LYMPHATIC.

876—℞ Tinct. iodi . . . . fᴣss.
Sig. Apply with a brush to the part. T. M. MARKOE.

877—℞ Iodi,
Terebinthinæ canadensis . . . . . āā ᴣj.
Collodii . . . . fᴣiv.—M.
Sig. Paint over diseased part. J. T. SHINN.

878—℞ Ungt. plumbi iodidi . . . . ᴣj.
Sig. Apply locally. BARTHOLOW.

878*bis.*—℞ Ungt. iodi comp. . . . . ᴣj.
Sig. Apply locally. H. B. SANDS.

879—℞ Potassii iodidi . . . . ᴣj.
Cerati simplicis. . . . . ᴣj.—M.
Sig. Apply to tumor. GOLDBERG.

880—℞ Pilocarpinæ hydrochloratis . . . . . gr. j.
Aquæ . . . . q. s. ad fᴣj.—M.
Sig. Teaspoonful three times a day. (*In early stage of acute inflammation.*)

881—℞ Barii iodidi . . . . gr. iv.
Adipis . . . . ᴣj.—M.
Sig. Apply to scrofulous tumors. BIETT.

882—℞ Hydrargyri biniodidi . . . . gr. vij.
Potassii iodidi . . . . ᴣj.
Adipis . . . . ᴣj.—M.
Sig. Apply to enlargement. C. C. HILDRETH.

883—℞ Hydrargyri protiodidi . . . . gr. vj.
Morphinæ acetatis . . . . gr. vij.
Adipis . . . . ᴣj.—M.
Sig. Apply to swelling. PELLETAN.

884—℞ Syr. ferri iodidi . . . . f ℨj.
Sig. Five to forty minims, according to age, well diluted, after meals, internally.   BARTHOLOW.

885—℞ Ichthyol,
    Ungt. hydrarg.,
    Ungt. belladon. . . . . āā ℨj.
    Ungt. petrolei . . . . ℥iv.—M.
Sig. Use locally night and morning.   HORWITZ.

886—℞ Calcii sulphidi . . . . gr. vj.
In pil. no. xxiv div.
Sig. One pill every four to six hours.   RINGER.

887—℞ Hydrarg. cum cretâ . . . . gr. iv.
    Sacch. lactis . . . . ℨj.—M.
In pulv. no. xx div.
Sig. One every two hours. (*In acute stage, tonsillitis, parotiditis, etc.*) .   BARTHOLOW.

GLEET. (See Gonorrhœa.)

GOITRE.

888—℞ Iodoform . . . . 1 part.
    Sulphuric ether . . . . 7 parts.
    Olive oil . . . . 7 parts.—M.
Sig. Inject into gland one-quarter to one drachm. C. GABRE.

889—℞ Unguenti iodi compositi,
    Unguenti belladonnæ . . . . . . āā ℨj.—M.
Sig. Rub in well once daily.   DA COSTA.

890—℞ Ungt. hydrarg. iodi rubri . . . . . . ℨj.
Sig. Rub in a piece the size of a pea, and expose to sun's rays.   RINGER.

891—℞ Extracti glandularis thyreoidi . . . . . ℨij.
Fiant tabellæ compressæ no. lx.
Sig. One to three tablets after each meal. (*Used in simple hypertrophic enlargement of thyroid.*)

892—℞ Potassii iodidi . . . . ℨiss.
    Vini pepsini . . . . f ℥viij.—M.
Sig. Dessertspoonful to tablespoonful in water after meals. (*Used in simple goitre.*)

893—℞ Ichthyol. . . . . ℨij.
    Ext. belladonnæ . . . . ℨj.
    Adipis . . . . ℥v.—M.
Sig. Apply twice a day.   J. C. WILSON.

894—℞ Tincturæ iodi . . . . f ℨj.
Sig. Inject ℳxxx into the substance of the gland once a week for the first two or three weeks, and, after, once a fortnight as long as necessary. Give iodide of potassium internally.   MORELL MACKENZIE.

895—℞ Iodi . . . . gr. ij.
    Potassii iodidi . . . . ℨiv.
    Aquæ menthæ piperitæ . . . . f ℥vj.
Fiat solutio.
Sig. A teaspoonful thrice daily.   MAGENDIE.

896—℞ Potassii bromidi . . . . ℨss.
In pulv. no. xii div.
Sig. A powder in a half-tumblerful of water three times daily. (*In exophthalmic goitre.*)   JON. HUTCHINSON.

GONORRHŒA.

897—℞ Creolin . . . . gtt. xxx.
    Extr. fluid. hydrast. canad. . . . . f ℥iiss.—M.
Sig. Two teaspoonfuls in a pint of warm water to be used at one injection. (*Vaginal.*)   LUTAUD.

898—℞ Protargoli . . . . gr. xl
      Aquæ . . . . f ʒiv.—M.
Sig. After urinating inject about two drachms, retain for fifteen minutes, allow fluid to escape, and again inject and retain for same period of time. (*For acute urethritis.*)

899—℞ Potassii permanganatis . . . . gr. j-iij.
      Aquæ destillatæ . . . . f ʒj.—M.
Sig. Use as injection. (*In gleet.*)   VAN BUREN AND KEYES.

900—℞ Liq. plumbi subacet. dil. . . . . f ʒj.
      Ext. opii aquosi. . . . . gr. vj.—M.
Sig. Use as injection two to four times daily.
                       VAN BUREN AND KEYES.

901—℞ Zinci sulpho-carbolatis . . . . gr. xx.
      Aquæ destillatæ . . . . f ʒviij.—M.
Sig. Inject a half-ounce two or three times a day.   RINGER.

902—℞ Zinci sulphatis . . . . gr. j-iij.
      Liq. plumbi subacet. dil. . . . . f ʒj.—M.
Sig. Shake, and inject three or four times daily, or

903—℞ Zinci sulphatis . . . . ʒj.
      Aluminis . . . . ʒiij.—M.
Sig. Dissolve a teaspoonful in one pint of water, and inject three times a day. (*In females.*)   RINGER.

904—℞ Zinci sulphatis . . . . gr. xv.
      Plumbi acetatis . . . . gr. xxx.
      Extracti krameriæ fluidi . . . . f ʒiij.
      Vini opii . . . . f ʒiij.
      Aquæ destillatæ . . . . q. s. ad f ʒvj.—M.
Sig. Use as injection two to four times daily after urinating.

905—℞ Saloli . . . . ʒij.
      Olei santali . . . . f ʒij.
      Oleoresinæ cubebæ . . . . f ʒij.
      Extracti pancreati . . . . ʒj.—M.
Pone in capsulas no. xxiv.
Sig. One capsule two hours after meals. (*Used in subacute and chronic gonorrhœa.*)

906—℞ Methylene blue . . . . gr. xxiv.
Fiant tabellas compressæ no. xxiv.
Sig. One three times daily. (*Acute gonorrhœa.*)

907—℞ Olei copaibæ,
      Olei cubebæ,
      Olei santali flavi . . . . āā ʒj.
      Magnesiæ . . . . ʒij.
Misce et fiant pilulæ no. lx.
Sig. Two pills every four hours.   BARTHOLOW.

908—℞ Methyl violet (blue pyoktanin) . . . . . ʒj.
      Water . . . . f ʒvj.—M.
Sig. Use three times a day as an injection.   J. C. WILSON.

909—℞ Zinci sulphatis,
      Acidi tannici . . . . āā gr. xv.
      Aquæ rosæ . . . . f ʒvj.—M.
Sig. A half-ounce as an injection two or three times daily.
(*In gleet.*)   RICORD.

910—℞ Zinci chloridi . . . . gr. j-ij.
      Aquæ destillatæ . . . . f ʒvj.
Solve.
Sig. Inject once or twice daily.   R. J. LEWIS.

911—℞ Bismuthi subnitratis,
      Glycerini . . . . āā ʒss.
      Aquæ destillatæ . . . . f ʒiij.—M.
Sig. Inject twice daily. (*In chronic cases and gleet.*)   RINGER.

912—℞ Hydrarg. chlor. corros. . . . . gr. ⅙.
　　　Zinci sulphocarbolat. . . . . ℨss.
　　　Acid. borici . . . . ℨij.
　　　Acid. carbolici . . . . ℳxv.
　　　Boroglyceride (25 per cent.). . . . . . . f ℨij.
　　　Aquæ . . . . q. s. ad f ℨvj.—M.
Sig. Use as an injection twice daily, after urinating. Dilute
if painful. (*Chronic gonorrhœa.*)　　　*Jefferson Hospital.*

913—℞ Hydrastinæ . . . . ℨj.-
　　　Mucilaginis acaciæ . . . . f ℨiv.—M.
Sig. A half-ounce as an injection. (*In chronic gonorrhœa and
gleet.*)　　　　　　　　　　　　　BARTHOLOW.

914—℞ Liquoris potassæ . . . . f ℨj.
　　　Balsami copaibæ . . . . f ℨss.
　　　Tincturæ cubebæ . . . . f ℨvj.
　　　Liquoris morphinæ sulphatis . . . . . f ℨj.
　　　Aquæ camphoræ . . . . q. s. ad f ℨvj.—M.
Sig. A tablespoonful four times a day.　　D. HAYES AGNEW.

915—℞ Ferri persulph. . . . . ℨss.
　　　Aquæ . . . . f ℨvj.—M.
Sig. Use as injection. (*In gleet.*)　　　　BUMSTEAD.

916—℞ Balsami copaibæ . . . . ℨss.
　　　Tinct. ferri mur.,
　　　Tinct. cantharidis . . . . āā f ℨij.
　　　Glycerini . . . . f ℨss.
　　　Syrupi . . . . q. s. ad f ℨiv.—M.
Sig. A tablespoonful after meals.　　　　BUMSTEAD.

917—℞ Balsami copaibæ,
　　　Spts. ætheris nitrosi,
　　　Spts. lavandulæ comp. . . . . āā f ℨss.
　　　Liq. potassæ . . . . f ℨj.
　　　Mucil. acaciæ . . . . q. s. ad f ℨiv.—M.
Sig. Shake, and take one tablespoonful. ("*Lafayette Mix-
ture.*")　　　　　　　　　Charity Hospital, N.Y.

918—℞ Aquæ rosæ . . . . f ℨij.
　　　Vini rubri . . . . f ℨj.—M.
Sig. Use as injection. (*In gleet.*) Gradually increase the red
wine until pure wine can be used.　　　RICORD.

919—℞ Thallin. sulphatis . . . . ℈j.
　　　Aquæ destillatæ . . . . f ℨij.—M.
Ft. injectio.
Sig. Use as an injection three or four times daily.
　　　　　　　　　　　　　　KREIS AND GOLL.

920—℞ Quininæ sulphatis . . . . gr. x.
　　　Glycerini . . . . f ℨss.
　　　Aquæ . . . . ad f ℨij.—M.
Sig. Use as injection.　　　　　　　LEDSSON.

921—℞ Liq. hydrarg. chlor. corros. (1-1000) . . Oj.
Sig. Distend the vagina with a speculum and cleanse thoroughly with the above solution. Then dust over and rub
in iodoform, and tampon the vagina with iodoform gauze.
　　　　　　　　　　　　　　SCHWARZ.

922—℞ Argenti nitratis . . . . ℨj.
　　　Aquæ destillatæ . . . . f ℨij.—M.
Sig. Wipe the vagina and cervix, and apply thoroughly by
means of a tubular speculum.　　　　GRANDIN.

923—℞ Olei gaultheriæ . . . . f ℨij.
　　　Mucil. acaciæ . . . . . . q. s. ut ft. emulsio.
　　　Syr. simplicis . . . . f ℨj.
　　　Aquæ . . . . ad f ℨiij.—M.
Sig. A teaspoonful three times daily. (*In gonorrhœal rheuma-
tism.*)　　　　　　　　　R. W. TAYLOR.

924—℞ Olei santali . . . . ℨj.
Sig. Fifteen or twenty drops on sugar, or in capsules (five-
drop), after meals.　　　　　　　LATZEL.

925—℞ Ext. colchici acetici,
    Ext. aloes,
    Pulv. ipecac.,
    Hydrarg. chlor. mit. . . . . āā gr. j.
    Ext. nucis vomicæ . . . . gr. ¼-ss.—M.
Ft. pil. no. i.
Sig. To be taken every four hours until it purges.   LOOMIS.

926—℞ Vini colchici seminis . . . . f3iij.
    Spiritus ammoniæ aromatici . . . . . . f3xiij.—M.
Sig. A teaspoonful every three hours until some physiological
effect is produced.   BARTHOLOW.

927—℞ Benzoic acid,
    Sodium borate . . . . āā gr. v.
    Water . . . . f3j.—M.
Sig. To be taken every two hours. (For dysuria due to uric
acid.)   Canada Lancet.

928—℞ Extracti colchici acetici,
    Extracti rhei,
    Extracti aloes socotrinæ . . . . . . āā gr. vj.
    Extracti belladonnæ . . . . gr. j.
Misce et fiant pilulæ no. vi.
Sig. One pill at bedtime twice a week.   A. B. GARROD.

929—℞ Pulveris colchici seminis . . . . 3ss.
    Hydrargyri chloridi mitis,
    Extracti colocynthidis . . . . āā gr. viij.
    Pulveris digitalis,
    Quiniæ sulphatis . . . . āā gr. xv.
Misce et fiat massa, in pilulas no. xx dividenda.
Sig. From one to four pills a day.   TROUSSEAU ET REVEIL.

930—℞ Aceti colchici . . . . f3j-ij.
    Magnesiæ . . . . gr. xv-xx.
    Magnesii sulphatis . . . . 3j-ij.
    Syrupi simplicis . . . . f3j.
    Aquæ cinnamomi . . . . f3ix.
Fiat haustus.
Sig. Repeat in three hours if necessary.   SCUDAMORE.

931—℞ Extracti colchici acetici . . . . gr. x.
    Pulveris ipecacuanhæ compositi,
    Pulveris digitalis,
    Extracti colocynthidis compositi . . āā gr. xij.
Misce et fiant pilulæ no. xii.
Sig. One pill twice or thrice a day.   HENRY HALFORD.

932—℞ Tincturæ colchici seminis . . . . ℳxv.
    Magnesii carbonatis . . . . gr. vj.
    Magnesii sulphatis . . . . gr. xxx.
    Aquæ menthæ piperitæ . . . . q. s. ad f3j.
Fiat haustus.
Sig. Repeat pro ne rata.   University Hospital.

933—℞ Piperazini . . . . 3j.
Pone in phialas no. xxxii.
Sig. Dissolve the contents of a vial in about a pint of water
and take a wineglassful every two hours through the
day.

934—℞ Chloroform,
    Spts. ammoniæ aromatici . . . . . āā f3ij.
    Spts. ætheris comp.,
    Tinct. opii camph. . . . . āā f3ss.
    Mucil. acaciæ. . . . . f3ss.—M.
Sig. A teaspoonful at once.   HARTSHORNE.

935—℞ Magnesii sulphatis . . . . 3j.
    Magnesiæ optimæ . . . . 3ij.
    Vini colchici radicis . . . . f3j.
    Aquæ menthæ pip. . . . . f3x.—M.
Sig. A tablespoonful every hour until it operates.
                                 SCUDAMORE.

GOUT (Continued).

936—℞ Potassii iodidi . . . . gr. v.
    Potassii bicarb. . . . . gr. x.
    Mist. ammoniaci . . . . ʃꝫj.—M.
Ft. haustus.
Sig. To be taken thrice daily.   FOTHERGILL.

937—℞ Potassii bromidi . . . . gr. xx.
    Tinct. hyoscyami . . . . ʃꝫss.
    Tinct. lupuli . . . . ʃꝫj.
    Aquæ camphoræ . . . . ʃꝫj.—M.
Ft. haustus.
Sig. Take at bedtime. (*For gouty insomnia.*)   FOTHERGILL.

938—℞ Sodii salicylatis . . . . ꝫij.
    Syr. aurantii cort. . . . . ʃꝫj.
    Aquæ . . . . ad ʃꝫiv.—M.
.Sig. A tablespoonful three times daily, in conjunction with
rest. Joints involved are wrapped in cotton wool.
                           JACCOUD.

939—℞ Lithii benzoatis . . . . ꝫij.
    Aquæ cinnamomi . . . . ʃꝫliss.—M.
Sig. A teaspoonful in a wineglassful of water every four or
six hours (*During intervals.*)   JACCOUD.

940—℞ Gran. efferv. lithii benzoatis . . . . . . ꝫiv.
Sig. A teaspoonful in water two or three times daily.
                      R. V. MATTISON.

941—℞ Gran. efferv. lithii citratis . . . . . . ꝫiv.
Sig. One or two teaspoonfuls in water three times daily.
                      R. V. MATTISON.

942—℞ Syrupi ferri iodidi . . . . ʃꝫiv.
    Olei morrhuæ . . . . ʃꝫj.—M.
Pone in capsulas no. xxiv.
Sig. One capsule two hours after meals, to be increased to
two capsules after meals. (*Used in chronic gout with anæmia.*)

943—℞ Lithii carbonatis vel citratis . . . . . . ꝫv.
    Aquæ destillatæ . . . . ʃꝫxx.—M.
Sig. Apply by means of lint, especially if the skin is broken.
                      GARROD.

944—℞ Veratrinæ . . . . ꝫj.
    Adipis . . . . ꝫj.—M.
Sig. Apply to painful joint *at onset.* (*Not when the skin is
broken.*)   TURNBULL.

GRAVES' DISEASE. (Exophthalmic Goitre.)

945—℞ Ext. belladonnæ . . . . gr. v.
In pil. no. xxx div.
Sig. One pill three or four times a day.   J. C. WILSON.

946—℞ Antipyrin . . . . ꝫj.
In chartulas no. xx div.
Sig. One powder three or four times a day.   J. C. WILSON.

947—℞ Extracti glandulæ suprarenalis . . . . ꝫiv.
Pone in capsulas no. lx.
Sig. One to two capsules three times a day. (*Used in true exophthalmic goitre with lowered arterial tension. The remedy
must be continued in moderate doses over a long period.*)

948—℞ Cannabin . . . . gr. ivss.
    Sacchari lactis . . . . q. s.—M.
Ft. pil. no. v.
Sig. To be taken in twenty-four hours.   VALIERI.

949—℞ Cannabin . . . . gr. ivss.
    Aquæ destillatæ . . . . ꝫiij.
    Syr. aurantii flor. . . . . ꝫj.—M.
Sig. To be taken in teaspoonful doses in twenty-four hours.
                      VALIERI.

GUMS, INFLAMED OR BLEEDING.

950—℞ Glyceriti acidi tannici . . . . ꝫj.
Sig. Apply with a camel's-hair brush. (*For spongy or bleeding
gums.*)   BARTHOLOW.

951—℞ Tincturæ benzoini compositæ . . . . . f℥j.
  Listerinæ . . . . f℥j.—M.
Sig. Apply to gums with camel's-hair brush three times a day.

952—℞ Chloral. hydratis,
  Tinct. cochleariæ (Ph. P.) . . . . . āā ℥iss.—M.
Sig. Apply to the gums, by means of a pledget of cotton, every
 day or two. (*For the gingivitis of pregnancy.*) PINARD.

953—℞ Chloroformi . . . . gr. lx.
  Acidi tannici . . . . gr. xxx.
  Menthol . . . . gr. xxx.
  Tinct. krameriæ . . . . f℥j.
  Aquæ dest. . . . . q. s. ad Oj.—M.
Sig. Locally.   VIAN.

— ℞ —

HÆMATEMESIS.

954—℞ Tinct. hamamelidis . . . . f℥ss.
Sig. Two to four drops every two or three hours. RINGER.

955—℞ Ergotini (Bonjean) . . . . gr. xij.
  Aquæ destillatæ . . . . f℥j.—M.
Sig. Five to ten minims hypodermically every three or four
 hours.   RINGER.

956—℞ Liquoris ferri subsulphatis . . . . gtt. xx.
  Aquæ destillatæ . . . . f℥ij.—M.
Sig. A teaspoonful every half-hour or hour, in ice-water,
 allowing the patient to swallow cracked ice. BARTHOLOW.

957—℞ Plumbi acetatis . . . . ℥ss.
  Hydrargyri chloridi mitis . . . . gr. v.
  Confectionis rosæ . . . . q. s.
Misce et fiant pilulæ no. x.
Sig. One pill every two to four hours. (*From ulcer.*) ELLIS.

958—℞ Acidi tannici . . . . gr. xx.
  Pulveris opii . . . . gr. v.
  Glycerini . . . . q. s.
Fiat massa, in pilulas no. x dividenda.
Sig. One pill every hour or two.   ELLIS.

959—℞ Acidi gallici . . . . gr. x.
  Acidi sulphurici dil. . . . . ℩₵x.
  Aquæ . . . . f℥j.—M.
Ft. haustus.
Sig. To be repeated in four or six hours if necessary.
            BRINTON.

960—℞ Ferri et ammonii sulphatis . . . . . . ℈ij.
  Aquæ cinnamomi . . . . f℥iv.—M.
Sig. A tablespoonful every two or three hours. BARTHOLOW.

961—℞ Aluminis . . . . ℥iss.
  Syrupi krameriæ . . . . f℥ij.
  Aquæ destillatæ . . . . f℥vj.—M.
Sig. The one-fourth part to be given every half-hour.
         TROUSSEAU ET REVEIL.

HÆMATURIA.

962—℞ Acidi gallici . . . . ℥ss.
  Acidi sulphurici dil. . . . . f℥j.
  Tinct. opii deodoratæ . . . . f℥j.
  Infusi digitalis . . . . f℥iv.—M.
Sig. A tablespoonful every four hours.   DRUITT.

963—℞ Ergotin . . . . ℥j.
  Gallic acid . . . . ℥ss.
  Turpentine . . . . f℥j.
  Aromatic elixir . . . . f℥iv.—M.
Sig. One or two teaspoonfuls every two or three hours.

964—℞ Olei terebinthinæ . . . . f℥ss.
    Mucil. acaciæ . . . . q. s.
    Syr. simplicis . . . . ad f℥iij.
    Olei gaultheriæ . . . . gtt. vij.—M.
Ft. emulsio.
Sig. One to three teaspoonfuls every two to four hours.
                          JOHN HUNTER.

965—℞ Tinct. ferri muriatis . . . . ℳxxx.
    Tinct. digitalis . . . . ℳxv.
    Aquæ menthæ pip. . . . . f℥iss.—M.
Ft. haustus.
Sig. To be repeated every four hours.   AITKEN.

HÆMOPTYSIS.

966—℞ Ext. ergotæ fld. . . . . f℥j.
    Tinct. opii deodoratæ . . . . f℥ij.—M.
Sig. Twenty drops in half an ounce of cold water every half-
hour, watching the effect.   J. C. WILSON.

967—℞ Ferri acetatis . . . . ℈ij.
    Aquæ . . . . q. s.
Sig. Make the solution distinctly but not disagreeably sour,
and let the patient constantly sip.   RINGER.

968—℞ Sodii chloridi . . . . ℈ij.
Sig. Take a half-teaspoonful dry. Repeat till nausea occurs.
                          RINGER.

969—℞ Gallic acid . . . . gr. xxx.
    Ergotin . . . . gr. xv.—M.
Make into twenty pills.
Sig. Take five or more each day.

970—℞ Plumbi acetatis . . . . gr. xx.
    Pulv. digitalis . . . . gr. x.
    Pulv. opii . . . . gr. v.—M.
Ft. massa et in pil. no. x div.
Sig. One pill every four hours.   BARTHOLOW.

971—℞ Infusi digitalis . . . . f℥iv.
Sig. A tablespoonful every hour until the pulse is reduced.
                         BRINTON.

972—℞ Pulv. aluminis . . . . ℈j.
    Sacchari albi . . . . ℈ss.
    Pulv. ipecac. comp. . . . . ℈j.—M.
In pulv. no. vi div.
Sig. One powder every two hours.   SKODA.

973—℞ Morphinæ sulphatis . . . . gr. ⅙.
Sig. Use hypodermically and repeat *pro re nata.* J. C. WILSON.

HAIR, FALLING OF THE. (See also Alopecia.)

974—℞ Acidi acetici . . . . f℥iv.
    Glycerini . . . . f℥ij.
    Aquæ coloniensis . . . . f℥j.—M.
Ft. linimentum.
Sig. Rub in daily. (*Syphilitic alopecia.*)

975—℞ Sodii biboratis . . . . ℈iv.
    Aquæ ammoniæ . . . . f℥j.
    Spts. myrciæ . . . . f℥ij.
    Aquæ rosæ . . . . ℥xiij.—M.
Sig. Shampoo hair-wash.   POTTER.

976—℞ Tinct. cantharidis . . . . f℥iv.
    Tinct. capsici . . . . f℥j.
    Ol. ricini . . . . f℥ss–f℥j.
    Alcoholis . . . . q. s. ad f℥iv.—M.
Sig. Rub thoroughly into the scalp.   STELWAGON.

977—℞ Tinct. cantharidis . . . . f℥j.
    Aceti destillati . . . . f℥iss.
    Glycerini . . . . f℥iss.
    Spts. rosmarini, ... f℥iss.
    Aquæ rosæ . . . . ad f℥viij.—M.
Sig. Hair-tonic. To be well sponged on to the scalp night and morning.   TILBURY FOX.

978—℞ Liquor. hydrogenii peroxidi (10 vol.) . . f℥iv.
Sig. Apply locally with a sponge or a soft brush. (*To bleach the hair.*)   ERASMUS WILSON.

HAY FEVER.

979—℞ Pulveris ipecacuanhæ compositi . . . . gr. xv-xx.
Fiat chartula.
Sig. One dose. (*For temporary relief in attacks of dyspnœa.*)
    HYDE SALTER.

980—℞ Antipyrin. . . . . ℥ss.
    Syr. aurantii cort. . . . . f℥j.
    Aquæ . . . . ad f℥iij.—M.
Sig. A teaspoonful one to three times daily.   CHEATHAM.

981—℞ Cocain. muriatis . . . . gr. v.
    Aquæ destillatæ . . . . f℥j.
Sig. Apply with a camel's-hair brush to the nasal passages.
    SAJOUS.

982—℞ Resorcini . . . . gr. xv.
    Glycerini . . . . f℥iv.
    Aquæ . . . . q. s. ad f℥iv.—M.
Sig. Use as spray once or twice daily.

983—℞ Quininæ hydrochloratis . . . . gr iv-vij.
    Aquæ destillatæ . . . . f℥j.—M.
Sig. Apply with large camel's-hair brush, or spray-producer, to nares and fauces.   BARTHOLOW.

984—℞ Tincturæ iodi. . . . . ℥j.
    Acidi carbolici . . . . gr. x.
    Aquæ destillatæ . . . . f℥iv.—M.
Sig. Apply to fauces and nares.   BARTHOLOW.

985—℞ Tincturæ aconiti radicis . . . . f℥iss.
    Glycerini . . . . f℥iss.—M.
Sig. Apply to outside of nose.   RINGER.

986—℞ Liquoris hydrogenii peroxidi (10 vol.) . f℥j.
    Aquæ ferventis . . . . ad f℥iv.—M.
Sig. Inject into the naso-pharynx with a post-nasal syringe.
    S. W. INGRAHAM.

987—℞ Atropinæ sulphatis . . . . gr. ⅛.
    Morphinæ sulphatis . . . . gr. viiss.
    Aquæ destillatæ . . . . f℥v.—M.
Sig. Five to fifteen minims hypodermically two or three times daily (five minims = atropine gr. $\frac{1}{360}$ and morphine gr. ⅛).   S. N. BISHOP.

988—℞ Boric acid,
    Salicylate of sodium . . . . āā gr. xxx.
    Hydrochlorate of cocaine . . . . . . gr. iii.—M.
Sig. Use by insufflation.

989—℞ Syr. acidi hydriodici . . . . f℥iv.
Sig. A teaspoonful every two hours.   JUDKINS.

990—℞ Potassii arsenitis . . . . gr. xv.
    Aquæ destillatæ . . . . f℥j.
Solve.
Sig. Unsized white paper to be thoroughly moistened with this solution, cut into twenty equal parts, and each part rolled into a cigarette, two or three of which may be smoked daily.   TROUSSEAU.

991—℞ Potassii iodidi . . . . ʒj.
    Liquoris potassii arsenitis . . . . fʒj.
    Aquæ destillatæ . . . . fʒiv.—M.
Sig. A teaspoonful every four or six hours.   SMITH.

HEADACHE.

992—℞ Tinct. belladonnæ . . . . fʒss.
Sig. Six drops every three hours. (*In congestive headache.*)
                                       RINGER.

993—℞ Crotonchloralis . . . . ʒj.
Pone in capsulas no. xii.
Sig. One capsule every four hours. (*Used in neuralgia of fifth nerve, not due to decayed tooth.*)

994—℞ Tinct. nucis vomicæ . . . . fʒss.
Sig. One drop frequently. (*In bilious headache with nausea.*)
                                         RINGER.

995—℞ Sparteine sulphate . . . . gr. ¼.
    Caffeine . . . . gr. iss.
    Antipyrin . . . . gr. viss.—M.
Sig. Taken at intervals of two hours until four have been taken, even though the pain has disappeared. ARITZMAN.

996—℞ Pulveris guaranæ . . . . gr. x-xv.
    Sacchari albi . . . . q. s.
Misce et fiat pulvis.
Sig. To be taken once or oftener in the day. (*In migraine or periodical headache.*)
                                         S. WILKS.

997—℞ Sodii bromid. . . . . gr. v-x.
    Ext. cannabis indica fl. . . . . ♏x-xv.—M.
Sig. Give in headache of eye-strain.   G. DE SCHWEINITZ.

998—℞ Sodii chloridi . . . . ʒj.
    Spiritus camphoræ . . . . fʒj.
    Aquæ ammoniæ . . . . fʒiss.
    Aquæ . . . . Oj.
Misce et fiat lotio.
Sig. "*Eau sédatif.*" For external use.   RASPAIL.

999—℞ Acetanilid. . . . . gr. viij.
    Caffein. citrat. . . . . gr. iv.
    Sodii bromid. . . . . gr. x.
M. et ft. in chart. iv.
Sig. One every hour.   HARE.

1000—℞ Ætheris,
    Spiritus ammoniæ aromatici . . . āā fʒj.
    Aquæ camphoræ . . . . fʒx.
    Tincturæ cardamomi compositæ . . . fʒj.
Misce pro haustu.
Sig. Two to three times a day. (*In nervous headache.*)
                                   BRANDE.

1001—℞ Pulv. capsici . . . . gr. xij.
    Ext. colocynth. comp. . . . . gr. iv.
    Ext. gentianæ . . . . gr. xxiv.—M.
Ft. massa et in pil. no. xii div.
Sig. One pill three times daily. Twenty-five grains of sodium bromide to be taken at night. (*In congestive headache.*)
                                    DA COSTA.

1002—℞ Potassii citratis . . . . ꝺj.
    Spts. juniperi . . . . ʒj.
    Spts. ætheris nitrosi . . . . ♏xx.
    Inf. scoparii . . . . fʒj.—M.
Sig. To be taken thrice daily. (*In uræmic form.*) W. H. DAY.

1003—℞ Ext. belladonnæ . . . . gr. v.
Sig. To be rubbed into the affected temple every night. (*In nervous form, migraine, clavus, etc.*)   W. H. DAY.

1004—℞ Ext. aconiti ale. . . . . 3j.
Adipis . . . . 3ij.—M.
Ft. ungt.
Sig. Rub into the affected temple every night. (*In nervous form, migraine, etc.*) W. H. DAY.

1005—℞ Gran. efferv. bromo-caffeini . . . . . . 3iv.
Sig. A teaspoonful in a half-glassful of cold water. Repeat in half an hour if necessary. (*In nervous form.*)
R. V. MATTISON.

1006—℞ Antipyrin. . . . . gr. iiss.
Sodii bicarb. . . . . .ᐟ. gr. iiss.
Caffein. citrat. . . . . gr. ss.—M.
Sig. Take at one dose and repeat every twenty or thirty minutes until relief is obtained. J. C. WILSON.

1007—℞ Ammonii chloridi . . . . 3ij.
Morphinæ acetatis . . . . gr. j.
Caffeinæ citratis . . . . 3ss.
Spts. ammoniæ aromatici . . . . . . f 3j.
Elix. guaranæ . . . . f 3iv.
Aquæ rosæ . . . . f 3iv.—M.
Sig. A dessertspoonful every quarter-hour until relieved. (*In bilious form.*) CARPENTER.

1008—℞ Zinci phosphidi . . . . gr. iij.
Ext. nucis vomicæ . . . . gr. x.
Confect. rosæ . . . . q. s.—M.
Ft. massa et in pil. no. xxx div.
Sig. One after each meal. (*In nervous form.*)
FORDYCE BARKER.

1009—℞ Potassii acetatis . . . . 3vj.
Infusi digitalis . . . . f 3vj.—M.
Sig. A tablespoonful every third hour. (*In uræmic headache.*)
A. A. SMITH.

1010—℞ Chloroformi . . . . f 3j.
Sig. Ten drops, stirred in a wineglassful of cold water, four or five times a day. (*For habitual headache.*) J. C. WILSON.

HEART-BURN. (See Acidity.)

HEART-DISEASE.

1011—℞ Tincturæ digitalis . . . . f 3j.
Sig. Ten minims three times daily. (*In irritable heart, with palpitation.*) DA COSTA.

1012—℞ Glandulæ suprarenalis dessicatæ . . . 3j.
Pone in capsulas no. xxx.
Sig. One three times a day. (*In cardiac enfeeblement with arterial relaxation.*)

1013—℞ Pulveris scillæ. . . . . gr. x.
Pulveris ferri,
Pulveris digitalis (English),
Quininæ sulphatis . . . . āā 9j.
Misce et fiant pilulæ no. xx.
Sig. One pill three or four times a day. (*In fatty degeneration; dilatation of cavities, especially the right; mitral regurgitation, with anæmia.*) BARTHOLOW.

1014—℞ Extracti veratri viridis . . . . f 3j.
Saechari lactis . . . . 3iss.
Alcohol . . . . q. s.
Fiant tabellæ triturationes no 1x.
Sig. One tablet every two hours. (*Used in cardiac hypertrophy with strong irregular heart.*) H. A. HARE.

1015—℞ Tincturæ digitalis . . . . ℥x.
Spiritus chloroformi . . . . ℥xxv.
Infusi buchu . . . . f 3j.
Fiat haustus.
Sig. To be taken three times a day. (*In simple cardiac debility.*)
FOTHERGILL.

1016—℞ Pulv. digitalis . . . . gr. xxx.
      Ferri sulph. exsiccati . . . . gr. xv.
      Pulv. capsici . . . . gr. xl.
      Pil. aloe et myrrhæ . . . . ℨij.—M.

Fiat massa et in pil. no. lx div.
Sig. One pill morning and night. (*Chronic heart-disease,
with gastric catarrh and constipation.*)   FOTHERGILL.

1017—℞ Potassii iodidi . . . . ℨj.
      Potassii bicarb. . . . . ℨiij.
      Infusi buchu . . . . ad f℥xij.—M.

Sig. Two tablespoonfuls three or four times daily. (*Cardiac
hypertrophy and increased arterial tension.*)   FOTHERGILL.

1018—℞ Pulv. fol. digitalis . . . . ∋j.

In pulv. no. x div.
Sig. A powder every three hours. (*In great dilatation and
hypertrophy.*)   RINGER.

1019—℞ Pulveris digitalis . . . . gr. ij.
      Aquæ . . . . f℥j.—M.

Sig. One tablespoonful *twice only.* (*In cardiac dropsy.*)
             NIEMEYER.

1020—℞ Tincturæ digitalis . . . . ℥lx-xx.
      Tincturæ calumbæ . . . . f℥j.
      Aquæ camphoræ . . . . f℥x.

Fiat haustus.
Sig. One dose, twice daily. (*In nervous palpitation.*)   PARIS.

1021—℞ Infusi digitalis . . . . f℥iv.
      Potassii acetatis   . . . . ℨij.
      Spiritus ætheris nitrosi . . . . f℥ij.
      Aquæ cassiæ . . . . f℥iss.—M.

Sig. A tablespoonful every fourth hour. (*With pericardiac
effusion.*)   KILGOUR.

1022—℞ Infusi digitalis . . . . f℥viiss.
      Potassii nitratis . . . . : . . ℨij.
      Acidi hydrocyanici diluti . . . . . . ℥lxiv.
      Syrupi aurantii corticis . . . . f℥ij.—M.

Sig. A tablespoonful every two hours. (*In hypertrophy.*)
             COPLAND.

1023—℞ Pulveris digitalis . . . . gr. v.
      Pulveris scillæ . . . . gr. x.
      Pilulæ hydrargyri . . . . ℨss.

Fiat massa et divide in pilulas x.
Sig. One pill three times daily. (*In palpitation with anasarca.*)
             BAILLIE.

1024—℞ Cocain. hydrochloratis . . . . gr. vj.
      Aquæ destillatæ . . . . f℥iij.—M.

Sig. A teaspoonful three times daily. (*In nervous cardiac
debility.*)   ROSENBACH.

1025—℞ Iodi carbolati . . . . f℥ss.
Sig. Fifteen or twenty drops on cotton, or in an inhaler. To
be inhaled several times daily. (*In endocarditis.*) McCLUN.

1026—℞ Gran. efferv. caffeini citratis . . . . . ℨiv.
Sig. Three to five teaspoonfuls several times daily, gradually
increased. (*In intermittent heart.*)   NOTHNAGEL.

1027—℞ Sodii iodidi,
      Potassii iodidi . . . . āā ℨss.
      Aquæ . . . . ad f℥j.—M.

Sig. One drop three times daily for fifteen days; then substitute—

1028—℞ Sol. nitro-glycerin. (1 per cent.) . . . . f℥j.
Sig. Take two to four drops three times daily for fifteen days,
and then revert to iodides. Alternate for one, two, or
three years. (*For atheromatous condition of the heart.*)
             HUCHARD.

1029—℞ Strychninæ sulphatis . . . . gr. j.
Aquæ fontanæ . . . . f ʒj.—M.

Ft. sol.
Sig. Eight to fifteen minims hypodermically. (*For exhausted
heart-muscle and its nerves.*) HABERSHON.

1030—℞ Vini cocæ . . . . Oj.
Sig. A wineglassful three or four times daily. (*In overstrain
of heart.*) BEVERLEY ROBINSON.

1031—℞ Infusi digitalis . . . . f ʒij.
Liq. potassii citratis . . . . f ʒiss.
Acetí scillæ . . . . f ʒss.—M.
Sig. A tablespoonful every four hours. (*In cardiac complica-
tions of acute rheumatism.*) OPPOLZER.

1032—℞ Tinct. strophanthi (1-20) . . . . . . f ʒj.
Sig. Five to fifteen drops three times daily. (*In fatty heart
and valvular disease.*) FRASER.

1033—℞ Extracti aconiti radicis fluidi . . . . . f ʒss.
Vini antimonii . . . . f ʒss.—M.
Sig. From ten to fifteen drops three times a day. (*In peri-
carditis with great pain.*) RUST.

1034—℞ Pulveris opii . . . . gr. ij.
Hydrargyri chloridi mitis . . . . gr. xvj.
Misce et fiant chartulæ no. viij.
Sig. One powder three times a day. (*In endocarditis.*)
BUDD.

1035—℞ Potassii citratis . . . . ʒij.
Tincturæ stramonii . . . . f ʒj.
Tincturæ colchici seminis . . . . f ʒij.
Infusi digitalis . . . . f ʒiij.
Aquæ menthæ piperitæ . . . . f ʒviij.—M.
Sig. Two tablespoonfuls three times a day. (*In violent palpi-
tation.*) HAZARD.

1036—℞ Tincturæ veratri viridis . . . . f ʒss.
Sig. Five drops. (*To reduce heart's action.*) HAZARD.

1037—℞ Extracti cimicifugæ fluidi,
Syrupi acaciæ . . . . āā f ʒss.
Aquæ amygdalæ amaræ . . . . f ʒiij.—M.
Sig. A teaspoonful every three hours. (*In fatty degeneration.*)
ELLIS.

HEMICRANIA. (See Headache.)

HEMIPLEGIA. (See Paralysis.)

HEMORRHAGE.

1038—℞ Ergotæ,
Ferri subcarb. . . . . āā ʒiss.
Quininæ sulph. . . . . ʒss.
Ext. digitalis . . . . gr. xv.
Misce et in pil. no. c div.
Sig. Two to be taken at each meal. Intermit the medicine
every three days. GALLARD.

1039—℞ Ergotoli . . . . f ʒiv.
Sig. Teaspoonful by mouth or thirty drops hypodermically.
Smaller doses repeated as required until uterus is firmly
contracted. (*Used in post-partum hemorrhage.*)

1040—℞ Ext. ipecac. fld. . . . . f ʒij.
Ext. ergotæ fld. . . . . f ʒiv.
Ext. digitalis fld. . . . . ad f ʒj.—M.
Sig. One-half to one teaspoonful, repeated as required. (*Ex-
cellent anti-hemorrhagic combination.*) BARTHOLOW.

1041—℞ Olei terebinthinæ . . . . f℥ij.
     Extracti digitalis fluidi . . . . f℥j.
     Mucilaginis acaciæ . . . . f℥ss.
     Aquæ menthæ piperitæ . . . . f℥j.—M.
Sig. A teaspoonful every three hours. (*In passive hemor-rhage.*)   BARTHOLOW.

1042—℞ Argenti nitratis fusæ . . . . q. s.
Sig. Wipe the wound dry and apply locally. (*In leech-bites.*)   RINGER.

1043—℞ Acidi acetici diluti . . . . f℥vj.
Sig. Apply locally. (*For leech-bites, piles, cuts, etc.*)   RINGER.

1044—℞ Tinct. hamamelidis . . . . f℥iv.
Sig. Use pure or diluted (1 to 8). (*In cuts, leech-bites, oozing from wounds, etc.*) Also, internally, one to three minims every two or three hours.   RINGER.

1045—℞ Tinct. opii . . . . f℥j.
     Spts. vini gallici . . . . f℥j.—M.
Fiat haustus.
Sig. To be taken at once. (*In flooding after delivery, with uterine exhaustion.*)   RINGER.

1046—℞ Ammonii carbonatis . . . . ℥ij.
     Tincturæ opii deodoratæ . . . . . . f℥iss.(!)
     Extracti glycyrrhizæ fluidi . . . . . . f℥vj.
     Aquæ destillatæ . . . . q. s. ad f℥vj.—M.
Sig. A tablespoonful every two hours. (*After hemorrhage ad deliquium.*)   CARSON.

1047—℞ Acidi carbolici . . . . ℥j.
     Aquæ destillatæ . . . . f℥iij.—M.
Sig. Apply to bleeding part. (*Does not prevent union by first intention.*)

1048—℞ Potassii carbonatis . . . . ℥ij.
     Saponis . . . . ℥i-ij.
     Alcoholis . . . . f℥iij.—M.
Sig. ("Pancoast's Styptic.") Use as a styptic, especially for operations about the face.   JOS. PANCOAST.

1049—℞ Ergotini . . . . 10.00 grammes.
     Aquæ destillatæ . . . . 70.00 "
     Glycerini . . . . 20.00 "
     Acidi salicylici . . . . 0.20 " M.
Sig. One teaspoonful in three teaspoonfuls of water, for rectal injection. (*Uterine hemorrhage.*)   REINSTADIER.

HEMORRHAGE, POST-PARTUM, AND UTERINE.
(See Menorrhagia.)

HEMORRHOIDS.

1050—℞ Cocain. hydrochloratis . . . . gr. iv.
     Aquæ . . . . f℥j.—M.
Sig. Apply locally. (*In ulcerated piles.*)   J. C. WILSON.

1051—℞ Ext. belladonnæ . . . . ℥j.
     Cerati simplicis . . . . ℥j.—M.
Ft. ungt.
Sig. Use as an ointment. (*In painful piles.*)   HARTSHORNE.

1052—℞ Acidi tannici . . . . gr. xx-xxx.
     Aquæ . . . . f℥vj.—M.
Sig. To be injected, after being cooled with ice, into the rectum. (*In bleeding piles.*)   HARTSHORNE.

1053—℞ Acidi nitrici . . . . f℥ss-j.
     Aquæ . . . . f℥viij.—M.
Ft. lotio.
Sig. Apply as a wash. (*In bleeding piles.*)   RINGER.

1054—℞ Tincturæ hamamelidis . . . . f℥iv.

Sig. Inject into the rectum one-half to one teaspoonful in an ounce of cold water daily before rising. Also take internally two to five minims three times daily. RINGER.

1055—℞ Potassii bromidi . . . . ℨj.
Glycerini . . . . f℥v.—M.

Sig. Apply to ease pain. RINGER.

1056—℞ Extracti ergotæ fluidi . . . . f℥j.
Tincturæ nucis vomicæ . . . . f℥j.—M.

Sig. A teaspoonful every four hours. (*In bleeding piles.*)
BARTHOLOW.

1057—℞ Iodoformi . . . . ℨj-iij.
Adipis benzoatis . . . . ℨj.—M.

Ft. unguentum.
Sig. Apply locally, after washing with cold water.
BARTHOLOW.

1058—℞ Pulv. gallæ . . . . gr. xx.
Pulv. opii . . . . gr. x.
Ungt. plumbi subacetatis . . . . gr. xl.
Ungt. simplicis . . . . ℨj.—M.

Ft. unguentum.
Sig. Use locally. OESTERLEN.

1059—℞ Ferri subsulph. . . . . gr. iij.
Plumb. acet. . . . . gr j
Mass. hydrarg. . . . . gr. ss.—M.
Ol. theobrom., q. s. ut. ft. suppos. j.

Sig. Introduce one morning and evening. HORWITZ.

1060—℞ Sulphuris loti . . . . ℨiss.
Confectionis sennæ . . . . ℨij.
Potassii nitratis . . . . ℨj.
Syrupi aurantii corticis . . . . q. s.

Misce et fiat confectio.
Sig. One or two drachms twice a day. ELLIS.

1061—℞ Solid extract of ergot . . . . gr. ij.
Extract of opium,
Extract of nux vomica,
Cocaine hydrochlorate . . . . . āā gr. ¼.—M.
Ol. theobroma to make a suppository.

1062—℞ Potassii sulphatis . . . . ℨss.
Sulphuris sublimati . . . . ℨij.
Confectionis sennæ . . . . ℨij.
Syrupi simplicis . . . . q. s.

Misce et fiat electuarium.
Sig. A dessertspoonful at night. AINSLIE.

1063—℞ Pulveris opii . . . . ℨij.
Unguenti picis liquidæ . . . . ℨj.

Fiat unguentum.
Sig. Apply once or twice daily. ELLIS.

1064—℞ Pulveris teucrii scordii . . . . ℨij.
Unguenti petrolei . . . . ℨj.—M.

Sig. Apply after each action of the bowels. R. B. CRUICE.

1065—℞ Plumbi tannatis . . . . ℨj.
Unguenti simplicis . . . . ℨj.—M.

Sig. Apply twice daily. MACDONALD.

1066—℞ Hydrargyri chloridi mitis . . . . ℨij.
Unguenti petrolei . . . . ℨj.—M.

Sig. Apply twice daily. I. BARTLETT.

1067—℞ Iodoformi . . . . ℨij.
Unguenti simplicis . . . . ℨj.—M.

Sig. Apply twice daily. BARTHOLOW.

1068—℞ Olei theobromæ . . . . 3ss.
Extracti krameriæ . . . . ℈ij.
Pulveris opii . . . . gr. v.
Misce secundum artem, et fiunt suppositoria no. x.
Sig. Use one morning and night.   J. PANCOAST.

1069—℞ Unguenti belladonnæ . . . . 3ij.
Camphoræ . . . . 3j.
Tincturæ camphoræ compositæ . . . . f3j.
Misce et fiat unguentum.
Sig. Apply to painful piles.   NELIGAN.

1070—℞ Morphinæ sulphatis . . . . gr. ij.
Vitell. unius ovi,
Olei anthemidis,
Olei papaveris . . . . āā f3j.
Misce et fiat injectio.
Sig. Inject, in painful piles.   BRERA.

1071—℞ Chrysarobin . . . . gr. xvj.
Iodoform . . . . gr. vj.
Extract of belladonna . . . . gr. xij.
Vaseline . . . . 3vj.—M.
Sig. A small quantity to be applied to the tumor several times
a day, the parts having previously been washed with a
solution of carbolic acid 1 to 50, or of creolin 1 to 100.
(*External piles.*)   KOSSOBUDSKI.

1072—℞ Chrysarobin,
Iodoform . . . . āā gr. iss.
Extract of belladonna . . . . gr. ¼.
Cacao butter . . . . gr. xxx.—M.
Make one suppository.
Sig. Use at bedtime. (*Internal piles.*)   KOSSOBUDSKI.

1073—℞ Acidi carbolici . . . . 3ij.
Acidi tannici . . . . 3j.
Alcoholis . . . . f3iv.
Glycerini . . . . f3j.—M.
Sig. Hypodermic injection for piles.   GIRARD.

1074—℞ Ceræ flavæ . . . . ℈viij.
Resinæ . . . . ℈iv.
Adipis . . . . 3ss.
Olei sassafras . . . . ℳxl.—M.
Sig. Melt wax, resin, and lard together; when the mixture
shows signs of stiffening, add the oil of sassafras and stir
until cold. Apply locally.   *Charity Hospital, N.Y.*

1075—℞ Ext. colocynth. comp. . . . . 3ss.
Ext. nucis vomicæ . . . . gr. vj.
Hydrarg. chlor. mit.,
Ext. hyoscyami . . . . āā gr. xij.
Ft. massa et in pil. no. xii div.
Sig. One as required. (*For sluggish bowels.*)   BARKER.

1076—℞ Ferri subsulphatis . . . . 3ss.
Adipis . . . . 3j.—M.
Ft. unguentum.
Sig. Apply every morning locally.   ELLIS.

1077—℞ Creolin . . . . ℳxxiv.
Olei theobromæ . . . . q. s.—M.
Ft. suppositoria no. xii.
Sig. One at night.   J. C. WILSON.

1078—℞ Ext. opii . . . . gr. viij.
Ext. belladonnæ . . . . gr. ij.
Olei theobromæ . . . . q. s.—M.
Ft. massa et in suppositoria no. viii div.
Sig. One to be introduced into the bowel every four or six
hours.   LEVIS.

1079—℞ Ext. hydrastis fld. . . . . f3iv.
Sig. Use as a lotion externally; also take internally the following:

1080—℞ Tinct. hydrastis can. . . . . f3j.
Sig. Five minims three times daily, internally. PHILLIPS.

HERPES. (See Skin Diseases.)

HICCOUGH.

1081—℞ Apomorphinæ muriatis . . . . gr. ⅒.
    Aquæ destillatæ . . . . ℥x.—M.
Sig. Inject hypodermically.   RINGER.

1082—℞ Amyli nitritis . . . . f ℥j.
Sig. Three to five drops on handkerchief by inhalation.

1083—℞ Pulv. sinapis . . . . ℥j.
    Aquæ bullientis . . . . f ℥iv.—M.
Ft. infusum.
Sig. Take at one draught.   RINGER.

1084—℞ Sodii bicarb. . . . . ℥j.
    Tinct. nucis vom. . . . . f ℥j.
    Tinct. cardamomi . . . . . q. s. ad f ℥iij.—M.
Sig. Teaspoonful before each meal. (*Due to indigestion.*)
             HARE.

1085—℞ Pilocarpinæ muriatis . . . . gr. ⅒.
    Aquæ destillatæ . . . . ℥x.—M.
Sig. Inject hypodermically.   ORTILLE.

1086—℞ Zinci valerianatis . . . . gr. ix.
    Ext. belladonnæ . . . . gr. iij.—M.
Ft. massa et in pil. no. xii div.
Sig. One every six hours as required.   DANET.

HOOPING-COUGH. (See Whooping-Cough.)

HYDROCEPHALUS.

1087—℞ Potassii iodidi . . . . ℥ss-j.
    Syr. aurantii cort. . . . . ℥j.
    Aquæ . . . . ad f ℥iv.—M.
Sig. A teaspoonful every two hours to an infant of six
months.   J. LEWIS SMITH.

1088—℞ Potassii iodidi . . . . gr. xvj.
    Iodi . . . . gr. iv.
    Aquæ . . . . ℥j.—M.
Sig. A teaspoonful every four hours. Used in connection
with—

1089—℞ Syrupi ferri iodidi . . . . f ℥j.
Sig. Three to five drops three times a day, according to age
of child.

1090—℞ Unguenti hydrargyri . . . . ℥j.
Sig. Rub on head, and take—

    ℞ Potassii iodidi . . . . gr. xij.
    Aquæ destillatæ . . . . f ℥ss.—M.
Sig. A teaspoonful three times a day.   HAZARD.

1091—℞ Olei tiglii . . . . ℥ij.
    Mucilaginis acaciæ . . . . f ℥j.
    Aquæ destillatæ . . . . f ℥j.—M.
Sig. The fourth part every four hours. (*To remove fluid from
ventricles.*)   DUNGLISON.

1092—℞ Pulv. digitalis,
    Hydrargyri chloridi mitis,
    Pulv. ipecac. . . . . āā gr. ij.
    Sacchari albi . . . . gr. x.—M.
In pulv. no. xii div.
Sig. A powder every three or four hours. (*In subacute form.*)
            CONDIE.

1093—℞ Pulveris digitalis . . . . gr. vj.
      Hydrargyri chloridi mitis . . . . gr. xij.
      Sacchari albi . . . . gr. xviij.
Misce et fiant chartulæ no. xii.
Sig. One powder every six hours.   HAZARD.

1094—℞ Collodii cum cantharide . . . . f ʒiv.
Sig. Paint back of neck every few days.   HARTSHORNE.

HYDROPS PERICARDII. (See Dropsy and Heart-Disease.)

HYDROTHORAX. (See Dropsy.)

HYPOCHONDRIA.

1095—℞ Morphinæ sulphatis . . . . gr. j-ij.
      Sacchari-lactis . . . . gr. x.—M.
In pulv. no. xii div.
Sig. A powder three times daily for at least two months. The
dose should never be large enough to induce sleep.
                W. A. HAMMOND.

1096—℞ Liq. potassii arsenitis . . . . ℥xl.
      Tinct. opii . . . . f ʒss-j.
      Aquæ menthæ pip. . . . . ad f ʒiiss.—M.
Sig. A teaspoonful three times daily. (In the aged.)
                LEMARE-PICQUOT.

1097—℞ Liquoris potassii arsenitis . . . . f ʒss.
      Tincturæ opii deodoratæ . . . . . . f ʒj.
      Aquæ cinnamomi . . . . f ʒxivss.—M.
Sig. A teaspoonful three times a day.   LEMARE-PICQUOT.

1098—℞ Tincturæ opii deodoratæ . . . . f ʒss.
Sig. Five to ten drops three times a day.   KRAFFT-EBING.

1099—℞ Potassii bromidi . . . . ʒss.
      Syrupi simplicis . . . . f ʒj.
      Aquæ destillatæ . . . . q. s. ad f ʒiij.—M.
Sig. A dessertspoonful three times a day.   RINGER.

1100—℞ Auri chloridi . . . . gr. j-iss.
      Ext. gentianæ . . . . gr. xv.—M.
Ft. massa et in pil. no. xxx div.
Sig. One pill thrice daily. (In anæmic subjects.) BARTHOLOW.

1101—℞ Mist. asafœtidæ . . . . f ʒiv.
Sig. One to two tablespoonfuls three or four times daily.
                BARTHOLOW.

1102—℞ Extracti ergotæ . . . . ʒj.
      Extracti cannabis indicæ . . . . gr. vj.
      Potassii bromidi . . . . ʒij.—M.
Pone in capsulas no. xxiv.
Sig. One capsule three times a day.

HYSTERIA.

1103—℞ Liq. potassii arsenitis . . . . f ʒss.
Sig. Three to five drops thrice daily, after meals.
                BARTHOLOW.

1104—℞ Spts. ætheris comp.,
      Tinct. valerianæ ammon. . . . . . . āā f ʒj.—M.
Sig. A teaspoonful in water every fifteen minutes until relieved.   BARTHOLOW.

1105—℞ Pulveris camphoræ,
      Extracti eucalypti . . . . āā gr. xij.
Misce et fiant pilulæ no. xii.
Sig. One pill every three hours. (In debilitated subjects.)
                BARTHOLOW.

1106—℞ Ammonii bromidi . . . . ʒij.
Spts. ammoniæ aromat. . . . . f̃ʒj.
Aquæ . . . . f̃ʒiv.—M.
Sig. A dessertspoonful thrice daily.　　HARTSHORNE.

1107—℞ Ferri citratis . . . . ʒij.
Syr. simplicis . . . . f̃ʒss.
Aquæ aurantii florum . . . . . . ad f̃ʒvj.—M.
Sig. A tablespoonful three times daily. (*In anæmic cases.*)
HARTSHORNE.

1108—℞ Iron lactate . . . . ʒij.
Iron arsenate . . . . gr. iij.
Extract of nux vomica . . . . gr. vij.
Extract of gentian . . . . gr. xlv.—M.
Divide into 100 pills.
Sig. Two pills to be taken three times daily.
Journal de Méd. de Paris.

1109—℞ Camphoræ,
Asafœtidæ . . . . āā ʒj.
Extracti belladonnæ . . . . ʒss.
Extracti opii aquosi . . . . gr. x.
Misce et fiant pilulæ no. xl.
Sig. One pill night and morning.　　HAZARD.

1110—℞ Sodium bromid. . . . . ʒj.
Solution of potassium arsenite . . . . f̃ʒiss.
Extract of ergot . . . . f̃ʒj.
Camphorated tincture of opium . . . f̃ʒj.
Water . . . . q. s. ad f̃ʒiv.—M.
Sig. One teaspoonful in water after meals.　　POPE.

1111—℞ Zinci valerianatis . . . . gr. ix.
Pulveris tragacanthæ. . . . . ʒss.
Misce et divide in pilulas no. xii.
Sig. One pill night and morning. (*With headache.*)　　DEVAY.

1112—℞ Zinci valerianatis,
Quininæ valerianatis . . . . āā gr. xv.
Extracti gentianæ . . . . q. s.
Fiant pilulæ no. xv.
Sig. One pill every hour. (*In the epileptoid form.*)　　MARTINI.

1113—℞ Tincturæ opii deodoratæ . . . . f̃ʒj.
Tincturæ nucis vomicæ. . . . . . . f̃ʒij.—M.
Sig. Three drops three or four times a day. (*In middle-aged people with flatulence, flushings, weight on head, etc.*)
RINGER.

1114—℞ Tincturæ avenæ concentratæ . . . . . f̃ʒss.
Sig. Fifteen drops in a fluidounce of hot water at bedtime.
(*Nervous tonic.*)　　WAUGH.

1115—℞ Ext. conii fld.,
Ext. hyoscyami fld. . . . . āā ℳvij.
Chloral. hydratis . . . . gr. x.
Aquæ . . . . ad f̃ʒj.—M.
Ft. haustus.
Sig. To be taken at a single dose and repeated as required.
MADIGAN.

1116—℞ Ext. salicis nigræ,
Elixiris simplicis . . . . āā f̃ʒj.—M.
Sig. A teaspoonful three times daily.　　HUTCHINSON.

1117—℞ Paraldehyd. . . . . ℳxxx-l.
Syr. simplicis . . . . f̃ʒss.
Aquæ menthæ pip. . . . . f̃ʒj.—M.
Fiat haustus.
Sig. To be taken at a draught. (*To produce sleep.*)

1118—℞ Apomorphinæ muriatis . . . . gr. j.
Syr. simplicis . . . . f̃ʒiv.
Aquæ . . . . ad f̃ʒx.
Sig. A teaspoonful as required. Repeat in a few hours if necessary.　　RINGER.

HYSTERIA (Continued).

1119—℞ Ergotini . . . . gr. lx.
Extracti cannabis ind. . . . . gr. iv.
Strychninæ . . . . gr. ⅜.—M.
In pil. no. xlviii div.
Sig. Two pills three times a day, after meals.　J. C. WILSON.

ICHTHYOSIS. (See Skin Diseases.)

IMPETIGO. (See Skin Diseases.)

IMPOTENCE.

1120—℞ Zinci phosphidi . . . . gr. ij.
Confectionis rosæ . . . . ɔj.—M.
Ft. massa et in pil. no. xxiv div.
Sig. One to three pills three times daily.　BARTHOLOW.

1121—℞ Ferri arseniatis . . . . gr. v.
Extracti ergotæ aquosi . . . . ꜱss.
Misce et fiant pilulæ no. xxx.
Sig. One pill night and morning. (*With spermatorrhœa.*)
BARTHOLOW.

1122—℞ Arsenauro . . . . f℥ss.
Sig. Five drops in water three times daily.　H. TUCKER.

1123—℞ Pulveris cantharidis . . . . gr. xviij.
Pulveris opii,
Pulveris camphoræ . . . . āā gr. xxxvj.
Confectionis rosæ . . . . q. s.
Misce et fiant pilulæ no. xxxvi.
Sig. One pill at night. (*From general debility.*)　HAZARD.

1124—℞ Phosphori . . . . gr ss.
Ætheris . . . . f℥ss.
Solve, et adde—
Tincturæ cantharidis,
Tincturæ nucis vomicæ . . . . . . āā f℥ss.—M.
Sig. Thirty drops three or four times a day.
VOGT.

1125—℞ Extracti cannabis indicæ,
Extracti nucis vomicæ . . . . . , āā gr. xv.
Extracti ergotæ aquosi . . . . ℥j.
Misce et divide in pilulas no. xxx.
Sig. One pill morning and evening.　DA COSTA.

1126—℞ Tinct. phosphori . . . . f℥iss.
Tinct. cantharidis . . . . f℥iiiss.
Elixiris simplicis . . . . ad f℥v.—M.
Sig. One teaspoonful three or four hours before retiring　Increase the dose carefully.　VAN BUREN AND KEYES.

1127—℞ Pulv. sanguinariæ . . . . gr. ij.
Ext. ergotæ . . . . ɔj.—M.
Ft. massa et in pil. no. xx div.
Sig. One pill thrice daily.　S. O. POTTER.

1128—℞ Phosphori . . . . gr. j.
Alcoholis absoluti . . . . f℥v.
Glycerini . . . . f℥iss.
Alcoholis . . . . f℥ij.
Spts. menthæ pip. . . . . f℥j.—M.
Sig. One-half to one teaspoonful three times daily. (*For old people.*)　J. A. THOMPSON.

INCONTINENCE OF URINE.

1129—℞ Syrupi belladonnæ . . . . f℥ij.
Syrupi tolutani,
Syrupi althææ . . . . āā f℥j.—M.
Sig. A half-teaspoonful two to eight times a day.
DESCROIZILLES.

96

I

1130—℞ Ext. belladonnæ . . . . gr. vj.
Pulv. acaciæ,
Pulv. althææ . . . . āā q. s.—M.

Fiant pilulæ no. xl.
Sig. One to fifteen to be taken daily, according to the severity
of the case.   DESCROIZILLES.

1131—℞ Atropini . . . . gr. ⅓.
Sacchari albi . . . . ℨiij.—M.

Fiant pulveres no. xl.
Sig. Two to four to be taken daily.   DESCROIZILLES.

1132—℞ Potassii bromidi . . . . ℨiss.
Aquæ cinnamomi . . . . fℨij.
Syrupi,
Syrupi aurantii amari cort. . . . . āā fℨj.—M.

Sig. A half-teaspoonful one to four times a day.
DESCROIZILLES.

1133—℞ Potassii citratis . . . . ℨss.
Spt. ætheris nitrosi . . . . f℥vj.
Aquæ . . . . q. s. ad f℥j.—M.

Sig. Dessertspoonful every four hours in equal quantity of
water.   HARE.

1134—℞ Syrupi ferri iodidi . . . . f℥ss.

Sig. Fifteen to twenty drops, well diluted, three times a
day. (*In pale, delicate, and strumous children.*)
BARTHOLOW.

1135—℞ Atropinæ sulphatis . . . . gr. j.
Aquæ destillatæ . . . . f℥j.—M.

Sig. Four to eight drops in water. (*For children.*)
BARTHOLOW.

1136—℞ Tinct. belladonnæ . . . . f℥j.

Sig. Ten to twenty drops thrice daily.   RINGER.

1137—℞ Santonini . . . . gr. xvj.
Olei ricini . . . . f℥j.—M.

Sig. One or two teaspoonfuls before breakfast, for two or three
mornings.   RINGER.

1138—℞ Strychninæ . . . . gr. j.
Acidi acetici . . . . gtt. ij.
Sacchari albi . . . . ℨij.
Aquæ destillatæ . . . . f℥ij.

Fiat solutio.
Sig. Fifteen to thirty drops for a child six to twelve years of
age.   MAGENDIE.

1139—℞ Acidi benzoici . . . . ℨij.
Aquæ cinnamomi . . . . f℥vj.—M.

Sig. A tablespoonful thrice daily.   HARTSHORNE.

1140—℞ Syrupi ferri bromidi,
Syrupi simplicis . . . . āā f℥ss.—M.

Sig. A half-teaspoonful three times a day. (*Child six to ten
years old.*)   DA COSTA.

1141—℞ Tinct. ferri muriatis . . . . f℥j.
Decocti uvæ ursi . . . . f℥vj.—M.

Sig. A tablespoonful two or three times daily.   WILLIS.

1142—℞ Collodii . . . . f℥j.

Sig. Pull forward the prepuce and smear over to form a cap.
Continue for a fortnight. Is easily picked off with finger-
nail.   D. CORRIGAN.

1143—℞ Spiritus ætheris nitrosi . . . . f℥vj.
Syrupi . . . . f℥iv.
Liquoris potassii citratis . . . . . . f℥viij.—M.

Sig. Tablespoonful in water every two hours.

1144—℞ Ext. rhois aromaticæ fld. . . . . . . f℥j.

Sig. Five minims at two years of age; ten minims at age of
two to six years; fifteen minims for older children. To be
given in sweetened water.   UNNA.

g

1145—℞ Tincturæ cantharidis . . . . ♏ij.
Tincturæ hyoscyami . . . . ♏v.
Aquæ destillatæ . . . . f℥x.
Fiat haustus.
Sig. Repeat the dose four times a day. (*For middle-aged and old women.*) GREGORY.

1146—℞ Chloral. hydratis . . . . gr. viiss.
Aquæ destillatæ . . . . f℥ss.
Fiat haustus.
Sig. Take at bedtime. VECCHIZETTI.

1147—℞ Tinct. ferri chlor. . . . . f℥ij.
Ext. ergotæ fld. . . . . f℥v.
Spts. chloroformi . . . . f℥ij.
Tinct. quassiæ . . . . ad f℥iv.—M.
Sig. A teaspoonful in a wineglassful of water thrice daily. (*For children.*) S. O. POTTER.

1148—℞ Linimenti cantharidis . . . . f℥ss.
Sig. Paint, high up, over the nape of the neck, a space three inches by two inches, till blistered. HARKIN.

1149—℞ Chloral. hydratis . . . . 3j.
Syr. tolutani . . . . f℥iiss.—M.
Sig. A teaspoonful thrice daily. (*For infantile incontinence.*) DA COSTA.

INDIGESTION. (See Dyspepsia.)

INFLAMMATION. (See the names as applied to the particular organs inflamed, Heart-Disease, Pleurisy, Synovitis, etc.)

INFLUENZA. (See Catarrh and Hay Fever.)

INGROWING TOE-NAIL.

1150—℞ Liquoris potassæ . . . . f℥ij.
Aquæ . . . . f℥j.—M.
Sig. Apply on cotton to the margin of the nail at the ulcerated surface, to soften the nail, BARTHOLOW.

1151—℞ Liquoris potassæ . . . . f℥ij.
Aquæ destillatæ . . . . f℥j,—M.
Sig. Apply with pledgets of cotton-wool. NORTON.

1152—℞ Acidi tannici . . . . 3j.
Aquæ destillatæ . . . . f℥vj.—M.
Sig. Paint the soft parts twice daily. MIALL.

1153—℞ Pulv. plumbi acetatis . . . . 3j.
Tinct. opii . . . . f℥j.
Aquæ . . . . ad f℥viij.—M.
Sig. Shake well, and apply constantly until the inflammation is reduced and pain alleviated; then separate the granulating surface from the nail and insert a small pledget of cotton; then use—

1154—℞ Argenti nitratis . . . . gr. xxx.
Aquæ destillatæ . . . . f℥j.—M.
Ft. lotio.
Sig. Apply two or three times daily with a brush. DAVIDSON.

INSOMNIA.

1155—℞ Antimonii et potassii tartratis . . . . gr. j-ij.
Morphinæ sulphatis . . . . gr. iss.
Aquæ laurocerasi . . . . f℥j.—M.
Sig. A teaspoonful every two, three, or four hours. (*In the delirium and wakefulness of fevers.*) BARTHOLOW.

INSOMNIA (Continued).

1156—℞ Amyl. hydratis . . . . gr. xlv.
 Syr. aurantii cort.. . . . . f℥ss.
 Aquæ . . . . f℥j.—M.

Ft. haustus.
Sig. To be taken at bedtime. Half as much more may be given when by enema. VON MERING.

1157—℞ Tincturæ hyoscyami . . . . f℥ij.
Sig. From one to four drachms. (*Where opium is not borne.*) CAMPBELL.

1158—℞ Hyoscinæ hydrobromatis . . . . gr. ⅛
 Camphoræ monobromatæ . . . . ℨj.—M.

Fiant capsulæ no. xv.
Sig. One capsule at bedtime and repeat in six hours if required. (*Used to induce sleep in melancholia, neurasthenia, and mania.*)

1159—℞ Chloral. hydratis . . . . ℨj.
 Potassii bromidi . . . . ℨij.
 Syrupi aurantii corticis. . . . . f℥ss.
 Aquæ caryophylli . . . . . . q. s. ad f℥vj.—M.
Sig. A tablespoonful three times a day in a wineglassful of water. QUAIN.

1160—℞ Ext. piscidiæ erythrin. fid. . . . . f℥j.
 Syr. simplicis . . . . f℥j.
 Aquæ aurantii flor. . . . . ad f℥iv.—M.
Sig. A teaspoonful to a tablespoonful at bedtime. (*For nervous cases that do not bear opiates well.*) PAYNE.

1161—℞ Antimonii et potass. tart. . . . . gr. iij-iv.
 Tinct. opii . . . . ℳxxxvj-l.
 Syr. simplicis . . . . f℥ss.
 Aquæ . . . . ad f℥iij.—M.
Sig. A teaspoonful every two hours till tranquil or asleep. (*In wakefulness or delirium of fevers.*) GRAVES.

1162—℞ Codeinæ . . . . gr. iss.
 Aquæ laurocerasi . . . . f℥iss. .
 Syrupi simplicis . . . . f℥j.
 Aquæ florum tiliæ . . . . f℥ij.—M.
Sig. A tablespoonful every half-hour. (*For sleeplessness due to pain.*) TROUSSEAU ET REVEIL.

1163—℞ Pulv. opii . . . . gr. iv-viij.
 Pulv. camphoræ . . . . gr. xij.
 Ext. hyoscyami . . . . ℨj.—M.
Ft. massa et in pil. no. xii div.
Sig. One or two pills at night. (*A good calmative.*) HARTSHORNE.

1164—℞ Chloral. hydratis . . . . gr. xxv.
 Tincturæ cardamomi compositæ . . . f℥ss.
 Syrupi simplicis . . . . f℥ij.
 Infusi caryophylli . . . . . . q. s. ad f℥iss.
Fiat haustus.
Sig. Use *pro re nata*. (*When due to mental overwork, anxiety, or physical fatigue.*) PRIESTLEY.

1165—℞ Trionalis . . . . ℨj.
Fiant chartulæ no. iii.
Sig. One powder in hot milk. H. TUCKER.

1166—℞ Potassii bromidi . . . . ℨiv.
 Chloral. hydratis . . . . ℨij.
 Syr. pruni virgin. . . . . f℥j.
 Aquæ . . . . ad f℥ij.—M.
Sig. A dessertspoonful in a wineglassful of water at bedtime.

1167—℞ Paraldehyd . . . . f℥iss.
 Alcoholis (90 per cent.) . . . . f℥iss.
 Tinct. vanillæ . . . . f℥ss.
 Aquæ . . . . f℥j.
 Syr. simplicis . . . . ad f℥iv.—M.
Sig. A teaspoonful or two every hour till sleep is obtained. YVON.

INSOMNIA (Continued).

1168—℞ Methylal . . . . ʒj.
Syr. aurantii flor. . . . . ad f ℥iv.—M.
Sig. A tablespoonful at bedtime. May be increased to four tablespoonfuls. RICHARDSON.

1169—℞ Urethan. . . . . ʒss.
Aquæ aurantii flor. . . . . f ℥ij.—M.
Sig. One to four teaspoonfuls at bedtime. (*In nervous cases not bearing opiates.*) ANDREWS.

1170—℞ Sulphonalis . . . . ʒj.
Fiant chartulæ no. vi.
Sig. One in cup of hot water, and repeat in four hours if required. (*Insomnia of drunkards.*)

1171—℞ Morphinæ sulph. . . . . gr. j.
Ext. valerianæ fld. . . . . f ʒj.
Elix. humuli . . . . f ʒj.—M.
Sig. One or two teaspoonfuls, as required. (*In insomnia of delirium tremens.*)

1172—℞ Morphinæ sulph. . . . . gr. ij.
Aquæ camphoræ . . . . f ℥ij.—M.
Sig. One to two teaspoonfuls at bedtime. SMITH.

INTERMITTENT FEVER. (See Fever.)

INTERTRIGO. (See Skin Diseases.)

INTESTINAL CATARRH. (See Catarrh.)

INTESTINAL PARASITES. (See Worms.)

INTUSSUSCEPTION.

1173—℞ Lobeliæ . . . . ʒss.
Aquæ bullientis . . . . Oj.
Fiat infusio.
Sig. Inject one-fourth or one-half, and repeat if permissible. BARTHOLOW.

1174—℞ Sodii bicarbonatis . . . . ∋ij–ʒij.
Aquæ . . . . f ℥vj.
Solve et fiat enema.
Sig. Inject, and follow immediately with—

1175—℞ Acidi tartarici pulverizati . . . . . gr. xxxv–xlvij.
Aquæ. . . . . f ℥iv.
Solve et fiat enema.
Sig. Inject immediately after the foregoing. (*The effervescence will cause the bowel suddenly to distend.*) BARTHOLOW.

1176—℞ Fellis bovini . . . . gr. x–xxx.
Aquæ ferventis . . . . Oj–iv.—M.
Sig. Inject slowly into the bowel until it is fully distended. (*Knee-chest position is the best.*) HAWKINS.

1177—℞ Ext. belladonnæ. . . . . gr. iv.
Aquæ ferventis . . . . Oj.—M.
Ft. solutio.
Sig. Inject into the rectum. WARING.

1178—℞ Hydrogenii . . . . cong. ij.
Sig. Inject slowly into the bowel from rubber bag with rectal tube. Patient should be under an anæsthetic, and buttocks raised and head lowered while the injection is being made. (*Used during first or second day; never later than fourth day.*)

IRITIS.

1179—℞ Atropinæ sulphatis . . . . gr. iv.
Aquæ destillatæ . . . . ƒ 3j.—M.

Sig. A drop or two in the eye two or three times daily. Use with hot water, bathing for fifteen minutes every hour till pain is relieved. CHILTON.

1180—℞ Scopolaminæ . . . . gr. ss.
Aquæ destillatæ . . . . ƒ 3j.—M.

Sig. One drop in eye morning and night. (*Used in cases where atropine causes irritation.*)

1181—℞ Extracti belladonnæ . . . . 3j.
Ungt. hydrargyri . . . . 3vj.—M.

Sig. For inunction to the brow. LEVIS.

1182—℞ Emplastri cantharidis . . . . 1 in. × 1 in.

Sig. Apply behind the ear, and poultice when blistered. HARTSHORNE.

1183—℞ Atropinæ sulphatis . . . . gr. j-iij.
Morphinæ sulphatis . . . . gr. iv.
Zinci sulphatis . . . . gr. ij-viij.
Aquæ destillatæ . . . . ƒ 3j.—M.

Sig. Apply as a lotion. BARTHOLOW.

1184—℞ Hydrarg. chlor. corros. . . . . gr. j.
Potassii iodidi . . . . 3j.
Tinct. calumbæ . . . . ƒ 3ij.
Aquæ destillatæ . . . . ad ƒ 3vj.—M.

Sig. A dessertspoonful in a wineglassful of water two or three times daily. LAWSON.

1185—℞ Hydrargyri chloridi mitis . . . . gr. x.
Extracti glycyrrhizæ . . . . q. s.

Misce et fiant pilulæ no. xx.
Sig. Two pills twice a day. NIEMEYER.

1186—℞ Sulphate of quinine . . . . gr. ij.
Protiodide of mercury . . . . gr. ¼-½.
Ext. of hyoscyamus . . . . gr. ¼.

Make one pill.
Sig. Take one pill three to six times daily. (*Syphilitic plastic iritis.*) DE SCHWEINITZ.

1187—℞ Hydrargyri biniodidi . . . . gr. ij.
Potassii iodidi . . . . 3iij.
Solve in—
Aquæ destillatæ . . . . ƒ 3ss.
Dein adde—
Syrupi stillingiæ compositi . . . . . . ƒ 3iiss.—M.

Sig. A teaspoonful after each meal. KEYSER.

1188—℞ Unguenti hydrargyri . . . . 3ij.

Sig. One drachm as an inunction at night. (*Used in plastic iritis; when gums are touched, discontinue.*)

1189—℞ Duboisiæ sulphatis . . . . gr. j.
Aquæ destillatæ . . . . ƒ 3j.—M.

Ft. collyrium.
Sig. One drop into the eye once or twice daily. TWEEDY.

1190—℞ Olei terebinthinæ . . . . ƒ 3j.
Mucil. acaciæ . . . . q. s. ut ft. emulsio.
Syr. simplicis . . . . ƒ 3j.
Aquæ menthæ pip. . . . . ad ƒ 3iv.—M.

Sig. A dessertspoonful three times daily. HOGG.

ITCH. (See **Skin Diseases and Lice.**)

JAUNDICE. (See **Biliousness, Catarrh, and Calculi.**)

JOINTS, DISEASES OF. (See **Synovitis.**)

KERATITIS, PHLYCTENULAR.

1191—℞ Hydrarg. oxid. flav. . . . . gr. j.
Petrolat. albi . . . . ℥ij.—M.

Sig. Rubbed into the eye well at night.   DE SCHWEINITZ.

1192—℞ Hydrarg. chloridi corrosivi . . . . . . gr. j.
Ammonii chloridi . . . . gr. vj.
Tinct. belladonnæ . . . . f℥ij.
Aquæ destillatæ . . . . f℥viij.—M.

Ft. collyrium.
Sig. A teaspoonful in a wineglassful of tepid water, to be applied frequently with a pledget of lint on the closed lids.
TURNBULL.

1193—℞ Syrupi ferri iodidi . . . . f℥vij.
Liquoris potassii arsenitis . . . . . . f℥j.—M.

Sig. Three to ten drops internally in a half-glass of water after meals. (*Tonic for strumous children.*)

1194—℞ Duboisiæ sulphatis . . . . gr. j.
Aquæ destillatæ . . . . f℥j.—M.

Ft. collyrium.
Sig. One or two drops in the eye two or three times daily.
THOMPSON.

1195—℞ Acidi carbolici . . . . gr. xl.
Aquæ . . . . f℥viij.—M.

Ft. collyrium.
Sig. Any trace of ulceration or granulation on the cornea, or any pustule on the conjunctiva, is scraped bare by a delicate eye-scraper. The cornea, lids, and conjunctival sac are washed with the above solution, and the cornea and conjunctival sac are dredged with—

1196—℞ Pulv. iodoformi . . . . ℈ss.

Sig. Use as a dredge; then moisten and paint the skin of the eyelids and eyebrows with solid nitrate of silver. Dredge with iodoform, and bandage.   TEALE.

KIDNEYS, DISEASES OF. (See Albuminuria, Nephritis, and Uræmia.)

LABOR.

1197—℞ Morphiuæ sulphatis . . . . gr. ij.
Aquæ destillatæ . . . . ℥j.—M.

Sig. Five to ten minims hypodermically, repeated if necessary. (*In protracted labor due to rigid os.*)   RINGER.

1198—℞ Morphiuæ sulphatis . . . . gr. j-ij.
Olei theobromæ . . . . ℥ij.—M.

Ft. massa et in suppositoria no. iv div.
Sig. One as required. (*In precipitate labor.*)   LEISHMAN.

1199—℞ Antimonii et potassii tartratis . . . . . gr. ij.
Tincturæ opii deodoratæ . . . . . . ℳxx.
Aquæ destillatæ . . . . f℥vj.—M.

Sig. A tablespoonful every hour, until nausea or vomiting supervenes. (*In rigid os.*)   HARDY.

1200—℞ Tincturæ opii deodoratæ . . . . . . gtt. xlv.
Tincturæ lactucarii,
Syrupi papaveris . . . . āā f℥iij.
Aquæ aurantii florum . . . . f℥iss.—M.

Sig. The one-third part. (*In protracted labor due to irregular tetanic pains.*)   VELPEAU.

1201—℞ Vini opii . . . . gtt. xl-lx.

Sig. Inject with a little starch-water, in two or three doses, in the course of a couple of hours. (*To prevent premature labor.*)   CAZEAUX.

1202—℞ Ext. ergotæ fld. . . . . ℥j.
Olei gaultheriæ . . . . gtt. iv.—M.

Sig. A teaspoonful every four hours, only if os is dilated and soft parts not rigid. (*In protracted labor from atony of uterus.*)
LEISHMAN

- K -

-L-

LABOR (Continued).

1203—℞ Ext. kolæ fl. . . . . f℥ij.

Sig. One-half drachm at a dose, and repeat once if necessary.
(*For lingering labor.*) B. C. HIRST.

1204—℞ Tincturæ nucis vomicæ. . . . . ℳv.
Extracti ergotæ fluidi. . . . . ℳxxx.
Elixiris simplicis . . . . f℥iij.

Fiat haustus.
Sig. Repeat every three hours. (*In retained placenta.*)
LOMBE ATTHILL.

1205—℞ Pulveris ergotæ . . . . ℨss.
Syrupi simplicis. . . . . f℥ss.
Aquæ menthæ piperitæ . . . . f℥j.—M.

Sig. One-third part every twenty minutes. (*In lingering labor.*)
SOUBEIRAN.

1206—℞ Antimonii et potassii tartratis. . . . . gr. iij.
Magnesii sulphatis . . . . ℨj.
Syrupi zingiberis . . . . f℥ss.
Infusi sennæ . . . . f℥viiss.—M.

Sig. Two tablespoonfuls every hour or half-hour. (*In rigid os.*)
HULL.

1207—℞ Chloral. hydratis . . . . ℨij.
Syr. aurantii cort. . . . . f℥j.
Aquæ aurantii flor. . . . . f℥iv.—M.

Sig. A tablespoonful every twenty minutes for three doses;
perhaps a fourth, after an hour's interval. PLAYFAIR.

1208—℞ Chloroformi . . . . f℥iv.

Sig. Let the patient inhale, but not to complete anæsthesia,
lest uterine action be interrupted. SIMPSON.

1209—℞ Quininæ sulphatis. . . . . ℈ij.
Acidi sulph. aromat. . . . . . q. s. ut ft. sol.
Syr. zingiberis . . . . f℥j.
Aquæ . . . . ad f℥ij.—M.

Sig. A tablespoonful at once, and a dessertspoonful every
four hours afterwards. (*In atony of the uterus.*) RINGER.

1210—℞ Amyl. nitritis . . . . ℨj.

Sig. Three to five drops to be inhaled from a handkerchief.
(*In hour-glass contraction of the uterus.*) BARNES.

LARYNGISMUS STRIDULUS.

1211—℞ Antipyrin. . . . . gr. xxx.
Syrupi acaciæ . . . . f℥ss.
Aquæ . . . . f℥iiss.—M.

Sig. A teaspoonful every hour or two. J. C. WILSON.

1212—℞ Potassii bromidi . . . . ℨij.
Chloral. hydratis . . . . ℨss.
Syr. tolutani . . . . f℥ss.
Aquæ . . . . f℥iss.—M.

Sig. A teaspoonful every half-hour. BARTHOLOW.

1213—℞ Chloroformi . . . . f℥j.
Sig. A few drops inhaled from a handkerchief. BARTHOLOW.

1214—℞ Syr. ipecacuanhæ . . . . f℥ij.
Sig. A teaspoonful every ten or fifteen minutes until free
emesis occurs. BARTHOLOW.

1215—℞ Chloral. hydratis . . . . ℨss.
Potassii bromidi . . . . ℨj.
Syrupi tolutani . . . . f℥ss.
Aquæ destillatæ . . . . f℥iss.—M.

Sig. A teaspoonful every half-hour. BARTHOLOW.

1216—℞ Thymoli . . . . gr. xx.
Alcohol . . . . f℥ij.—M.

Sig. Evaporate tablespoonful in room every hour. (*Used to
relieve laryngeal spasm.*)

1217—℞ Quininæ sulphatis . . . . gr. vj.
　　　Acidi sulphurici diluti . . . . ♏vj.
　　　Tincturæ aurantii,
　　　Syrupi zingiberis . . . . āā f℥ij.
　　　Aquæ destillatæ . . . . f℥ij.—M.
Sig. A teaspoonful three times a day. (*In rickety, cachectic children.*) OKE.

1218—℞ Syrupi scillæ compositi . . . . f℥j.
Sig. Thirty drops every quarter- or half-hour as an emetic, or ten drops every three hours as an expectorant. (*For a child two years old.*) COXE.

1219—℞ Syrupi ipecacuanhæ . . . . f℥j.
Sig. A teaspoonful every fifteen minutes. MEIGS.

1220—℞ Potassii citratis . . . . ℨj.
　　　Syr. ipecac. . . . . f℥ij.
　　　Tinct. opii deod.. . . . . gtt. xij.
　　　Syr. simplicis . . . . f℥j.
　　　Aquæ . . . . f℥iss.—M.
Sig. A teaspoonful every two hours at two years of age. (*In severe form.*) MEIGS AND PEPPER.

1221—℞ Atropinæ sulphatis . . . . gr. ₁₆.
　　　Aquæ destillatæ . . . . f℥j.—M.
Sig. Mix in a gobletful of water (*sixty doses*), of which give a teaspoonful every hour or half-hour. A. A. SMITH.

1222—℞ Tinct. aconiti radicis . . . . f℥ss.
Sig. One drop in a teaspoonful of water every hour for three or four doses; then every two hours. RINGER.

1223—℞ Ferri citratis . . . . ℨij.
　　　Aquæ aurantii flor. . . . . f℥vss.
　　　Syr. simplicis . . . . f℥ss.—M.
Sig. From a teaspoonful to a tablespoonful thrice daily between the paroxysms. (*For the anæmic condition.*) HARTSHORNE

LARYNGITIS.

1224—℞ Potassii iodidi . . . . ℨj-℥ij (!).
　　　Aquæ destillatæ. . . . . f℥vj.
Solve.
Sig. A dessertspoonful every four hours. (*In rapidly destructive syphilitic form.*) BARTHOLOW.

1225—℞ Sol. cocain. muriatis (15–20 per cent.) . f℥ss.
Sig. Apply locally to the larynx before and, if much pain, after the following:

1226—℞ Acidi lactici . . . . ℨss.
Sig. Apply locally to all infiltrations and ulcerations in the larynx. (*In tuberculous laryngitis.*) HERING.

1227—℞ Argenti nitratis . . . . gr. ss-v.
　　　Aquæ destillatæ . . . . f℥j.—M.
Sig. Apply by means of atomizer. (*In chronic form.*) RINGER.

1228—℞ Hydrargyri biniodidi . . . . gr. ij.
　　　Potassii iodidi . . . . ℨij.
　　　Extracti sarsaparillæ fluidi . . . . . . f℥ij.—M.
Sig. A teaspoonful three times a day. Follow in five or six days with—

1229—℞ Potassii iodidi . . . . ℨiss.
　　　Aquæ destillatæ. . . . . f℥ij.—M.
Sig. A teaspoonful three times a day. (*In syphilitic form.*) HAZARD.

1230—℞ Potassii permanganatis . . . . gr. ij.
　　　Aquæ destillatæ. . . . . f℥j.—M.
Sig. Use with atomizer several times daily. (*In fetid variety of chronic laryngitis.*) SAJOUS.

1231—℞ Sodii biboratis . . . . gr. viij.
     Aquæ . . . . f℥ij.
     Aquæ coloniensis . . . . gtt. x.—M.
Sig. Use frequently as a spray with atomizer. (*Chronic form.*)
                      SAJOUS.

1232—℞ Tinct. aconiti radicis . . . . f℥ss.
Sig. One drop every hour in water. Best results when following a dose of castor oil. When it has existed some days, then give—

1233—℞ Vini cocæ . . . . Oj.
Sig. A wineglassful every three hours, with absolute rest of voice. (*In acute laryngitis.*)   SAJOUS.

1234—℞ Tincturæ aconiti radicis . . . . . . ℔xxx.
     Syrupi limonis . . . . f℥ss.
     Liquoris ammonii acetatis . . . . . f℥ij.—M.
Sig. A dessertspoonful every three hours. (*In acute form.*)
                      R. P. THOMAS.

1235—℞ Acidi sulphurosi . . . . partem j.
     Aquæ destillatæ . . . . partes ij.-M.
Sig. Apply twice daily by means of atomizer. (*In chronic form.*)   BIETT.

1236—℞ Acidi benzoici . . . . gr. ss.
     Sodii biboratis . . . . gr. iss.
     Acaciæ, sugar, or currant-paste . . . . q. s.—M.
Ft. trochiscum no. i.
Sig. One every hour. (*In acute laryngitis.*)   SAJOUS.

1237—℞ Hydrargyri protiodidi . . . . gr. iij.
     Potassii iodidi . . . . ℥ij.
     Tincturæ gentianæ comp.,
     Syrupi sarsaparillæ comp. . . . . . āā f℥ij.—M.
Sig. A teaspoonful three times daily. (*In follicular laryngitis and ulcerations of the epiglottis.*)   HORACE GREEN.

1238—℞ Argenti nitratis . . . . gr. lx.
     Aquæ destillatæ . . . . f℥j.—M.
Sig. Apply locally on cotton after using—

1239—℞ Sol. cocain. muriatis (10 per cent.) . . f℥j.
Sig. Apply locally to the larynx. (*In chronic form.*)   SEILER.

1240—℞ Menthol. . . . . gr. xxv-c.
     Olei olivæ . . . . f℥j.—M.
Sig. Apply locally to the ulcerations. (*In tuberculous laryngitis.*)   M. A. ROSENBERG.

1241—℞ Iodol. . . . . ℥j.
Sig. Apply a small portion to the larynx by insufflation once daily, or two or three times a week. (*In tuberculous laryngitis.*)   LUBLINSKI.

1242—℞ Hydrarg. cyanidi . . . . gr. ij.
     Sacch. lactis . . . . gr. xv.
     Mucil. acaciæ . . . . q. s. ut ft. massa.—M.
Ft. massa et in pil. no. xx div.
Sig. One pill twice daily. (*In syphilitic laryngitis.*)
                  MORELL MACKENZIE.

1243—℞ Hydrarg. chloridi corrosivi . . . . . gr. j.
     Potassii iodidi . . . . ℥ij.
     Aquæ cinnamomi . . . . ℥iij.—M.
Sig. A teaspoonful three times daily. (*In syphilitic laryngitis.*)
                  L. ELSBERG.

1244—℞ Hydrarg. chloridi corrosivi . . . . . . gr. j-ij.
     Aquæ destillatæ . . . . ℥ij.—M.
Sig. Inhale from an atomizer several times daily. (*In syphilitic laryngitis.*)   DEMARQUAY.

LEAD POISONING. (See Colic.)

LEPRA. (See Skin Diseases.)

1245—℞ Quininæ sulphatis . . . . ʒi.
　　　Ferri sulphatis exsiccatæ . . . . . . ʒiss.
Fiat massa, in pilulas no. xxx dividenda.
Sig. Four or five pills during the day. (*Ague cake.*)
BARTHOLOW.

1246—℞ Extracti glandulæ suprarenalis . . . ʒij.
Pone in capsulas no. xxiv.
Sig. One capsule two hours after each meal.

1247—℞ Acidi arseniosi . . . . gr. j.
　　　Pilulæ ferri carbonatis . . . . ʒj.
　　　Quinidinæ sulphatis . . . . ʒj.
Misce et divide in pilulas xl.
Sig. Two pills three times a day.　　　DA COSTA.

1248—℞ Acidi nitro-muriatici dil. . . . . . . fʒj.
Sig. Ten to twenty drops in a wineglassful of water thrice
　daily.　　　　　　　　　　　　HARTSHORNE.

1249—℞ Olei eucalypti . . . . gtt. c.
　　　Piperini,
　　　Ceræ albæ . . . . āā ʒj.
　　　Pulv. althææ . . . . ʒij.—M.
Ft. massa et in pil. no. c div.
Sig. Three to five pills thrice daily.　　　MOSLER.

1250—℞ Pulveris aloes socotrinæ,
　　　Ferri sulphatis exsiccatæ . . . . . āā ʒj.
　　　Mastiches . . . . gr. x.
　　　Pulveris capsici . . . . ʒj.
　　　Syrupi simplicis . . . . q. s.
Fiat massa, in pilulas xx dividenda.
Sig. One pill every four hours,　　　COPLAND.

LEUCORRHŒA.

1251—℞ Sodii biboratis . . . . ʒij.
Sig. A teaspoonful in a pint of water as a vaginal wash. (*For
leucorrhœa of pregnancy.*)　　　PARVIN.

1252—℞ Potassii chloratis . . . . ʒij.
Sig. A teaspoonful to a pint of water as a vaginal injection.
(*In simple cases.*)　　　PARVIN.

1253—℞ Potassii permanganatis . . . . ʒss.
　　　Aquæ . . . . fʒxv.
Sig. For vaginal injection. (*In fetid discharges.*)
BARTHOLOW.

1254—℞ Iodoformi . . . . ʒj.
　　　Acidi tannici . . . . ʒj.—M.
Sig. Pack a sufficient quantity in the dry state around the
　cervix uteri.　　　　　　　　　BARTHOLOW.

1255—℞ Extracti hydrastis fluidi . . . . fʒj.
Sig. Apply topically to cervix uteri. (*When due to ulcerations
and erosions.*)　　　　　　　　BARTHOLOW.

1256—℞ Tannic acid . . . . grs. dcccc.
　　　Pure alcohol,
　　　Creasote . . . . āā grs. ccccl.
　　　Distilled water . . . . ʒviiss.—M.
Sig. From three to four injections a day are to be taken, for
　each of which a dessertspoonful of the solution is to be di-
　luted with a pint of warm water.　　　LIROLA.

1257—℞ Acidi arsenosi . . . . gr. ¼.
　　　Ferri reducti . . . . gr. v.
　　　Quininæ sulph. . . . . ʒj.—M.
Ft. pil. xx.
Sig. One pill three times a day after meals. (*Leucorrhœa of
anæmia.*)　　　　　　　　　　H. A. HARE.

1258—℞ Creolini . . . . fʒj.
Sig. Half a teaspoonful in two quarts of hot water as a douche.
J. C. WILSON.

LEUCORRHŒA (Continued).

1259—℞ Creasoti . . . . ♏xij.
　　　　 Mucilaginis tragacanthæ . . . . ℨij.
　　　　 Aquæ ferventis . . . . f℥xiv.

Fiat mistura.
Sig. After washing out the vagina with warm water, use the injection. (*In vitiated discharges from puerperal fever.*)
　　　　　　　　　　　　　　　　　　MACKENZIE.

1260—℞ Acidi tannici . . . . ℨiv.
　　　　 Glycerini . . . . f℥xvj.—M.

Sig. A tablespoonful to a quart of tepid water, used as a vaginal injection for five minutes, night and morning, by means of a Davidson's or a fountain syringe.
　　　　　　　　　　　　　　　　T. GAILLARD THOMAS.

1261—℞ Zinci sulphatis . . . . ℨiss.
　　　　 Aluminis sulphatis . . . . ℨiss.
　　　　 Glycerini . . . . f℥vj.—M.

Sig. A tablespoonful to a quart of water, as a vaginal injection.
　　　　　　　　　　　　　　　　T. GAILLARD THOMAS.

1262—℞ Liquoris sodæ chlorinatæ . . . . f℥j.
　　　　 Aquæ . . . . f℥x.—M.

Sig. Inject once or twice daily.　　　　　TROUSSEAU.

1263—℞ Aristol. . . . . ℨj.

Sig. Apply freely as a dusting-powder, by means of a speculum, every second or third day.　　　J. C. WILSON.

1264—℞ Argenti nitratis . . . . gr. xxx.
　　　　 Aquæ . . . . f℥j.—M.

Sig. Apply to cervix daily with swab. (*In ulceration of cervix.*)

1265—℞ Sodii bicarbonatis . . . . ℨj.
　　　　 Tinct. belladonnæ . . . . ℨij.
　　　　 Aquæ . . . . Oj.—M.

Sig. Use as a vaginal wash. (*In over-secretion of the glands about the os uteri, with pain.*)　　　　RINGER.

1266—℞ Ext. belladonnæ . . . . gr. x-xx.
　　　　 Acidi tannici . . . . ℈iij-iv.
　　　　 Olei theobromæ . . . . ℨx.—M.

Ft. massa et in suppositoria no. x div.
Sig. Introduce one into the vagina, place in contact with the os, and retain with a small tampon. Renew as required. (*In ulcerated and painful os, and leucorrhœa.*)　　TROUSSEAU.

LICE.

1267—℞ Vinegar . . . . 500 parts.
　　　　 Sublimate . . . . 1 part.—M.

Sig. Apply night and morning. (*For pediculi pubis.*)　BROCQ.

1268—℞ Johnson's ethereal soap . . . . f℥iv.

Sig. Apply freely with hand twice daily and then bathe with warm water.

1269—℞ Pulv. cocculi indici . . . . ℈iv.
　　　　 Adipis . . . . ℨj.—M.

Ft. ungt.
Sig. Apply locally, rubbing in well.　　HARTSHORNE.

1270—℞ Acidi carbolici . . . . ℨj-ij.
　　　　 Glycerini . . . . ℨj.
　　　　 Aquæ . . . . ad f℥viij.—M.

Ft. lotio.
Sig. Apply as a wash. (*To destroy lice or relieve pruritus.*)
　　　　　　　　　　　　　　　　HARTSHORNE.

1271—℞ Hydrargyri chloridi corrosivi . . . . . gr. iv.
　　　　 Alcoholis . . . . f℥vj.
　　　　 Ammonii chloridi . . . . f℥ss.
　　　　 Aquæ rosæ . . . . q. s. ad f℥vj.—M.

Sig. Apply once daily. (*In scabies and head lice.*)
　　　　　　　　　　　　　　　　TILBURY FOX.

107

LICE (Continued).

1272—℞ Acidi carbolici . . . . ℨj.
    Potass. caustic. . . . . ℨss.
    Aquæ . . . . f℥vj.—M.
Sig. Dilute with two parts of water and apply locally.
                                    J. C. WILSON.

1273—℞ Storacis . . . . f℥j.
    Spiritus vini rectificati . . . . f℥ij.
Misce, et adde—
    Olei olivæ . . . . f℥j.
Sig. Rub the whole body carefully except the head; repeat in twenty-four hours. (In scabies.)   McCALL ANDERSON.

1274—℞ Hydrarg. chlor. corros. . . . . gr. vjss.
    Aquæ . . . . ℥xvj.—M.
Sig. Apply locally. (Crab lice.)
Followed by—

1275—℞ Dalmatian insect powder . . . . ℨss.
Sig. Dusting powder.   H. TUCKER.

1276—℞ Olei rosmarini . . . . f℥ss.
    Olei olivæ . . . . f℥iss.—M.
Sig. Apply once daily. (In head and body lice.) RINGER.

1277—℞ Manganesii oxidi nigri . . . . ℨij.
    Adipis . . . . ℨj.
Misce et fiat unguentum.
Sig. Apply once or twice daily. (In scabies.) BARTHOLOW.

1278—℞ Sodii hyposulphitis . . . . ℨiij.
    Acidi sulphurosi diluti . . . . f℥iv.
    Aquæ . . . . q. s. ad f℥xvj.—M.
Sig. Apply once daily. (In scabies and head lice.) STARTIN.

1279—℞ Tinct. delphinii,
    Aquæ coloniensis . . . . āā f℥ij.—M.
Sig. Apply night and morning. (For pediculi pubis.)
                                     J. C. WILSON.

LICHEN. (See Skin Diseases.)

LIVER, DISEASES OF. (See Biliousness, Colic, and Catarrh.)

LOCOMOTOR ATAXIA. (See also Sclerosis.)

1280—℞ Strychninæ sulphatis . . . . gr. iss.
    Syr. hypophosphiti . . . . f℥xij.—M.
Sig. A teaspoonful thrice daily. (When the system is saturated with silver.)   DA COSTA.

1281—℞ Argenti nitratis . . . . gr. x.
    Confect. rosæ . . . . ℈j.—M.
Ft. massa et in pil. no. xl div.
Sig. One or two pills thrice daily. Cease giving after a few weeks, to prevent argyria.   DA COSTA.

1282—℞ Extracti physostigmatis . . . . gr. x.
    Pulveris zingiberis . . . . ℈j.
Misce et fiant pilulæ no. xx.
Sig. One pill three times a day.   RINGER.

1283—℞ Antipyrin. . . . . ℨj.
    Syr. zingiberis . . . . f℥j.
    Aquæ cinnamomi . . . . ad f℥iv.—M.
Sig. A teaspoonful every one to four hours for three to six doses. (In lightning-pain of locomotor ataxia.) GERMAIN SÉE.

1284—℞ Liquoris potassii arsenitis . . . . . . f℥j.
Sig. One drop in water three times a day after meals, and increase until œdema below eyes; then reduce to smaller dose.

1285—℞ Antifebrin. . . . . ℥j.

Dispensa in capsulas no. xv.
Sig. One or two capsules every half-hour for two doses, if
necessary; then one every four or six hours if required.
(*For pains of locomotor ataxia.*)   DUJARDIN-BEAUMETZ.

LUMBAGO.

1286—℞ Aquæ destillatæ . . . . f℥j.
Sig. Thirty to sixty minims hypodermically.   BARTHOLOW.

1287—℞ Phenazoni . . . . gr. iij.
Aquæ destillatæ . . . . f℥j.—M.
Sig. Inject deeply with long hypodermic needle into painful
area. (*Used in obstinate cases.*)

1288—℞ Empl. belladonnæ (6 in. × 4 in.).
Sig. Apply locally. (*For persistent remains, affecting a small
spot.*)   RINGER.

1289—℞ Pulv. potassii nitratis . . . . ℨij.
In pulv. no. xii div.
Sig. A powder in a half-tumblerful of water every hour or
two. (*When urine is scanty and high-colored.*)   RINGER.

1290—℞ Atropinæ sulphatis . . . . gr. j½.
Morphinæ sulphatis . . . . gr. xvj.
Aquæ destillatæ . . . . f℥j.—M.
Sig. Five minims injected deep into the muscular tissues.
DA COSTA.

1291—℞ Extracti cimicifugæ fluidi,
Syrupi acaciæ . . . . āā f℥ss.
Aquæ amygdalæ amaræ . . . . . . f℥iij.—M.
Sig. A teaspoonful every three hours.   BARTLETT.

1292—℞ Potassii iodidi,
Potassii carbonatis . . . . āā ℨj.
Tincturæ aconiti radicis . . . . f℥ij.
Aquæ destillatæ . . . . f℥x.—M.
Sig. Apply locally every few hours.   ERICHSEN.

1293—℞ Potassii iodidi . . . . ℨss.
Tincturæ opii deodoratæ . . . . f℥j.
Spiritus lavandulæ compositi . . . . . f℥j.
Spiritus ætheris nitrosi . . . . f℥ss.
Aquæ destillatæ . . . . f℥xij.—M.
Sig. Two tablespoonfuls twice daily.   B. BRODIE.

1294—℞ Olei terebinthinæ . . . . f℥ij-iij.
Mucilag. acaciæ . . . . q. s. ut fl. emulsio.
Syr. zingiberis . . . . f℥j.
Aquæ . . . . ad f℥iij.—M.
Sig. A tablespoonful every four to six hours, carefully, lest
strangury and nephritis intervene. (*When urine is clear
and abundant, and bowels regular.*)   WARING.

1295—℞ Antipyrin. . . . . ℨj.
Syr. tolutani . . . . f℥j.
Aquæ menthæ pip. . . . . ad f℥iv.—M.
Sig. A teaspoonful every one to four hours for three to six
doses.   GERMAIN SÉE.

1296—℞ Methyl. chloridi . . . . ℨss.
Sig. Use locally, applying carefully.   DEBOVE.

1297—℞ Potassii iodidi . . . . ℨiv.
Vini colchici sem. . . . . f℥j.
Syr. sarsaparillæ comp. . . . . f℥j.
Aquæ . . . . q. s. ad f℥iij.—M.
Sig. A teaspoonful in a wineglassful of water every four
hours.   J. M. LEEDOM.

1298—℞ Tinct. iodi . . . . f℥ij.
Tinct. aconiti rad. . . . . f℥ij.
Chloroformi . . . . f℥iv.
Linimenti saponis comp. . . . . . ad f℥iij.—M.
Sig. Apply every few hours locally.   *Bellevue Hospital, N.Y.*

1299—℞ Resorcin. . . . . ʒiiss.
Vaselini . . . . ʒv.—M.
Ft. ungt.
Sig. Apply locally. (*In all forms of lupus.*) BERTARELLI.

1300—℞ Phosphori concisi . . . . gr. ij.
Glycerini . . . . fʒj.
Solve cum leni calore.
Sig. Ten minims three times a day. CREWCOUR.

1301—℞ Salicylic acid . . . . ʒiiss.
Creasote . . . . ʒv.
Simple cerate . . . . ʒiiiss.
White wax . . . . gr. lxxv.
Sig. Use externally. UNNA.

1302—℞ Arsenici iodidi . . . . gr. ⅛.
Hydrargyri biniodidi . . . . gr. ¹⁄₁₂.
Confectionis rosæ . . . . q. s.
Fiat pilula.
Sig. Two pills daily after meals. (*In lupus exedens.*)
A. T. THOMPSON.

1303—℞ Acidi pyrogallici . . . . ʒj.
Adipis . . . . ʒj.—M.
Sig. Apply thickly twice a day, watching effect. J. C. WILSON.

1304—℞ Lotion. calaminæ . . . . f ʒij.
Zinci carbonatis . . . . gr. xx.
Zinci oxidi . . . . gr. xv.—M.
Sig. Apply locally. After the inflammation has subsided and
cicatrization has begun the parts are painted with the fol-
lowing, for protection:

1305—℞ Acid. salicylic. . . . . gr. x.
Collodii flexilis . . . . f ʒj.—M.
Sig. Apply locally. STELWAGON.

1306—℞ Sol. acidi lactici (80 per cent.) . . . . ʒss.
Sig. To be applied locally, after poulticing to detach scabs.
(*In lupus of nasal cavities.*) MOSETIG.

1307—℞ Vitelli ovi,
Acidi acetici dil. . . . . . āā partes æquales.—M.
Sig. Apply over the affected surface. (*In erythematous lupus.*)
BROCQ.

1308—℞ Zinci sulphatis exsiccatæ . . . . ʒj.
Sig. Dust over diseased part. BARTHOLOW.

1309—℞ Acidi chromici . . . . ʒv.
Aquæ destillatæ . . . . f ʒiij.—M.
Sig. Apply to diseased part. WOOSTER.

1310—℞ Liquoris potassii arsenitis . . . . . . f ʒj.
Aquæ destillatæ . . . . f ʒj.
Fiat lotio. (*In mild cases.*) HOOPER.

1311—℞ Formaldehydi (40 per cent. sol.) . . . f ʒj.
Sig. Apply to diseased area with small cotton swab, first co-
cainizing the part. (*As cauterant. To be applied every second
or third day after removing scales by poultices.*)

1312—℞ Acidi pyrogallici . . . . ʒj.
Cerati simplicis . . . . ʒix.—M.
Sig. Apply locally. (*In lupus of eyelids and skin.*) KAPOSI.

1313—℞ Acidi lactici puri . . . . ʒj.
Sig. Soak moderately a pledget of absorbent cotton, and
apply to the ulcer. Cover with oiled silk and bandage. If
the surrounding tissue be quite normal, protect it with
grease or collodion. WICHMANN.

1314—℞ Sat. sol. cocain. muriatis . . . . . . ʒij.
Sig. Apply locally. FOWLER.

LUPUS (Continued).

1315—℞ Acidi arseniosi . . . . ℈j.
  Hydrarg. sulphureti rubri . . . . . . ℨj.
  Ungt. simplicis . . . . ℨj.—M.
Ft. ungt.
Sig. Spread thickly on cloth, and apply to the patch for two or three days, until the lupus nodules and points are blackish and destroyed. "Cosmes' Paste" modified by
                Hebra.

MALARIA. (See Fever.)

MAMMARY INFLAMMATION. (See also Abscess.)

1316—℞ Ext. gelsemii fld. . . . . f℥vj-viij.
  Syr. limonis . . . . f℥j.
  Aquæ . . . . ad f℥iij.—M.
Sig. A teaspoonful two or three times daily. Increase the dose until the patient has dilated pupil, drooping eyelids, and a feeling of languor.   Bartholow.

1317—℞ Atropinæ sulphatis . . . . gr. viij.
  Aquæ rosæ . . . . f℥ij.—M.
Ft. lotio.
Sig. Apply locally, but discontinue in case of dilatation of pupils or dryness of throat.   L. Starr.

1318—℞ Ammonii carbonatis . . . . ℨj.
  Aquæ . . . . Oj.—M.
Ft. lotio.
Sig. Apply locally.   L. Starr.

1319—℞ Ammonii chloridi . . . . ℨj.
  Aquæ . . . . Oj.—M.
Sig. Apply locally by means of compresses frequently renewed.   J. C. Wilson.

1320—℞ Extracti belladonnæ . . . . ℈j.
  Aquæ . . . . f℥iv.
Ft. lotio.   Druitt.

1321—℞ Boric acid . . . . ℨj.
  Glycerin . . . . f℥j.
  Water . . . . Oj.—M.
Sig. Locally.

1322—℞ Ext. phytolaccæ decandræ fld. . . . . f℥j.
Sig. Ten drops in water every hour for three or four doses, then gradually lengthen the intervals. The breast may be bandaged, but not poulticed or rubbed. Give a brisk purgative. (*In threatened mastitis.*)   Todd.

1323—℞ Ungt. belladonnæ . . . . ℨj.
  Pulv. camphoræ . . . . ℨss.—M.
Sig. Apply locally, supporting the breast with a bandage.
              Neligan.

1324—℞ Linimenti camphoræ . . . . f℥viij.
Sig. Apply locally, rubbing gently from the circumference toward the nipple. (*In incipient mastitis.*)   Parry.

1325—℞ Hydrarg. chloridi mitis,
  Pulv. jalapæ . . . . āā gr. x.—M.
Ft. pulv. no. i.
Sig. Take at once. (*Brisk purge for incipient mastitis.*) Rush.

1326—℞ Morphinæ . . . . gr. x.
  Hydrargyri oleatis . . . . ℨss.
  Acidi oleici . . . . ℨixss.—M.
Sig. Anoint three times a day.   Marshall.

1327—℞ Tincturæ belladonnæ . . . . f℥ij.
  Linimenti saponis camphorati . . . . f℥viij.
Fiat linimentum.   Neligan.

1328—℞ Liquoris plumbi subacetatis,
  Tincturæ opii . . . . āā f℥ij.—M.
Sig. Add to one quart of water, and keep constantly applied to breast on soft cloths.

1329—℞ Tinct. digitalis,
        Aquæ cinnamomi . . . . āā f℥j.—M.
Sig. One to two teaspoonfuls three times daily. (*Watch pulse.*)
                               MAUDSLEY.

1330—℞ Hyoscyaminæ sulphatis . . . . gr. j.
        Aquæ destillatæ . . . . f℥xij.—M.
Sig. Five to twelve minims hypodermically.
              Ward's Island Insane Asylum, N.Y.

MANIA, ACUTE.

1331—℞ Extracti gelsemii fluidi . . . . f℥ij.
        Syrupi acidi citrici . . . . f℥j.
        Aquæ destillatæ . . . . f℥xj.—M.
Sig. A teaspoonful every two hours until physiological effects
are produced. (*With great motor excitement.*) BARTHOLOW.

1332—℞ Hypnal . . . . ℥iss.
        Syr. aurantii . . . . f℥j.
        Aquæ destillatæ . . . . q. s. f℥ij.—M.
Sig. Tablespoonful at bedtime   H. TUCKER.

1333—℞ Methylal . . . . f℥ij.
        Syr. aurantii corticis . . . . f℥j.
        Aquæ . . . . ad f℥iv.—M.
Sig. From a teaspoonful to a tablespoonful, repeated if necessary, to produce quietness or sleep.
             MAIRET AND COMBEMALE.

1334—℞ Potassii bromidi . . . . ℥j.
        Tinct. cannabis indicæ . . . . f℥j.
        Syr. simplicis . . . . f℥j.
        Aquæ . . . . q. s. ad f℥iv.—M.
Sig. A tablespoonful thrice daily. (*In periodical mania and
senile mania.*)   CLOUSTON.

1335—℞ Potassii bromidi . . . . gr. xxv.
        Tincturæ hyoscyami . . . . ℥ss.
        Spiritus chloroformi . . . . ℳx.
        Aquæ destillatæ . . . . q. s. ad f℥iss.
Fiat haustus.
Sig. At once.   TYLER SMITH.

1336—℞ Chloral. hydratis . . . . gr. xxv.
        Tincturæ cardamomi compositæ . . . ℥ss.
        Syrupi simplicis . . . . f℥j.
        Infusi caryophylli . . . . . . q. s. ad f℥iss.
Misce et fiat haustus.
Sig. To be repeated in an hour if necessary. PRIESTLEY.

1337—℞ Amyl. hydratis . . . . ℥j.
Sig. Forty to seventy-five minims, in sweetened water, as
required.   VON MERING.

1338—℞ Trional . . . . ℥vj.
Fiant in chartulæ no. xii.
Sig. At bedtime. Repeat once or twice according to indica-
tion.   H. TUCKER.

1339—℞ Ext. conii fld.,
        Ext. hyoscyami fld. . . . . āā ℳvij.
        Chloral. hydratis . . . . gr. x.
        Aquæ . . . . f℥ij.—M.
Ft. haustus.
Sig. To be taken at a draught, and repeated if required.
              MADIGAN.

1340—℞ Paraldehyd. . . . . f℥ss.
Sig. Thirty to fifty minims in an ounce or two of water, by
the rectum.   RINGER.

1341—℞ Pulv. tragacanthæ comp. . . . . ℥j.
        Syr. aurantii corticis . . . . f℥iv.
        Paraldehyd. . . . . f℥j.
        Spts. chloroformi . . . . ℳxv.
        Aquæ . . . . ad f℥iij.—M.
Ft. haustus.
Sig. To be taken at one draught.   HODGSON.

MANIA, ACUTE (Continued).

1342—℞ Tinct. digitalis,
　　　 Aquæ cinnamomi . . . . āā f3j.—M.

Sig. One or two teaspoonfuls three times daily. (*Watch pulse for intermittence.*)　　　MAUDSLEY.

1343—℞ Hyoscin. hydrobromatis . . . . gr. 1⁄40.

Sig. This dose in pill or hypodermically cautiously repeated at intervals of four or six hours.　　　J. C. WILSON.

MANIA, CHRONIC.

1344—℞ Tincturæ ferri chloridi . . . . f3ij.
　　　 Syrupi zingiberis . . . . f3j.
　　　 Aquæ destillatæ . . . . f3vij.—M.

Sig. A tablespoonful three or four times a day. (*In anæmic cases.*)　　　BUCKNILL.

1345—℞ Tinct. ferri chloridi,
　　　 Tinct. nucis vomicæ . . . . āā 3j.
　　　 Aquæ . . . . q. s. ad 3vj.—M.

Sig. A teaspoonful thrice daily, after meals.
　　　　Ward's Island Insane Asylum, N.Y.

1346—℞ Tincturæ ferri chloridi . . . . f3ij.
　　　 Spiritus ætheris nitrosi . . . . f3ss.
　　　 Infusi quassiæ . . . . q. s. ad f3vj.—M.

Sig. A tablespoonful three times a day. (*In debilitated cases.*)　　　TUKE.

1347—℞ Ergotini . . . . gr. lx.
　　　 Ext. cannabis indicæ . . . . gr. ij.
　　　 Strychninæ . . . . gr. 1⁄2.—M.

In pil. no. xx div.
Sig. One pill after each meal, and at bedtime.　　　J. C. WILSON.

1348—℞ Extracti ergotæ fluidi . . . . f3iss.
　　　 Syrupi aurantii corticis . . . . f3j.
　　　 Aquæ destillatæ . . . . f3iiiss.—M.

Sig. A tablespoonful three or four times a day.
　　　　CRICHTON BROWNE.

1349—℞ Caffeinæ citratis . . . . 3ss.
　　　 Syrupi acidi citrici . . . . f3ss.
　　　 Aquæ destillatæ . . . . f3iss.—M.

Sig. A teaspoonful three or four times a day.　　　BARTHOLOW.

MANIA, PUERPERAL.

1350—℞ Olei tiglii . . . . gtt. vj.
　　　 Micæ panis . . . . q. s. ut ft. massa.

Ft. massa et in pil. no. vi div.
Sig. One or two pills, as a purge. (*When cerebral congestion is present.*)　　　LEISHMAN.

1351—℞ Extracti cimicifugæ fluidi . . . . . . f3iss.
　　　 Mucilaginis acaciæ . . . . f3j.
　　　 Aquæ destillatæ . . . . f3iiiss.—M.

Sig. A tablespoonful every three hours.　　　RINGER.

1352—℞ Potassii bromidi . . . . 3ij.
　　　 Chloral. hydratis . . . . 3ss.
　　　 Syrupi aurantii corticis . . . . f3j.
　　　 Aquæ fœniculi . . . . q. s. ad f3vj.—M.

Sig. A tablespoonful every two hours.　　　QUAIN.

MARASMUS.

1353—℞ Syr. ferri iodidi . . . . f3j.

Sig. Three to five drops, in water, thrice daily after eating.
　　　　EUSTACE SMITH

1354—℞ Quininæ . . . . gr. viij.
　　　 Alcoholis . . . . f3j.
Fiat solutio. Dein adde—
　　　 Olei morrhuæ . . . . f3iv.

Solve cum leni calore.
Sig. From a half to one teaspoonful, according to age of child.　　　LYMAN.

MARASMUS (Continued).

1355—℞ Tinct. cinchonæ comp.,
    Tinct. gentianæ comp. . . . . . . āā f3j.—M.
Sig. Fifteen drops to a teaspoonful, in sweetened water, thrice
    daily.   J. L. SMITH.

1356—℞ Olei morrhuæ . . . . f3ij.
    Aquæ calcis . . . . f3iv.
    Syr. calcis lactophosphatis . . . . ad f3iv.—M.
Sig. A teaspoonful two or three times daily.   BOSLEY.

1357—℞ Pepsini saccharati . . . . 3j-iss.
In pulv. no. xx div.
Sig. A powder after each feeding.   BARTHEZ.

1358—℞ Quininæ sulphatis . . . . gr. ij-vj.
    Acidi sulphurici diluti . . . . gtt. ij-vj.
    Syrupi aurantii corticis . . . . f3j.
    Aquæ destillatæ . . . . f3ij.—M.
Sig. A teaspoonful three or four times a day.   COULSON.

1359—℞ Iodi . . . . gr. iss.
    Olei morrhuæ . . . . f3v.
Tere simul.
Sig. A half to one teaspoonful for a child.   FLEISCHMANN.

1360—℞ Syrupi ferri iodidi . . . . f3j.
    Syrupi acaciæ. . . . . f3vij.
    Aquæ fœniculi . . . . f3j.—M.
Sig.—A teaspoonful three times a day.   DUPASQUIER.

MEASLES. (See Fever.)

MELANCHOLIA. (See also Hypochondria.)

1361—℞ Tinct. ferri chloridi,
    Syr simplicis . . . . āā f3j.
Sig. Twenty or thirty drops, well diluted, thrice daily.
                            BARTHOLOW.

1362—℞ Olei phosphorati . . . . mxxiv.
    Olei morrhuæ . . . . f3j.—M.
Pone in capsulas no. xxiv.
Sig. One capsule two hours after meals. (*Used in debilitated
subjects.*)

1363—℞ Zinci valerianatis,
    Ferri valerianatis,
    Quininæ valerianatis . . . . . . āā 3ss.—M.
Ft. massa et in pil. no. xxx div.
Sig. One pill three times daily.   J. C. WILSON.

1364—℞ Moschi optimi,
    Pulveris camphoræ . . . . āā 3ss.
    Olei cajuputi . . . . mv.
Misce et divide in pilulas xii.
Sig. One pill every two or three hours.   HOOPER.

1365—℞ Paraldehydi . . . . f3j.
    Elixiris aromatici . . . . f3j.—M.
Sig. One to two teasponfuls in water at bedtime. (*Used for
relief of insomnia.*)

1366—℞ Potassii bromidi . . . . 3ij.
    Tinct. calumbæ . . . . f3ij.
    Spts. ammoniæ aromatici . . . . . . f3ij.
    Aquæ cinnamomi . . . . f3ij.
    Aquæ . . . . q. s. ad f3vij.—M.
Sig. A wineglassful two or three times daily.   LAWRENCE.

MENINGITIS.

1367—℞ Sodii bromidi . . . . 3ij.
    Chloral. hydratis . . . . 3j.
    Syr. aurantii corticis . . . . f3j.
    Aquæ . . . . q. s. ad f3iij.—M.
Sig. A dessertspoonful every hour or two until excitement
    abates.   HERRMANN.

1368—℞ Potassii bromidi. . . . . ᴣss.
     Syrupi simplicis. . . . . f ᴣss.
     Aquæ destillatæ. . . . . f ᴣj.

Sig. A teaspoonful every two hours. (*In after-remaining con-vulsions.*)
              RINGER.

1369—℞ Morphinæ sulphatis . . . . gr. ij.
     Aquæ destillatæ. . . . . f ᴣj.—M.

Sig. Five minims hypodermically every three to five hours, or oftener. (*In the cerebro-spinal form.*)   LEYDEN.

1370—℞ Olei tiglii . . . . ℩℩℩v.
     Saponis,
     Pulveris acaciæ . . . . āā ᴣj.

Misce et fiant pilulæ no. xx.
Sig. One to three pills. (*After effusion and in hydrocephalus.*)
              SUNDELIN.

1371—℞ Iodoformi . . . . gr. xv.
     Vaselini . . . . gr. lxxv.-M.

Ft. ungt.
Sig. Shave the scalp, and rub in night and morning the above quantity of ointment. Keep the head covered with an oiled-silk cap. (*In the tubercular variety.*) WARFVINGE.

1372—℞ Tincturæ opii deodoratæ,
     Extracti gelsemii fluidi . . . . . . āā f ᴣj.
     Syrupi limonis . . . . f ᴣij.
     Aquæ fœniculi . . . . f ᴣiss.—M.

Sig.—A teaspoonful every two hours.   BARTHOLOW.

1373—℞ Hydrarg. chloridi mitis,
     Pulv. jalapæ,
     Sacchari albi . . . . āā ᴣj.—M.

In pulv. no. x. div.
Sig. A powder every hour until free purgation occurs. (*In cerebro-spinal meningitis.*)   KOBERT.

1374—℞ Tincturæ digitalis . . . . f ᴣij.
     Extracti ergotæ fluidi . . . . f ᴣviij.—M.

Sig. Ten to thirty drops, according to age and idiosyncrasy, every six hours. (*Used during later stages with circulatory depression.*)   E. Q. THORNTON.

1375—℞ Acidi tannici . . . . ᴣj.

In capsulas no. xx div.
Sig. A capsule every three hours. With ice to the head. (*In simple meningitis.*)   LARDIER.

1376—℞ Morphinæ sulphatis . . . . gr. ss.
     Acidi sulphurici aromatici . . . . . . f ᴣj.
     Elixiris cinchonæ . . . . . . q. s. ad f ᴣiij.—M.

Sig. A teaspoonful every two hours for a child twelve years old. (*In the cerebro-spinal form.*) MEIGS AND PEPPER.

1377—℞ Tinct. ferri chloridi . . . . f ᴣij.
Sig. Twenty to thirty minims every two hours.   KLAPP.

1378—℞ Tinct. aconiti radicis . . . . f ᴣij.
     Tinct. opii deodoratæ. . . . . f ᴣv.—M.

Sig. Seven drops in water, every two hours, during the stage of excitement. (*In cerebral meningitis.*) BARTHOLOW.

1379—℞ Acidi hydrocyanici dil. . . . . ℩℩℩xx-xl.
     Sodii bicarbonatis . . . . ᴣij-v.
     Syr. simplicis,
     Aquæ . . . . q. s. ad f ᴣiss.—M

Sig. A teaspoonful every three or four hours for severe vomiting. (*In the cerebro-spinal form.*)   DELAFIELD.

MENINGITIS, CEREBRO-SPINAL. (See Meningitis.)

MENORRHAGIA.

1380—℞ Ext. ergotæ fld. . . . . f ᴣij.
Sig. A half to one teaspoonful thrice daily.   MEIGS.

1381—℞ Liq. ferri perchloridi . . . . f3iv.
    Aquæ . . . . f3xij.—M.

Sig. Inject slowly and carefully into the uterus with a David-son's syringe fitted with a long uterine tube. Avoid intro-ducing air. Allow a free outlet for the fluid. (*In post-partum hemorrhage.*)   R. BARNES.

1382—℞ Tinct. hamamelidis . . . . f3ij.
Sig. One-half to one teaspoonful thrice daily.   RINGER.

1383—℞ Pulv. potassii bromidi . . . . 5ij.
In pulv. no. xii div.
Sig. A powder in a wineglassful of water three times daily. Begin before the period, and continue till it is over.
    RINGER.

1384—℞ Tinct. sabinæ . . . . f3ss.

Sig. Five to ten drops in cold water every half-hour to every three hours.   PHILLIPS.

1385—℞ Chloralimidi . . . . 3iv.

Fiant chartulæ no. **xii.**
Sig. One powder in half-glass of water. (*Used in extreme rest-lessness and insomnia.*)

1386—℞ Tincturæ capsici,
    Tincturæ cubebæ . . . . āā f3j.
    Tincturæ cantharidis . . . . f3ss.
    Mucilaginis acaciæ . . . . . q. s. ad f3iv.—M.
Sig. A tablespoonful twice a day. (*When from debility.*)
    HAZARD.

1387—℞ Acidi gallici . . . . gr. xv.
    Acidi sulphurici aromatici . . . . . . ♏xv.
    Tincturæ cinnamomi . . . . f3ij.
    Aquæ destillatæ . . . . f3ij.—M.
Sig. One dose, to be taken every four hours until bleeding ceases. (*In profuse bleeding.*)   HAZARD.

1388—℞ Acidi arseniosi . . . . gr. j.
    Mastiches . . . . gr. x.
    Ferri sulphatis exsiccati,
    Pulveris capsici,
    Pulveris aloes socotrinæ . . . . . . āā 3j.
    Syrupi simplicis . . . . q. s.
Fiat massa, in pilulas xx dividenda.
Sig. One pill three or four times a day. (*In relaxed and debili-tated cases.*)   COPLAND.

1389—℞ Olei cinnamomi f3j
Pone in capsulas no. **xxx.**
Sig. One capsule after meals. (*Used in oozing hemorrhage.*)

1390—℞ Ext. gossypii fld.,
    Syr. simplicis . . . . āā f3j.—M.
Sig. A teaspoonful every four hours.   PARVIN.

1391—℞ Ext. geranii fld. . . . . f3iv.
Sig. A teaspoonful every hour for a few doses, then every three to four hours. May be used with advantage locally.
    SHOEMAKER.

1392—℞ Ext. rhois aromat. fld. . . . . f3j.
Sig. Fifteen to sixty minims thrice daily.   UNNA.

1393—℞ Ext. hydrastis can. fld. . . . . f3j.
Sig. Twenty drops four times daily.   R. W. WILCOX.

1394—℞ Acidi gallici . . . . 3ss.
    Acidi sulphurici dil. . . . . f3j.
    Tinct. opii deod. . . . . f3j.
    Inf. rosæ comp. . . . . f3iv.—M.
Sig. A tablespoonful every four hours or oftener.
    BARTHOLOW.

1395—℞ Tincturæ krameriæ,
  Extracti ergotæ fluidi . . . . āā f3j.
  Infusi digitalis . . . . f3ij.—M.
Sig. A tablespoonful *pro re nata.* (*In plethoric cases, and when due to mitral regurgitation.*)   BARTHOLOW.

1396—℞ Extracti ipecacuanhæ fluidi,
  Extracti digitalis fluidi . . . . . . āā f3ij.
  Extracti ergotæ fluidi . . . . f3ss.—M.
Sig. One-half to one teaspoonful at a dose, as required.   BARTHOLOW.

1397—℞ Ext. viburni fld. . . . . f3iij.
Sig. A teaspoonful in water every three or four hours in connection with local treatment.   J. C. WILSON.

1398—℞ Pulveris ergotæ,
  Pulveris sabinæ . . . . āā ɘij.
Misce et fiant chartulæ no. iv.
Sig. One powder morning and night. (*In atony of uterus.*)   RINGER.

MERCURIALISM. (See Ptyalism.)

METRITIS.

1399—℞ Tincturæ aconiti radicis . . . . gtt. xvj.
  Extracti gelsemii fluidi . . . . f3j.
  Extracti ergotæ fluidi . . . . f3vij.—M.
Sig. A teaspoonful every two to six hours. (*Also in uterine tumor.*)   BARTHOLOW.

1400—℞ Potassæ . . . . 3v.
  Calcis . . . . 3vj.
  Alcoholis . . . . q. s. ut fiat magma.
Sig. Apply locally with extreme caution. (*In induration of cervix and chronic metritis.*)   BENNETT.

1401—℞ Tinct. iodi comp. . . . . f3j.
Sig. Use locally on a probe wrapped with absorbent cotton, once or twice weekly. Two applications are made, and a glycerin tampon is left against the cervix. In the intervals let the patient use a gallon of hot water as a vaginal injection twice or thrice daily.   T. G. THOMAS.

MIGRAINE. (See also Headache.)

1402—℞ Quininæ valerianatis . . . . gr. xv.
  Ext. colchici . . . . gr. iv.
  Ext. digitalis . . . . gr. iv.
  Ext. aconiti . . . . gr. ij.—M.
Ft. pil. x.
Sig. One at night after dinner. (*Gouty migraine.*)   HIRTZ.

1403—℞ Caffeinæ citratis . . . . gr. xv.
  Phenacetin. . . . . gr. xxx.
  Sacchari albi . . . . gr. xv.
Fiat pulv. Dis. in capsulas no. x.
Sig. One capsule to be taken, in the intervals of the attacks, every two or three hours.   HAMMERSCHLAG.

MITRAL DISEASE. (See Heart-Disease.)

MORNING SICKNESS. (See also Vomiting.)

1404—℞ Cerii oxalatis . . . . gr. xxiv.
  Ext. hyoscyami . . . . gr. xxxvj.
Misce et fiat massa, in pil. no. xii div.
Sig. One pill twice daily.   GOODELL.

1405—℞ Cupri sulphatis . . . . gr. ij.
  Aquæ destillatæ . . . . f3ss.—M.
Sig. Six drops three times a day.   BARTHOLOW.

1406—℞ Liquoris potassii arsenitis . . . . f3ss.
Sig. One drop before meals. (*In bloody vomit.*)   BARTHOLOW.

1407—℞ Menthol . . . . gr. v.
   Elixir. pepsinæ . . . . 3j.
   Tinct. opii . . . . 3ij.—M.
Sig. Ten to twenty drops before meals.   LATAUD.

1408—℞ Tinct. cantharidis,
   Tinct. ferri muriatis . . . . āā f 3j.—M.
Sig. Twenty-five drops, well diluted, three times daily.
              HIGGINS.

1409—℞ Sodii bicarbonatis . . . . gr. iv.
   Acidi hydrocyanici dil. . . . . gtt. j.
   Syr. lactopeptini . . . . f 3j.—M.
Sig. To be given half an hour before meals. J. FREE.

1410—℞ Creasoti . . . . ℳiij.
   Pulveris hyoscyami . . . . gr. xij.
   Confectionis rosæ . . . . q. s.
Misce et fiant pilulæ no. xii.
Sig. One pill three times a day.   HAZARD.

1411—℞ Cerii oxalatis . . . . gr. xv.
   Extracti gentianæ . . . . gr. v.
Fiat massa, in pilulas x dividenda.
Sig. One pill an hour after each meal. J. Y. SIMPSON.

1412—℞ Cerii valerianatis . . . . gr. xv.
In pil. no. xx div.
Sig. Two to four pills daily.   MUNDÉ.

1413—℞ Cocain. hydrochloratis . . . . gr. j.
   Aquæ . . . . f 3j.—M.
Sig. A teaspoonful three times daily before meals. (*May be
given hypodermically.*)   PARVIN.

1414—℞ Extracti opii aquosi . . . . gr. x.
   Fellis bovini inspissati . . . . 3ij.
Misce et fiant pilulæ no. xl.
Sig. Two pills an hour before meals. CAZEAUX.

1415—℞ Diluted nitrohydrochloric acid . . . . f 3iss.
   Spirit of lemon . . . . f 3j.
   Simple syrup . . . . f 3ij.—M.
Sig. Give one teaspoonful in a wineglass of ice water three
times a day.   *Buffalo Med. and Surg. Jour.*

1416—℞ Cocain. muriatis . . . . gr. j.
   Ext. belladonnæ . . . . 3vj.—M.
Sig. Apply locally to the cervix uteri morning and evening.
              FENN.

1417—℞ Acidi phenici deliquesc. . . . . f 3j.
   Aceti opii . . . . f 3iij.—M.
Sig. Four drops in a little sweetened water five minutes
before meals thrice daily.

1418—℞ Tinct. nucis vomicæ . . . . f 3ss.
Sig. One drop every hour or two, in water. RINGER.

1419—℞ Atropinæ sulphatis . . . . gr. j.
   Morphinæ sulphatis . . . . gr. iv.
   Acidi sulphurici aromatici . . . . . . f 3iij.
   Aquæ . . . . f 3v.—M.
Sig. Ten to twenty drops, in water, thrice daily. BOYS.

1420—℞ Bismuthi subnitratis . . . . 3ij.
In pulv. no. xii div.
Sig. A powder thrice daily before meals. CAZEAUX.

MUMPS. (See also Fever.)

1421—℞ Lanolin.,
   Ungt. belladonnæ (10 per cent.),
   Ichthyol. (10 per cent.) . . . . . . āā 3ss.
Sig. Apply several times a day.   J. C. WILSON.

1422—℞ Hydrargyri cum cretâ . . . . gr. ij.
    Sacchari lactis . . . . gr. xx.

Misce et fiaut chartulæ no. vi
Sig. One powder three or four times a day.   RINGER.

1423—℞ Pilocarpinæ hydrochloratis . . . . . . gr. j.
    Sacchari lactis . . . . gr. xviij.
    Alcohol . . . . q. s.—M.

Fiant tabellæ triturationes no. xii.
Sig. One tablet every hour until mild salivation or diaphoresis. (*In acute stage.*)

MYALGIA.

1424—℞ Linimenti belladonnæ . . . . ʒiv.
Sig. Rub in well, several times daily.   BARTHOLOW.

1425—℞ Extracti xanthoxyli fluidi . . . . . . fʒj.
Sig. From fifteen minims to two drachms. (*In torticollis,
lumbago, etc.*)   BARTHOLOW.

1426—℞ Saloli . . . . ʒiv.
    Phenacetini . . . . ʒiv.—M.

Fiant chartulæ no. xxiv.
Sig. One powder after meals.

1427—℞ Tinct. belladonnæ . . . . fʒj.
    Tinct. aconiti . . . . fʒij.
    Tinct. opii . . . . fʒij.
    Liniment. saponis . . . . . . q. s. ad fʒvj.—M.

Sig. Poison. To be used externally only.   HARE.

NÆVUS.

1428—℞ Acidi chromici . . . . gr. c.
    Aquæ destillatæ . . . . fʒj.—M.
Sig. Apply locally with care.   BARTHOLOW.

1429—℞ Hydrargyri chloridi corrosivi . . . . . gr. j.
    Formaldehydi (40 per cent. sol.) . . . . fʒj.—M.
Sig. Apply with small cotton-wool swab every second or
third day. (*Used to remove small birth-marks.*)

1430—℞ Sodii ethylatis . . . . gr. vj.
    Alcohol absoluti . . . . fʒij.—M.
Sig. Paint over nævus freely, and after drying cover with
collodion. Allow to remain on for ten to twenty days.
(*Used to remove small birth-marks.*)

NECROSIS. (See Caries.)

NEPHRITIS. (See also Albuminuria.)

1431—℞ Ext. jaborandi fld. . . . . fʒj.
Sig. Five to ten minims every hour or half-hour, until free
diaphoresis is established. May be combined with digitalis.
(*In acute nephritis.*)   DA COSTA.

1432—℞ Pilocarpinæ muriatis . . . . gr. vj.
    Aquæ destillatæ . . . . fʒij.—M.
Sig. Five to ten minims by the stomach, or hypodermically
if uræmia is present. (*In acute nephritis.*)   RINGER.

1433—℞ Symphorolis . . . . ʒiv.
Fiant tabellæ compressæ no. xxiv.
Sig. One tablet three times a day. (*Used in chronic Bright's
disease with arterial relaxation and dropsy.*)

1434—℞ Tincturæ ferri chloridi . . . . fʒij.
    Acidi acetici diluti . . . . fʒiss.
    Syrupi simplicis . . . . fʒss.
    Liquoris ammonii acetatis . . q. s. ad fʒiv.—M.

Sig.—A dessertspoonful every three or four hours.   BASHAM.

1435—℞ Potassii acetatis . . . .   ӡss.
Infusi digitalis . . . .   f ӡvj.—M.
Sig. One teaspoonful every fourth hour to a child five years old. Used with the following:

1436—℞ Resinæ podophylli . . . .   gr. j.
Sacchari albi . . . .   ӡj.—M.
In pulv. no. viii–xii div.
Sig. Take one powder. Repeat if necessary. (*To produce catharsis.*)   J. LEWIS SMITH.

1437—℞ Potassii bitartratis . . . .   ӡij.
Aquæ ferventis . . . .   Oij.
Corticis limonis,
Sacchari . . . .   āā q. s. ad conciliandum gustum.
Sig. Use *ad libitum.*   JOY.

1438—℞ Extracti jaborandi fluidi . . . .   f ӡj.
Elixiris simplicis,
Syrupi simplicis . . . .   āā f ӡss.—M.
Sig. One to two teaspoonfuls. (*With uræmia.*)   BARTHOLOW.

1439—℞ Methyli cærulei (methyl blue) . . . .   gr. xij.
Pone in capsulas no. xxiv.
Sig. One capsule three times a day.

1440—℞ Scoparii flor . . . .   ӡviiss.
Juniperi . . . .   ӡiss.
Aquæ bullientis . . . .   f ӡxxxj.—M.
Ft. infusum et adde—
Syr. e quinque radicibus (Edinb., 1744)   f ӡiss.—M.
Sig. A wineglassful several times daily.   DUBIEF.

1441—℞ Potassii tartratis . . . .   ӡj.
Potassii nitratis . . . .   ӡss.
Mannæ . . . .   ӡj.
Decocti taraxaci . . . .   f ӡvj.—M.
Sig. A tablespoonful every hour or two. (*After scarlet fever.*)   PHOEBUS.

1442—℞ Potassii acetatis . . . .   ӡj.
Oxymellis scillæ . . . .   f ӡj.
Vini opii . . . .   ♏xv.
Aquæ florum tiliæ . . . .   f ӡss.
Syrupi althææ . . . .   f ӡj.—M.
Sig. A tablespoonful.   PIERQUIN.

1443—℞ Pulv. jalapæ comp. . . . .   ӡj.
In pulv. no. xii div.
Sig. A powder every four hours until free catharsis occurs. To be given after the patient has been rolled in blankets wrung out of hot water. (*In acute nephritis.*)   FOTHERGILL.

1444—℞ Sodii iodidi . . . .   gr. xv.
Sodii phosphatis . . . .   gr. xxx.
Sodii chloridi . . . .   gr. xc.—M.
Sig. Dissolve in water, and give in the course of the twenty-four hours, either alone or in milk.   SEMMOLA.

1445—℞ Mercuric chlorid. . . . .   gr. ⅛.
Potassium iodid. . . . .   ӡj.
Syrup . . . .   f ӡj.
Infusion of gentian . . . .   f ӡvij.—M.
Sig. One tablespoonful three times a day.   D. C. BLACK.

1446—℞ Acidi tannici,
Ext. cinchonæ . . . .   āā gr. xxx.
Fuchsin. . . . .   gr. xv.—M.
Ft. massa et in pil. no. xx div.
Sig. One pill morning and evening. (*In chronic cases.*)   MONIN.

NEPHRITIS (Continued).

1447—℞ Camphoræ . . . . gr. v.
Lanolini,
Ungt. belladounæ . . . . ā̄ā 3ss.—M.
Ft. unguentum.
Sig. Apply to the abdomen. (*For tympany occurring in chronic Bright's disease and due to peritoneal congestion.*)   DA COSTA.

NERVOUSNESS. (See Hysteria.)

NETTLERASH. (See Urticaria.)

NEURALGIA. (See also Sciatica.)

1448—℞ Butyl. chloral. . . . . gr. xl-lxxv.
Alcohol. rect. . . . . f3iiss.
Glycerini . . . . f3v.
Aquæ destillatæ . . . . f3iv.—M.
Sig. Two to four spoonfuls at once.   LEIBREICH.

1449—℞ Sol. nitro-glycerin. (1 per cent.) . . . . f3ss.
Sig. One or two drops on the tongue every four to six hours, as required. (*When pallor of face is present.*)   TRUSSEWITSCH.

1450—℞ Antipyrin. . . . . 3iss.
Aquæ destillatæ . . . . f3v.—M.
Sig. Twenty-five minims hypodermically every three or four hours till relieved.   DUJARDIN-BEAUMETZ.

1451—℞ Menthol,
Guaiacol . . . . ā̄ā 3j.
Alcohol. absolut. . . . . f3xviij.—M.
Sig. A drachm of this mixture is to be rubbed lightly into the affected part two or three times a day.   SABBATINI.

1452—℞ Ethoxycaffeini,
Sodii salicylatis . . . . ā̄ā gr. liiᵻ.
Cocainæ muriatis . . . . gr. iss.
Aquæ aurantii flor. . . . . f3xv.
Syr. simplicis . . . . f3v.—M.
Sig. To be taken at one dose at the commencement of the attack. (*For migraine.*)   DUJARDIN-BEAUMETZ.

1453—℞ Ext. cocæ fld. . . . . 3j.
Syr. aurantii flor. . . . . f3v.
Aquæ . . . . ad f3ij.—M.
Sig. A teaspoonful every hour till relieved. (*In gastralgia.*)
D'ARDENNE.

1454—℞ Liq. chloroformi aq. sat. . . . . f3xv.
Aquæ aurantii flor. . . . . f3xiv.
Tinct. anisi stellati . . . . f3j.—M.
Sig. A teaspoonful every quarter of an hour. (*In gastralgia.*)
DUJARDIN-BEAUMETZ.

1455—℞ Olei amygdalæ amari . . . . ℥xx.
Alcoholis . . . . f3iij.—M.
Sig. Ten drops three times a day.   HAZARD.

1456—℞ Extract of hyoscyamus,
Extract of valerian . . . . ā̄ā gr. iv.
Hydrochlorate of morphine . . . . . . gr. j.—M.
Sig. Make into four pills; take one to four in twenty-four hours.   *Revue de Thérapeutique.*

1457—℞ Quininæ valerianatis . . . . gr. x.
Tincturæ sumbuli . . . . f3ij.
Extracti taraxaci fluidi . . . . f3vj.
Infusi cascarillæ . . . . f3v.—M.
Sig. A dessertspoonful three times a day.   HAZARD.

1458—℞ Tincturæ aconiti (Fleming) . . . . . f3j.
Sodii carbonatis . . . . 3iss.
Magnesii sulphatis . . . . 3iss.
Aquæ destillatæ . . . . f3vj.
Fiat mistura.
Sig. A tablespoonful when pain is urgent. (*In gastralgia.*)
FLEMING.

1459—℞ Tincturæ cannabis indicæ . . . . . . f 3vj.
    Syrupi acaciæ . . . . f 3iss.
    Aquæ destillatæ . . . . q. s. ad f 3vj.—M.

Sig. A tablespoonful every four to six hours. (*In sciatica.*)
                               NELIGAN.

1460—℞ Ethylum chloridum in tuba.

Sig. Use as spray for freezing painful area. (*Used in neuralgia of superficial nerves.*)

1461—℞ Thein.,
    Sodii benzoatis . . . . āā 3j.
    Sodii chloridi . . . . gr. x.
    Aquæ destillatæ . . . . f 3j.—M.

Sig. Three to twenty drops, as required.   MAYS.

1462—℞ Thymoli . . . . 3j.
    Camphoræ . . . . 3j.
    Alcohol . . . . f 3j.—M.

Sig. Apply over painful area with brush. (*Used in neuralgia of superficial nerve.*)

1463—℞ Aconitinæ nitratis cryst. . . . . gr. ⅜.
    Quininæ hydrobromatis . . . . gr. lxxv.
    Syrupi . . . . q. s. ut ft. massa.—M.

Ft. massa et in pil. no. 1 div.
Sig. One pill every four hours until five or six are taken. The following day take at longer intervals if there be any disturbance of digestion or formication in the extremities.
                                 LABORDE.

1464—℞ Delphinii (alkaloid of staphisagria). . gr. xv.
    Ext. tritici repentis . . . . 3ss.
    Pulv. althææ . . . . q. s.—M.

Ft. massa et in pil. no. 1 div.
Sig. Four to six pills daily.   TURNBULL.

1465—℞ Tinct. conii . . . . 3j.
    Tinct. valerianæ,
    Tinct. opii camphoratæ,
    Aquæ laurocerasi . . . . āā f 3ij.—M.

Sig. Seven drops in a little milk when the pain appears. (*In gastralgia.*)   MONIN.

1466—℞ Sulphonal. . . . . 3j.

In chart. no. xii div.
Sig. One powder after each meal, and at bedtime. (*In neuralgic headaches of elderly people, with restlessness.*)
                         J. C. WILSON.

1467—℞ Ferri sulphatis exsiccati,
    Potassii carbonatis . . . . āā gr. ccl.

Misce et fiant pilulæ no. c.
Sig. Begin with three a day, and increase to six: take several hundred.   J. E. GARRETSON.

1468—℞ Codein. phosphat. . . . . gr. ¼.
    Bismuth. subnitrat. . . . . gr. v.
    Sacchari lactis . . . . gr. iij.—M.

Sig. To be taken every two hours. (*For gastralgia.*)
                                EWALD.

1469—℞ Strychninæ sulphatis . . . . gr. j.
    Morphinæ sulphatis,
    Acidi arseniosi . . . . āā gr. iss.
    Extracti aconiti . . . . gr. xv.
    Quininæ sulphatis . . . . 3j.

Misce et fiant pilulæ no. xxx.
Sig. One pill three times a day.   S. D. GROSS.

1470—℞ Chloroformi . . . . f 3j.
    Liq. vaselini . . . . f 3iv.—M.

Sig. Fifteen to thirty minims hypodermically at the seat of pain.   MEUNIER.

1471—℞ Extracti belladonnæ . . . . 3iss.
    Tincturæ opii . . . . ℳxl.
    Chloroformi . . . . f 3j.—M.

Sig. Apply locally.   HAZARD.

NEURALGIA (Continued).

1472—℞ Atropinæ sulphatis . . . . gr. ss.
    Aconitinæ . . . . gr. iss.
    Olei tiglii . . . . gtt. ij.
    Unguenti petrolei . . . . 3ij.
Misce accuratissime.
Sig. Apply to the affected part.   J. R. LUDLOW.

1473—℞ Tinct. momordicæ (balsam-apple). . . 3v.
    Tinct. aconiti . . . . f 3j.
    Chloroformi . . . . f 3ss.—M.
Sig. Soak a piece of flannel, lay it on the painful part, and
cover with oiled silk.   GUÉNEAU DE MUSSY.

1474—℞ Aconiti . . . . gr. iss.
    Spts. vini rectificati . . . . q. s.
    Adipis præparatæ . . . . 3ij.—M.
Ft. unguentum.
Sig. To be rubbed in three times daily.   BROCKES.

1475—℞ Carbonis bisulphidi . . . . 3iv.
    Pulv. camphoræ . . . . q. s.—M.
Ft. sol. saturat.
Sig. Apply with a brush to the painful region. (*For lumbo-
abdominal neuralgia.*)   (HÉRON.

1476—℞ Chloroformi . . . . ℥xx.
    Tincturæ aconiti radicis,
    Tincturæ opii . . . . āā f 3j.
    Linimenti saponis camphorati . . . . f 3ss.—M.
Sig. Apply to the painful part.   NELIGAN.

1477—℞ Veratrinæ,
    Morphinæ sulphatis . . . . āā gr. x.
    Adipis . . . . 3j.—M.
Sig. Rub in three times daily.   T. KENNARD.

1478—℞ Camphoræ,
    Chloral. hydratis . . . . āā 3ss.—M.
Sig. Apply frequently. (*In pleurodynia, toothache, and neuralgia about the head.*)   GEORGE BIRD.

1479—℞ Menthol. . . . . gr. xxiiss.
    Cocain. muriatis . . . . gr. viiss.
    Chloral. hydratis . . . . gr. ivss.
    Vaselini . . . . 3iiss.—M.
Ft. ungnentum.
Sig. Apply to the painful part and cover with a strip of court-
plaster. (*For supraorbital neuralgia.*)   GALEZOWSKI.

1480—℞ Methyl. chloridi pur. . . . . 3j.
Sig. Apply with a brush or an atomizer, or on pledgets of lint,
to the painful parts.   DEBOVE.

1481—℞ Camphoræ . . . . 3iss.
    Chloroformi . . . . f 3ss.
    Olei olivæ . . . . f 3ij.—M.
Sig. Apply frequently.   HAZARD.

NIPPLES, SORE. (See Fissure.)

NYMPHOMANIA.

1482—℞ Sodii arsenatis . . . . gr. ss.
    Hyoscinæ hydrobromatis . . . . . . gr. ⅛.
    Potassii bromidi . . . . 3j.—M.
Fiant tabellæ compressæ no. xxx.
Sig. One tablet after meals. (*All sources of local irritation
should be removed.*)

1483—℞ Potassii bromidi . . . . 3vj.
    Aquæ destillatæ . . . . f 3v.—M.
Sig. Three teaspoonfuls before dinner and four at bedtime.
    BROWN-SÉQUARD.

1484—℞ Pulveris camphoræ,
    Extracti lactucarii . . . . āā ℈iiss.
Misce et fiant pilulæ no. xx.
Sig. From four to six pills to be taken daily.   RICORD.

OBESITY.

1485—℞ Potassi permanganatis . . . . gr. iv-xvj.
Aquæ destillatæ . . . . f 3iv.—M.
Sig. A dessertspoonful three times a day.   BARTHOLOW.

1486—℞ Tabellas ext. gland. thyroid. . . . ââ gr. iiss.
No. xxv.
Sig. One after each meal, to be carefully increased and
stopped when untoward symptoms arise. Also—

1487—℞ Potassii iodidi . . . . 3ss.
Aquæ . . . . f 3ss.—M.
Sig. Five drops three times daily after meals, to be given with
No. 1486.   H. TUCKER.

ŒDEMA. (See Dropsy.)

ONYCHIA.

1488—℞ Thymol-diiodidi . . . . 3ij.
Sig. Apply freely and cover with antiseptic gauze, after removing diseased portion of matrix.

1489—℞ Unguenti hydrargyri . . . . 3ss.
Sig. Apply for ten minutes every hour, applying poultices at
other times.   RINGER.

1490—℞ Pulveris plumbi nitratis . . . . . . 3ss.
Detur in scatula.
Sig. Dust on the diseased tissue night and morning.
SCOTT AND MCCORMAC.

1491—℞ Acidi boracici,
Ceræ albæ . . . . ââ ɔiv.
Paraffini,
Olei amygdalæ dulcis . . . . . ââ ɔviij.—M.
Ft. ceratum.
Sig. To be used as a dressing, after the pus has been evacu-
ated. (For whitlow.)   SELLDÉN.

OPHTHALMIA.

1492—℞ Distilled water . . . . grammes 100.
Naphthol-α . . . . grammes 0.50.
Alcohol . . . . grammes 25.—M.
Sig. Instil in the eyes.   BUDIN.

1493—℞ Hydrarg. chloridi corrosivi . . . . . . gr. j.
Aquæ . . . . f 3xij.—M.
Sig. Irrigate the eye frequently with the solution.   CREDÉ.

1494—℞ Argenti nitratis . . . . gr. x.
Aquæ destillatæ . . . . f 3j.—M.
Ft. collyrium.
Sig. Bathe the eyes frequently, removing all the pus, and
apply the above locally, followed by a solution of sodium
chloride.   CREDÉ.

1495—℞ Hydrargyri chloridi corrosivi . . . . . gr. j.
Aquæ destillatæ . . . . f 3iv.—M.
Fiat collyrium. (In gonorrhœal ophthalmia.)   ELLIS.

1496—℞ Ferri sulphatis . . . . gr. ij.
Aquæ destillatæ . . . . f 3j —M.
Fiat solutio. (In the chronic form.)   HAZARD.

1497—℞ Acidi boracici . . . . gr. xvj.
Acidi salicylici . . . . gr. ij.
Glycerini . . . . ♏ xl.
Aquæ bullientis . . . . ad f 3j.—M.
Sig. Instil into the eye, after cauterizing trachoma follicles
with the thermo-cautery. (In trachoma.)   ARMAIGNAC.

1498—℞ Hydrarg. chloridi corrosivi . . . . . . gr. j.
Aquæ . . . . f 3j.—M.
Sig. Apply once daily to the lids with a brush. Use 1-7000
solution several times daily.   QUAITA.

1499—℞ Argenti nitratis . . . . ℈ss.
          Aquæ destillatæ . . . . f℥j.
Fiat collyrium.
Sig. One or two drops into the eye every second day. (*In Egyptian ophthalmia.*)   RIDGEWAY.

1500—℞ Argenti nitratis . . . . gr. iv.
          Aquæ destillatæ . . . . f℥j.
Fiat collyrium.
Sig. One drop to the eye every five or six hours. (*In catarrhal ophthalmia and superficial ulceration.*)   MACKENZIE.

1501—℞ Coniuæ . . . . partes ij.
          Alcoholis . . . . partes xij.
          Aquæ destillatæ . . . . partes cc.
Fiat solutio.
Sig. Drop in the eye and rub around the orbits several times a day. (*In scrofulous ophthalmia with photophobia.*)
        FRONMUELLER.

1502—℞ Pulv. acidi tannici . . . . ℥j.
          Pulv. acidi boracici . . . . ℥iij.—M.
Sig. Dust the lids. Cautery may precede it. (*In trachoma.*)
        WICHERKIEWICZ.

1503—℞ Pulveris aluminis . . . . gr. x.
          Aquæ rosæ . . . . f℥iij.
Misce et fiat collyrium.
Sig. Apply thrice daily. (*After the acute stage.*)   BRANDE.

1504—℞ Cocain. sulphatis . . . . gr. iv.
          Atropinæ sulphatis . . . . gr. ss.
          Vaselini . . . . ℈v.—M.
Sig. To be applied with a camel's-hair brush. The chemosis and pain are relieved instantly. (*In catarrhal ophthalmia.*)
        LEAHY.

1505—℞ Hydrarg. oxidi rubri . . . . gr. vj.
          Plumbi subacetatis cryst. . . . . . . gr. iij.
          Vaselini . . . . ℈v.—M.
Ft. ungt.
Sig. Apply to the free border of the eyelids once daily, after bathing the eyelids in hot water. (*In chronic blepharitis.*)
        PARINAUD.

1506—℞ Acidi tannici pulverizati . . . . . . ℈ij.
Detur in scatula.
Sig. Evert the lid and dust over. (*In the granular, phlyctenular, pustular, and chronic forms, and in pannus.*)   HAMILTON.

1507—℞ Eserinæ sulph. . . . . gr. j.
          Cocain. muriat. . . . . gr. v.
          Aq. destill. . . . . f℥j.—M.
Sig. Two drops as directed. (*Ulcerations in gonorrhœal ophthalmia.*)   DE SCHWEINITZ.

1508—℞ Hydrastinæ sulph.,
          Acid. boric.,
          Sodii biborat. . . . . āā gr. v.
          Tinct. opii deod. . . . . ℥ss.
          Aquæ dest. . . . . f℥j.
Mix and filter.
Sig. Inject under lids every hour and cleanse with boric solution. (*In infants.*)   SCOTT.

1509—℞ Iodoformi . . . . ℈ss.
          Sacchari lactis . . . . ℈iij.—M.
Sig. Evert the lids and dust over. (*In the granular form.*)

1510—℞ Hydrargyri chloridi mitis (lævigati) . ℈ij.
Detur in scatula.
Sig. Evert the lid and dust over once or twice daily. (*In the phlyctenular form.*)   BARTHOLOW.

1511—℞ Argenti nitratis . . . . gr. ij-x.
          Liquoris plumbi subacetatis . . . . . ℥x-xx.
          Cerati cetacei . . . . ℥j.—M.
Sig. The size of a pin's head to be put within the eyelids and repeated according to the degree of inflammation produced. (*In opacity of the cornea.*)   GUTHRIE.

OPHTHALMIA (Continued).

1512—℞ Glyceriti iodoformi (10 per cent.) . . . ʒss.
Sig. Instil into the eyes. (*In non-specific conjunctivitis in infants.*)　　　　　　　　HOGNER.

1513—℞ Iodi . . . . gr. j.
Potassii iodidi . . . . gr. iv.
Aquæ destillatæ . . . . ʒss.
Sig. Use as a spray. (*In chronic conjunctivitis*).　　BEDOIN.

1514—℞ Hydrargyri oxidi flavi . . . . gr. v.
Zinci sulphatis . . . . gr. x.
Adipis . . . . ʒj.—M.
Ft. ungt.
Sig. Smear on the everted eyelids, and on the free border of
the lids. (*In the chronic scrofutous form.*)　　DUPUYTREN.

OPIUM HABIT.

1515—℞ Spartein. sulphatis . . . . gr. j.
Aquæ destillatæ . . . . fʒj.—M.
Sig. Ten minims hypodermically, to tide the patient over the
period of collapse produced by withdrawing the drug.
　　　　　　　　　　　　　　　　BALL.

1516—℞ Strychninæ sulphatis . . . . gr. ⅓.
Tincturæ digitalis . . . . fʒj.
Aquæ destillatæ . . . . fʒij.—M.
Sig. Twenty drops hypodermically, to be repeated cautiously
if required. (*For depression and collapse, following with-
drawal of opiates.*)　　　　　E. Q. THORNTON.

1517—℞ Ext. cannabis indicæ (Squibb) . . . . fʒij.
Sig. A teaspoonful every hour or two, as required. (*For restlessness.*)

1518—℞ Tinct. nucis vomicæ . . . . gtt. xij.
Acidi phosphorici dil. . . . . gtt. xx.
Syr. pruni virginianæ . . . . fʒss.—M.
Sig. To be taken twice daily.　　　　MATTISON.

ORCHITIS.

1519—℞ Tinct. aconiti . . . . ℳj.
Morphinæ sulph. . . . . gr. ¼.
Antimonii tart. . . . . gr. 1/12.
Magnesii sulph. . . . . gr. xij.—M.
Sig. One dose. Repeat thrice daily.　　HORWITZ.

1520—℞ Tinct. iodi . . . . fʒj.
Sig. Apply locally to the swollen testicle after the acute
symptoms are over.　　　　　BARTHOLOW.

1521—℞ Ammonii chloridi . . . . ʒij.
Spiritus vini rectificati,
Aquæ destillatæ . . . . āā fʒij.—M.
Sig. Apply with moistened cloths frequently.　　BARTHOLOW.

1522—℞ Antimonii et potassii tartratis . . . . . gr. j.
Potassii nitratis . . . . ʒj.
Magnesii sulphatis . . . . ʒiss.
Aquæ destillatæ . . . . q. s. ad fʒvj.—M.
Sig. A tablespoonful every four to six hours. (*In the acute
form.*)　　　　　　　　ERICHSEN.

1523—℞ Tincturæ opii . . . . fʒiv.
Liquoris plumbi subacetatis . . . . . fʒiv.—M.
Sig. Add to pint of water and use locally.

1524—℞ Thymol . . . . gr. iv.
Sodii salicylat. . . . . gr. xxxj.
Ung. zinci oxid. benz. . . . . gr. ℈℈℈xiij.
Sig. Use locally.　　　　　　　　M.

1525—℞ Iodi . . . . gr. ij.
Potassii iodidi . . . . ʒj.
Aquæ destillatæ . . . . fʒiv.—M.
Fiat lotio.
Sig. Apply with a camel's-hair pencil. (*After the acute symp-
toms have subsided.*)　　　　　NIEMEYER.

1526—℞ Morphinæ sulphatis . . . . gr. viij.
    Hydrargyri oleatis (10 per cent.) . . . ℥j.—M.
Sig. Apply twice daily. (*For the subsequent induration.*)
                    MARSHALL.

1527—℞ Guaiacol . . . . ℥ij.
Sig. Apply a few drops over scrotum.   BALZER.

1528—℞ Tincturæ phytolaccæ (1–10) . . . . . . f℥j.
Sig. Ten drops every three or four hours.   J. C. WILSON.

OTITIS AND OTORRHŒA.

1529—℞ Creolin. . . . . gtt. x.
    Aquæ tepidæ . . . . Oj.—M.
Sig. Inject into the ear.   EITELBERG.

1530—℞ Acidi carboliei,
    Zinci sulphatis,
    Plumbi acetatis . . . . āā gr. x.
    Aquæ destillatæ . . . . f℥viij.—M.
Sig. Inject twice a day. (*When discharge is offensive.*)
                    HAZARD.

1531—℞ Lactis recentis,
    Aquæ calcis . . . . āā f℥j.
    Pulveris myrrhæ . . . . gr. xij.—M.
Sig. As an injection. (*In the acute form.*)   HAZARD.

1532—℞ Liquor. hydrogenii peroxidi (10 vol.) . f℥iv.
Sig. Syringe the ear carefully with one part of solution to two
parts of water, and when cleansed instil a few drops of the
above solution.   C. H. BURNETT.

1533—℞ Sol. boroglycerid. (50 per cent.) . . . . ℥j.
Sig. Instil a few drops into the ear, after cleansing it, twice
or thrice daily.   L. W. FOX.

1534—℞ Pulv. iodol. . . . . ℥ss.
    Spts. vini rectif. . . . . f℥iiss.
    Glycerini . . . . f℥viiiss.-M.
Sig. Use once or twice daily by instillation, after cleansing
the canal. (*In purulent otitis.*)   MAZZONI.

1535—℞ Tincturæ aconiti radicis . . . . f℥iss.
    Glycerini . . . . f℥iss.—M.
Sig. To be dropped into the ear.   SMITH.

1536—℞ Chloral,
    Camphor.,
    Acid. carbol. . . . . āā gr. x.
    Ol. ricini . . . . f℥ss.—M.
Sig. Some drops of this solution are put into the ear. The
solution must be warmed each time. (*For earache.*)

1537—℞ Morphinæ muriatis . . . . gr. v.
    Atropinæ sulphatis . . . . gr. j.
    Olei olivæ . . . . f℥j.
    Glycerini . . . . f℥iss.—M.
Sig. Three to five drops in the ear. Repeat every hour until
the pain is relieved. Place a small pledget of cotton in the
ear after introducing the drops. (*For otalgia.*)

1538—℞ Acidi carbolici . . . . ℥j.
    Glycerini . . . . f℥ix.—M.
Sig. Instil a few drops into the ear two or three times daily,
after cleansing.   HARTMANN.

1539—℞ Nosophen . . . . ℥ij.
Sig. Use as dusting powder after thorough cleansing.
W. H. KING.

1540—℞ Picis liquidæ . . . . ℈j.
Vaselini . . . . ℈v.
Sulphuris loti . . . . gr. vj.
Spts. camphoræ . . . . gr. iv.
Chloral. hydratis . . . . gr. ij.—M.
Ft. ungt.
Sig. Anoint the external ear and auditory canal, morning
and evening, after cleansing. Then twice weekly use—

1541—℞ Tinct. iodi . . . . ℔xxiv.
Glycerini,
Aquæ . . . . āā f℥j.
Potassii iodidi . . . . gr. vj.
Vini opii . . . . gr. xxiv.-M.
Sig. Bathe the whole surface of the auditory canal and the
external ear two or three times weekly. (*For eczematous
inflammation of the external ear.*) MIOT.

1542—℞ Unguenti hydrargyri nitratis rubri . . ℥ss.
Sig. Apply a small quantity to the integument. (*In chronic inflammation of the external meatus.*) BARTHOLOW.

1543—℞ Glyceriti acidi tannici . . . . ℥ss.
Sig. Fill the meatus and plug with cotton-wool. (*In the
chronic form.*) RINGER.

1544—℞ Pulv. iodol. . . . . ℥ss.
Sig. To be insufflated once or twice daily after thorough
cleansing and drying. (*In acute purulent cases.*) STETTER.

1545—℞ Pulv. iodoformi . . . . ℥ij.
Sig. Insufflate into the ear, after thoroughly cleansing and
drying it. (*For chronic cases, when discharge is slight.*)
BEZOLD

OXALURIA.

1546—℞ Acidi nitrohydrochlorici U. S. P. . . . f℥iv.
Sig. Three drops in half-glass of water after meals. (*Used in
hepatic torpor. To be taken through glass tube.*)

1547—℞ Acidi nitro-muriatici dil. . . . . ℥ij-iij.
Tinct. gentianæ comp.,
Tinct. cinchonæ comp. . . . . . . āā f℥j.
Elixir. curaçoæ . . . . ad f℥iij.—M.
Sig. A dessertspoonful in a wineglassful of water thrice daily.
RINGER.

1548—℞ Acidi hydrochlorici diluti . . . . f℥ss.
·Tincturæ ferri chloridi . . . . f℥ij.
Syrupi simplicis . . . . f℥iss.
Aquæ destillatæ . . . . f℥iij.—M.
Sig. A tablespoonful three times a day through a glass tube.
(*With anæmia and nervous atony.*) HAZARD.

1549—℞ Tincturæ aconiti foliorum . . . . . . ℔xxx.
Acidi nitro-hydrochlorici diluti . . . . f℥ij.
Tincturæ gentianæ . . . . f℥iij.
Syrupi aurantii corticis . . . . f℥j.
Infusi aurantii . . . . f℥viij.—M.
Sig. A tablespoonful three times a day. HAZARD.

OZÆNA.

1550—℞ Creolin . . . . gtt. iij-v.
Aquæ destillatæ . . . . Oj.
Sig. Use as a nasal douche. LICHTWITZ.

1551—℞ Acidi carbolici . . . . f 3iv.
Glycerini . . . . f 3iiss.
Alcoholis (90 per cent.) . . . . f 3x.
Aquæ . . . . f 3ix.—M.

Sig. A tablespoonful to a pint of tepid water, as a douche or spray. MOURE.

1552—℞ Resorcini . . . . 3ss.
Glycerini . . . . f 3ij.
Aquæ destillatæ . . . . q. s. ad f 3iv.—M.

Sig. Use as nasal spray every second day after using alkaline wash.

1553—℞ Alum. acet. tart., ... 3v-x.
Acidi borici . . . . 3iiss-iij.—M.

Sig. A coffeespoonful of this mixture to a quart of water.
MOURE.

1554—℞ Aqua cinnamom.,
Ext. hamamilid (colorless),
Hydrogen peroxid. . . . . āā f 3j.—M.

Sig. Use two teaspoonfuls as a nasal douche twice daily.
W. H. KING.

1555—℞ Salol. . . . . gr. lxxv.
Olei petrolei . . . . f 3v.—M.

Sig. Apply locally. MOURE.

1556—℞ Sodii biboratis,
Ammonii chloridi . . . . āā 9j.
Potassii permanganatis . . . . gr. x.

Sig. To be dissolved in one pint of tepid water, and used thrice daily with a syringe or douche. SAJOUS.

1557—℞ Syr. ferri iodidi . . . . 3j.

Sig. Five drops, increased to thirty drops, thrice daily after meals. SAJOUS.

1558—℞ Hydrargyri chloridi mitis . . . . gr. xv.
Sacchari albi . . . . 3iv.—M.

Sig. For insufflation. TROUSSEAU.

1559—℞ Hydrargyri ammoniati . . . . gr. ivss.
Sacchari albi . . . . 3ss.

Misce et fiat pulvis et detur in scatula.
Sig. After clearing the nose, snuff up twice or thrice daily.
TROUSSEAU.

1560—℞ Potassii permanganatis . . . . 3ss.
Tincturæ myrrhæ. . . . . f 3ij.
Aquæ destillatæ . . . . Oj.—M.

Sig. Use with a douche three times a day. HAZARD.

1561—℞ Sodii hyposulphitis . . . . 3iij.
Aquæ . . . . Oj.—M.

Sig. Use with a douche three times a day. HAZARD.

1562—℞ Ungt. hydrargyri nitratis . . . . 3ss.

Sig. Warm slightly and apply twice a day, after clearing the nose. (*In syphilitic ozæna of children.*) RINGER.

1563—℞ Glyceriti acidi tannici . . . . 3ss.

Sig. Apply with a camel's-hair brush two or three times daily, after clearing the nose. RINGER.

1564—℞ Extracti hydrastis fluidi,
Aquæ destillatæ . . . . āā f 3j.—M.

Sig.—Ten to twenty drops three times a day; also as injection into the nares. BARTHOLOW.

1565—℞ Bromi. . . . . 3ss.
Alcoholis . . . . f 3iv.—M.

Sig. Warm the wide-mouthed bottle in the hand, and snuff the vapor well into the nose. BARTHOLOW.

1566—℞ Pulv. carbonis ligni,
Pulv. quininæ sulphatis,
Pulv. myrrhæ . . . . āā partes æquales.

Sig. To be insufflated into the nares once or twice daily.
MEYER.

1567—℞ Plumbi nitratis . . . . ℈ij.
   Aquæ destillatæ. . . . . f℥iv.
Solve.
Sig. Inject into the nostril night and morning.   STILLÉ.

1568—℞ Iodi . . . . gr. ij-iv.
   Potassii iodidi . . . . gr. iv-viij.
   Aquæ destillatæ . . . . '. . . . f℥vj.
Fiat injectio.
Sig. Use twice daily.   NIEMEYER.

1569—℞ Iodol. . . . . ℥j.
   Ætheris . . . . ℥j.—M.
Sig. Use with an atomizer.   WOLFENDEN.

1570—℞ Pulv. saloli,
   Pulv. talci . . . . āā ℈ij.—M.
Sig. Insufflate the nose every two hours.   GEORGI.

PAIN. (See Neuralgia, Myalgia, Colic, etc.)

PALPITATION. (See Heart-Disease.)

PARALYSIS.

1571—℞ Ammonii iodidi . . . . ℥j.
   Ammonii carbonatis . . . . ℈ij.
   Liquoris ammonii acetatis . . . . . . ℥vj.—M.
Sig. A tablespoonful thrice daily. (*To absorb thrombi in incipient hemiplegic paralysis, due to endarteritis deformans.*)
            BARTHOLOW.

1572—℞ Strychninæ sulphatis . . . . gr. j.
   Aquæ destillatæ . . . . f℥x.
Fiat solutio.
Sig. For hypodermic use. Ten minims contain ₁⁄₁₀₀ gr. of strychnine sulphate. Inject in substance of paralyzed muscle. (*In diphtheritic paralysis; in local paralyses, such as facial, of the vocal cords, in lead palsy, paralysis of the sphincters ani and vesicæ; also in paraplegia when no structural alteration of cord, and in long-standing cases of hemiplegia.*)
            BARTHOLOW.

1573—℞ Phosphori . . . . gr. j.
   Ætheris . . . . ℏc.
   Glycerini . . . . f℥v.
   Aquæ destillatæ . . . . q. s. ad f℥xiiss.—M.
Sig. A teaspoonful three times a day. (*In paralysis agitans.*)
         S. M. BRADLEY.

1574—℞ Phosphori . . . . gr. ij.
   Alcoholis absoluti . . . . ℥xxiij.
   Tinct. vanillæ . . . . ℥ss.
   Olei aurantii cort. . . . . ℏxj.
   Alcoholis absoluti . . . . . . q. s. ad ℥iij.—M.
Sig. Twenty to forty minims two or three times daily. (*In cerebral softening and hysterical paralysis.*) HAMMOND.

1575—℞ Strychninæ sulphatis . . . . gr. j.
   Acidi arseniosi . . . . gr. ij.
   Extracti belladonnæ . . . . gr. v.
   Quininæ sulphatis,
   Pilulæ ferri carbonatis . . . . . . āā ℈ij.
   Extracti taraxaci . . . . ℈j.
Misce et fiant pilulæ no. xl.
Sig. One pill three times a day. (*In paralysis agitans.*)
          S. W. GROSS.

1576—℞ Coninæ.
   Acidi acetici fortioris . . . . . . āā f℥iij ℏxij.
Misce gradatim ad neutralizandum. Dein adde—
   Spiritus vini rectificati . . . . f℥j.
   Aquæ destillatæ . . . . . . q. s. ad f℥ij.—M.
Sig. For hypodermic use. Begin with one minim and gradually increase as necessary.   EULENBURG.

PARALYSIS (Continued).

1577—℞ Ext. physostigmatis . . . . gr. j.
Ext. gentianæ . . . . ℈j.—M
Ft. massa. et in pil. no. xxx div.
Sig. A pill every two hours. (*In general paralysis of the insane.*)
CRICHTON BROWNE.

1578—℞ Ext. physostigmatis . . . . gr. iij.
Ext. taraxaci . . . . gr. xxiv.-M.
Ft. massa et in pil. no. xxx div.
Sig. A pill every three hours. (*In paraplegia, locomotor ataxia, writer's cramp, and progressive muscular atrophy.*) MURRELL.

1579—℞ Extracti ergotæ aquosi . . . . gr. xv.
Syrupi aurantii corticis . . . . f ʒj.
Aquæ destillatæ . . . . f ʒiij.—M.
Sig. A tablespoonful three or four times a day. (*In paralysis of sphincter ani and sphincter vesicæ.*) BONJEAN.

1580—℞ Extracti buchu fluidi,
Extracti uvæ ursi . . . . āā f ʒij.
Syrupi acaciæ . . . . f ʒss.
Aquæ menthæ viridis . . . . f ʒj.—M.
Sig. A dessertspoonful every three hours. HAZARD.

1581—℞ Hyoscyaminæ sulphatis . . . . gr. ss.
Aquæ destillatæ . . . . ʒvj.—M.
Sig. Five minims hypodermically once daily, or by the stomach twice daily. (*In paralysis agitans.*) SÉGUIN.

PARTURITION. (See Labor.)

PEDICULI. (See Lice.)

PEMPHIGUS. (See Skin Diseases.)

PERICARDITIS. (See also Heart-Disease.)

1582—℞ Hydrarg. chloridi mitis,
Pulv. ipecac. . . . . āā gr. vj.
Potassii nitratis . . . . ʒss-j.—M.
In pulv. no. xii div.
Sig. A powder every three hours. HARTSHORNE.

1583—℞ Antimonii et potassii tart. . . . . . . gr. iv.
Tinct. opii . . . . f ʒj.
Aquæ camphoræ . . . . f ʒviij.—M.
Sig. A tablespoonful every two hours. (*In the acute form.*)
GRAVES.

1584—℞ Tinct. aconiti radicis . . . . f ʒss.
Sig. Half a drop to a drop in a teaspoonful of water every ten minutes or quarter of an hour for two hours; then every hour or two. RINGER.

1585—℞ Empl. cantharidis . . . . 2 in. × 3 in.
Sig. Apply over the præcordial space. Repeat at intervals after the skin is healed. (*In the chronic stage.*) TANNER.

PERIOSTITIS (NODES).

1586—℞ Potassii iodidi . . . . gr. ij-x.
Potassii bromidi . . . . gr. v-xx.
Ammonii carbonatis . . . . gr. v.
Spts. chloroformi . . . . ♏ xv.
Aquæ . . . . q. s. ad f ʒj.—M.
Sig. Take three times daily. BERKELEY HILL.

1587—℞ Iodi . . . . gr. ss.
Potassii iodidi . . . . ʒss.
Syr. papaveris . . . . f ʒss.
Infusi gentianæ comp. . . . . f ʒx.—M.
Sig. Take two tablespoonfuls thrice daily. Take a half-grain of morphine acetate at night. (*In weakly constitutions.*)
BRANSBY COOPER.

1588—℞ Cadmii iodidi . . . . ʒij.
Ichthyoli . . . . f ℥iv.
Adipis lanæ hydrosi . . . . . q. s. ad ʒij.—M.

Sig. Spread upon new cloth and apply to affected area.

1589—℞ Potassii iodidi . . . . ℈j.
Syrupi aurantii corticis . . . . f ʒj.
Aquæ aurantii florum . . . . f ℥v.—M.

Sig. Take a tablespoonful morning and night in hop-tea.
LISFRANC.

1590—℞ Potassii iodidi . . . . gr. xv.
Spiritus vini rectificati . . . . f ʒij.
Extracti dulcamaræ . . . . ʒij.
Pulveris glycyrrhizæ,
Aquæ destillatæ . . . . āā q. s.

Fiat massa in pilulas clxxx dividenda.
Sig. Take six pills two or three times a day. VOGT.

1591—℞ Potassii iodidi . . . . ʒij.
Ammonii iodidi . . . . ʒj.
Tinct. cinchonæ comp. . . . . f ʒiij.—M.

Sig. A teaspoonful, largely diluted with water, after eating.
VAN BUREN AND KEYES.

1592—℞ Hydrargyri biniodidi . . . . gr. vij.
Potassii iodidi . . . . ℈j.
Adipis . . . . ʒj.

Fiat unguentum. C. C. HILDRETH.

1593—℞ Iodi,
Terebinthinæ canadensis . . . . . āā ʒj.
Collodii . . . . f ℥iv.

Solve.
Sig. Paint over with a brush. J. T. SHINN.

1594—℞ Potassii iodidi,
Potassii carbonatis . . . . āā ʒij.
Spts. vini rectificati . . . . f ʒj.
Aquæ . . . . f ℥xj.—M.

Fiat lotio.
Sig. Apply twice daily (in the early stage), with the following
internally:

1595—℞ Potassii iodidi,
Potassii chloratis . . . . āā ʒj.
Potassii bicarbonatis . . . . ʒiij.—M.

In chartulas no. xii div.
Sig. One powder morning and evening in half a pint of milk.
ERICHSEN.

1596—℞ Barii iodidi . . . . gr. iv.
Adipis . . . . ℥j.

Fiat unguentum. BIETT.

1597—℞ Zinci iodidi . . . . ʒj.
Adipis . . . . ℥j.

Fiat unguentum.
Sig. Apply twice a day. URE.

1598—℞ Sodii iodidi . . . . ʒj.
Decocti sarsaparillæ comp. . . . . . . f ℥viij.—M.

Sig. One-sixth part three times daily. TANNER.

1599—℞ Cadmii iodidi . . . . ʒss.
Ætheris . . . . ℳxl.

Tere simul et adde—
Adipis . . . . ʒj.

Misce et fiat unguentum. A. B. GARROD.

1600—℞ Cadmii iodidi . . . . ʒj.
Adipis præparatæ . . . . ℥j.
Linimenti aconiti . . . . f ʒij.—M.

Fiat unguentum. TANNER.

1601—℞ Unguenti plumbi iodidi. . . . . ℥j.

Sig. Apply twice daily. (In chronic periosteal thickening)
HOOPER.

1602—℞ Potassii iodidi . . . . ℨj.
Aquæ bullientis . . . . f ℨj.
Vaselini . . . . ℨvij.—M.

Fiat unguentum.
Sig. Apply twice daily, and use the following:

1603—℞ Potassii iodidi . . . . ℨj-ij.

In pulv. no. xii div.
Sig. One powder, morning and evening, in a glassful of milk
RINGER.

1604—℞ Morphinæ . . . . gr. viij.
Hydrargyri oleatis (10-20 per cent.) . . . ℨj.—M.

Sig. Apply with a brush. MARSHALL.

PERITONITIS.

1605—℞ Hydrargyri chloridi mitis . . . . . . gr. ij.
Pulv. ipecacuanhæ et opii . . . . . gr. xvj.—M.

In pil. no. xvi div.
Sig. One every hour, watching the effect. J. C. WILSON.

1606—℞ Guaiacoli carbonatis . . . . gr. xxiv.

Pone in capsulas no. xxiv.
Sig. One capsule after each meal; the dose to be gradually
increased to three capsules. (*Used in tubercular peritonitis.*)

1607—℞ Tincturæ aconiti radicis . . . . f ℨij.
Tincturæ opii deodoratæ . . . . f ℨvj.—M.

Sig. Eight drops in water every hour or two. BARTHOLOW.

1608—℞ Pulveris opii . . . . gr. j.
Pulveris antimonialis . . . . gr. viij.
Hydrargyri chloridi mitis . . . . gr. iv.

Misce et divide in chartulas iv.
Sig. One powder every six hours with a saline effervescent
draught. (*At the commencement of the attack.*) GREGORY.

1609—℞ Linimenti hydrargyri . . . . f ℨiv.

Sig. Daily inunctions over abdomen and application of flannel abdominal binder, which is not to be changed when
soiled. (*Used in tubercular peritonitis.*)

1610—℞ Morphinæ sulphatis . . . . gr. viij.
Aquæ destillatæ . . . . f ℨiv.—M.

Sig. Begin with a dessertspoonful and wait two hours. If no
effect, give three teaspoonfuls and wait two hours. If still
no effect, give four teaspoonfuls and wait two hours. The
medicine should be increased gradually to produce these
effects: to allay pain, to produce gentle sleep, to reduce the
respirations to twelve per minute when aroused (may get
as low as eight, but should go no lower). Continue these
effects for two days, and then gradually diminish the dose;
but if the symptoms return, increase again.
ALONZO CLARK.

1611—℞ Olei terebinthinæ . . . . f ℨij.
Lactis asafœtidæ . . . . f ℨiij.
Aquæ ferventis . . . . f ℨiv.—M.

Sig. Use as an injection. LEVIS.

1612—℞ Tinct. aconiti folii . . . . f ℨv.
Ext. veratri viridis fld. . . . . f ℨj.—M.

Sig. Twelve drops every two hours. (*Where opium is inad-
missible.*) ELLIS.

1613—℞ Maguesii sulphatis . . . . ℨiss.

In pulv. no. xii div.
Sig. A powder in hot peppermint-water every hour until the
bowels are freely opened. (*In acute peritonitis, at the beginning of the attack.*) MUNDÉ.

1614—℞ Camphoræ, redactæ in pulverem . . . gr. v.
    Pulveris ipecacuanhæ compositi . . . gr. x.
    Potassii nitratis . . . . gr. xx.
Misce et fiant chartulæ ii.
Sig. One powder at bedtime.   SIMPSON.

1615—℞ Pulveris piperis,
    Pulveris zingiberis . . . . āā 3j.
    Sinapis nigræ contusæ . . . . ℔ss.
    Aquæ bullientis . . . . q. s.
Misce et fiat cataplasma. (*As a rubefacient.*)   ELLIS.

1616—℞ Acetphenetidin . . . . 3ij.
In pulv. no. xii div.
Sig. A powder stirred in a little water, as required. One-third to one-half the dose for children. (*For febrile condition.*)   KOBLER.

1617—℞ Acidi tannici . . . . gr. clxxx.
    Glycerini . . . . q. s. ad ℔ sol.—M.
Sig. To be taken in divided doses during the day. (*In localized peritonitis.*)   DEBOUÉ.

PERTUSSIS. (See Whooping-Cough.)

PHAGEDÆNA.

1618—℞ Potassii permanganatis . . . . 3ss.
    Aquæ . . . . Oj.—M.
Sig. Apply locally.   LEVIS.

1619—℞ Hydrargyri chloridi corrosivi . . . . . gr. j.
    Iodoformi,
    Ferri redacti . . . . āā 3j.
Misce et fiant pilulæ xx.
Sig. One pill three times a day. (*In sloughing phagedæna.*)
         BARTHOLOW.

1620—℞ Acidi salicylici . . . . 3ss.
Sig. Dust over the slough.   BARTHOLOW.

1621—℞ Ferri et potassii tartratis . . . . 3j-ij.
    Aquæ . . . . f3j.—M.
Ft. lotio.
Sig. Apply freely locally. (*When caustics cannot be used, as where large vessels are exposed, large surface, weak condition of patient, etc.*)   RICORD.

1622—℞ Acidi pyrogallici . . . . 3ij.
    Pulv. amyli . . . . 3j.—M.
Ft. pulv.
Sig. Dust over or insufflate the sores twice daily. The powder should be fresh, and kept in a tightly-corked bottle.
         TERRILLON.

1623—℞ Saloli . . . . gr. v-l.
    Amyli . . . . 3j.—M.
Ft. pulv.
Sig. Dust over locally.   SEIFERT.

1624—℞ Acidi nitrici diluti : . . . . ♏x.
    Extracti opii . . . . gr. v.
    Aquæ . . . . f3j.
Ft. lotio. (*In sloughing incised wounds.*)   ERICHSEN.

1625—℞ Iodoformi . . . . 3ijss.
    Thymoll . . . . 3v.
    Sacchari lactis . . . . gr. ij.—M.
Ft. pulv.
Sig. Dust over the sores.   HOWARD.

1626—℞ Acidi nitrici fort. . . . . f3j.
Sig. Apply thoroughly but carefully to the whole secreting surface, after drying it. Give the patient an anæsthetic if necessary, and a hypodermic of morphine later.
        VAN BUREN AND KEYES.

1627—℞ Aristol. . . . . 3j.
Sig. Apply lightly and cover with a poultice.   J. C. WILSON.

1628—℞ Pilocarpinœ muriatis . . . . gr. ij.
Aquæ,
Glycerini . . . . ãã f ʒj.—M.
Sig. A teaspoonful thrice daily. (*In atrophic or dry pharyngitis.*)
SAJOUS.

1629—℞ Tinct. guaiaci ammoniatæ . . . . . . f ʒj.
Sig. A teaspoonful in a half-glassful of milk, used as a gargle and swallowed every three hours. (*In rheumatic subjects.*)
SAJOUS.

1630—℞ Argenti nitratis . . . . gr. xl.
Aquæ destillatæ . . . . f ʒj.—M.
Sig. Apply to the throat after cleansing it. (*In chronic pharyngitis.*)
SAJOUS.

1631—℞ Olei vaselini . . . . ʒij.
Sig. Apply with a brush or an atomizer three or four times daily. (*Where astringents are not tolerated, in chronic pharyngitis.*)
SAJOUS.

1632—℞ Liq. potassii arsenitis . . . . f ʒj.
Sig. One or two drops in water, thrice daily. (*To remove the tendency to attacks of pharyngitis.*)
SAJOUS.

1633—℞ Menthol . . . . ʒss.
Oil of sweet almonds or liquid vaselin f ʒv.—M.
Sig. Apply locally with a brush.
Medical Record.

1634—℞ Sodii bicarb.,
Sodii biborat.,
Sodii chlorat.,
Potas. bicarb. . . . . ãã f ʒiv.—M.
Sig. A quarter of a teaspoonful in quarter of a glass of tepid water, and use by insufflation and gargle.
D. B. KYLE.

1635—℞ Potassii chlorat. . . . . ʒij.
Zinci sulphat. . . . . gr. x.
Tinct. myrrhæ . . . . f ʒj.
Syrup. simpl. . . . . f ʒj.
Aquæ destillatæ . . . . f ʒiv.—M.
Sig. Gargle.

1636—℞ Iodine . . . . gr. iij.
Potassium iodide . . . . gr. v.
Trichloracetic acid . . . . gr. vij.
Glycerin,
Water . . . . ãã f ʒss.—M.
Sig. To be applied locally. (*Follicular pharyngitis.*)
Tri-State Medical Journal.

1637—℞ Cocain. muriatis . . . . gr. x.
Aquæ destillatæ . . . . f ʒss.—M.
Sig. Cleanse the throat with a spray of chlorate of potassium solution (saturate). After drying it, apply the solution with a brush every two hours. A wineglassful of coca-wine every two hours also aids. (*In the acute form.*)
SAJOUS.

1638—℞ Tablet pilocarpine gran. efferves. . ãã gr. 1/100.
No. x.
Sig. One tablet every hour for three or four doses. (*Dry stage.*)
W. H. KING.

1639—℞ Ol. santali . . . . gr. iij.
Benzoinal . . . . f ʒj.—M.
Sig. Apply locally in spray or on cotton carrier two or three times a day.
W. H. KING.

1640—℞ Alpha-naphthol . . . . gr. xlv.
Alcohol . . . . f ʒx.—M.
Sig. A teaspoonful of this solution to be added to a quart of hot water which has been boil d.

1641—℞ Iodol.,
Glycerini . . . . ãã f ʒj.
Vaselini . . . . f ʒvij.—M.
Sig. Warm slightly and apply locally.
WOLFENDEN.

1642—℞ Phenacetini . . . . 3ij.
Fiant chartulæ no. xii.
Sig. One powder not oftener than every four hours. (*For relief of pain.*)

1643—℞ Acidi hydrochlorici diluti . . . . . . 3j.
Potassii chloratis . . . . 3ss.
Decocti hordei . . . . Oij.—M.
Sig. To be taken in divided doses during the day.
MACKENZIE.

1644—℞ Ext. hamamelidis fld. . . . . f3j.
Syr. simplicis,
Elixir. simplicis . . . . āā f3ss.—M.
Sig. One or two teaspoonfuls three or four times daily.
PRESTON.

1645—℞ Phenacetin. . . . . 3j.
In pilulas (compressas) no. xii div.
Sig. One tablet every three or four hours. (*For the relief of pain.*)
J. C. WILSON.

PHLEGMON. (See Carbuncle.)

PHTHISIS. (See also Bronchitis, Diarrhœa, Sweating, and Hæmoptysis.)

1646—℞ Creasote (of the beech) . . . . gr. xv.
Tincture of gentian . . . . f3j.
Pure alcohol . . . . f3viij.
Tokay wine . . . . f3xxij.—M.
Sig. A tablespoonful in water three times a day. GUTTMANN.

1647—℞ Creasoti . . . . ℳj-v.
Spiritus ammonii aromatici . . . . . ℳxv-f3j.
Aquæ destillatæ . . . . f3iss.
Fiat haustus. KESTEVEN.

1648—℞ Creasoti . . . . f3iiss.
Tinct. gentianæ . . . . f3j.
Spts. vini rectificati . . . . f3viij.
Vini xerici . . . . ad Oij.—M.
Sig. A tablespoonful in a wineglassful of water three times daily. (*In incipient tuberculosis.*) FRÄNTZEL.

1649—℞ Hydrarg. chloridi mitis . . . . gr. x.
Pepsini . . . . gr. lvi.
Tinct. opii . . . . gtt. xxx.
Ext. phellandrii . . . . q. s.—M.
Fiant pilulæ no. lx.
Sig. One or two daily. DOCHMANN.

1650—℞ Hydrarg. chloridi mitis . . . . gr. ij.
Glycerini . . . . ℳxv.
Aquæ . . . . ℳxv.—M.
Sig. Prepare freshly; shake thoroughly; inject deeply into gluteal or deltoid region once in five days. J. C. WILSON.

1651—℞ Morphinæ muriatis . . . . gr. j.
Acidi muriatici diluti . . . . ℳv.
Acidi hydrocyanici diluti . . . . . . ℳxxx.
Syrupi scillæ,
Aquæ destillatæ . . . . āā f3j.—M.
Sig. A teaspoonful when the cough is troublesome.
A. T. THOMPSON.

1652—℞ Tincturæ benzoini compositæ . . . . . f3j.
Aquæ bullientis . . . . Oss.—M.
Sig. Inhale twice daily. (*Eases cough and lessens expectoration.*)
RINGER.

1653—℞ Codeinæ . . . . gr. vj.
Acidi sulphurici diluti . . . . f3j.
Glycerini . . . . f3ss.
Aquæ laurocerasi . . . . f3j.
Syr. pruni virginianæ . . . . . q.s. ad f3iij.—M.
Sig. A teaspoonful occasionally for the relief of cough.
J. C. WILSON.

PHTHISIS (Continued).

1654—℞ Iodi . . . . gr. iij.
        Potassii iodidi . . . . gr. vj.
        Aquæ destillatæ . . . . f 3j.—M.

Sig. Ten drops three times a day in a draught of cold water.
(*With glandular disease.*)   S. G. MORTON.

1655—℞ Ferri sulphatis . . . . 3j.
        Magnesiæ . . . . gr. x.
        Sacchari albi . . . . 3j.
        Aquæ cinnamomi . . . . f 3viij.—M.

Sig. A tablespoonful every three hours. (*As an efficient tonic in phthisis.*)   DONOVAN.

1656—℞ Tincturæ ferri chloridi,
        Acidi nitrici diluti . . . . āā f 3j.
        Syrupi zingiberis . . . . f 3xiv.
        Aquæ menthæ viridis . . . . f 3iv.—M.

Sig. A tablespoonful every four hours. (*An astringent tonic.*)   R. BENNETT.

1657—℞ Calcii chloridi . . . . 3j.
        Extracti hyoscyami . . . . 3ss.
        Syrupi glycyrrhizæ . . . . f 3j.
        Aquæ destillatæ . . . . f 3vj.—M.

Sig. A tablespoonful to be taken four times a day. BEDDOES.

1658—℞ Extract. hydrast. canaden. fluid.,
        Extract. ergotæ fluid. . . . . āā f 3vj.—M.

Sig. Thirty to forty drops of this solution in a little water, four or five times a day, after food. (*Cough with muco-purulent expectoration.*)   Jour. de Méd. de Paris.

1659—℞ Olei delphinidæ (porpoise-oil). . . . . Oss.

Sig. A teaspoonful to a tablespoonful thrice daily, after meals. (*Aliment in phthisis.*)   WEST.

1660—℞ Sodii iodidi . . . . gr. lxxv.
        Sodii bromidi . . . . 3iss.
        Sodii chloridi . . . . 3v.
        Aquæ destillatæ . . . . f 3l.—M.

Sig. A teaspoonful every morning in a cupful of milk. "Summer Cod-Liver Oil." Contains the principal constituents of olei morrhuæ. (*Aliment in phthisis.*)   POTAIN.

1661—℞ Spts. vini gallici vel jamaicensis . . . f 3iss.
        Olei menthæ pip. . . . . ℳj.
        Glycerini . . . . f 3x.—M.

Sig.—To be taken in divided doses during the day. In cases which present no sign of abnormal excitability of the nervous system or heart, the dose of glycerin may be raised to twelve or fifteen ounces daily. (*Aliment, when patients cannot take olei morrhuæ.*)   JACCOUD.

1662—℞ Salviæ,
        Eupatorii . . . . āā 3ss.
        Cascarillæ . . . . 3j.
        Aquæ bullientis . . . . Oj.

Digere per horas duas et cola.
Sig. A wineglassful every three or four hours. (*In hectic.*)   ELLIS.

1663—℞ Acidi nitrici . . . . f 3j.
        Sacchari albi . . . . 3j.
        Aquæ . . . . Oij.

Fiat mistura.
Sig. One-eighth part daily in divided doses. (*Sometimes arrests colliquative sweats when other remedies fail.*) FERRIAR.

1664—℞ Codeine . . . . gr. iv.
        Dilute hydrochloric acid . . . . . . ℳxxx.
        Spirit of chloroform . . . . f 3iss.
        Syrup of lemon . . . . f 3j.
        Water sufficient to make . . . . . . f 3iv.—M.

Sig. One teaspoonful as occasion demands. (*For cough.*) MURRELL.

1665—℞ Acidi salicylici . . . . 3v.

Divide in partes æquales no. xl, et fiant pilulæ compressæ.
Sig. Two pills two or three times a day. (*For foul breath and offensive expectoration; also in pyrexia.*)   RINGER.

1666—℞ Plumbi acet. . . . . gr. x.
  Ext. gentianæ . . . . q. s.—M.
Ft. chart. xii.
Sig. Three to five powders daily. (*Night-sweats.*) Med. News.

1667—℞ Ext. ergotæ fld. . . . . f ʒj.
Sig. Twenty drops three times daily. (*To relieve diarrhœa and sweats.*) A. L. HODGSON.

1668—℞ Acetphenctidin. . . . . ʒiiss.
In pulv. no. xv div.
Sig. A powder stirred in a little water, two or three times daily. (*For hectic.*) HINSBERG AND KAST.

1669—℞ Antifebrin. . . . . ʒij.
  Spts. vini gallici . . . . f ʒiij.—M.
Sig. From a dessertspoonful to a tablespoonful two or three times daily. (*For hectic.*) FAUST.

1670—℞ Ammonii boratis . . . . ʒij.
  Syr. simplicis,
  Elix. simplicis. . . . . āā f ʒiss.—M.
Sig. A teaspoonful thrice daily. (*For expectoration and hectic.*) LASHKEVITCH.

1671—℞ Antipyrin. . . . . gr. lxxv.
  Spts. jamaicensis . . . . f ʒv.
  Syr. limonis . . . . f ʒviiss.
  Aquæ destillatæ. . . . . f ʒiiss.—M.
Sig. One to three tablespoonfuls once or twice daily. (*For hectic.*) VIGIER.

1672—℞ Acidi borici . . . . ʒiij.
  Misturæ acaciæ . . . . f ʒiv.
  Vini cocæ . . . . q. s. ad f ʒiij.—M.
Sig. Shake the vial. A dessertspoonful every four hours. (*For diarrhœa.*) J. C. WILSON.

1673—℞ Picrotoxini . . . . gr. ⅙.
  Sacchari lactis . . . . gr. xx.
  Alcohol . . . . q. s.—M.
Fiant tabellæ triturationes no. xii.
Sig. One tablet at bedtime. (*Used to prevent night-sweats.*)

1674—℞ Chloral. hydratis . . . . ʒij.
  Syrupi tolutani . . . . f ʒj.
  Aquæ destillatæ . . . . q. s. ad f ʒiij.—M.
Sig. A tablespoonful at bedtime. (*To procure sleep.*) WALSHE.

1675—℞ Chondri crispi electi,
  Aquæ . . . . āā q. s.
Coque ad f ʒvj, cola, et adde—
  Sodii phosphatis . . . . ʒiss.
  Syrupi papaveris . . . . f ʒij.—M.
Sig. A tablespoonful every two hours. (*In hæmoptysis.*) CLARUS.

1676—℞ Balsami copaibæ,
  Syrupi tolutani,
  Aquæ menthæ piperitæ,
  Spiritus vini rectificati . . . . . . āā f ʒj.
  Spiritus ætheris nitrosi . . . . f ʒj.—M.
Sig. Two teaspoonfuls every two to four hours. (*In obstinate hæmoptysis.*) NIEMEYER.

1677—℞ Tellurate of sodium . . . . gr. ij-iij.
  Alcohol (90 per cent. solution) . . . . f ʒij.
Sig. A small teaspoonful night and morning in a little sugar and water. (*Night-sweats.*) JOGET.

1678—℞ Sulphuris sublimati . . . . q. s.
Sig. In a close room burn two to five drachms of sulphur for each cubic yard of air-space; close and leave for twelve hours. Patient then enters the room and remains eight hours. This is repeated daily. SOLLARD.

1679—℞ Pilocarpinæ muriatis . . . . gr. iij.
Aquæ destillatæ . . . . f3ij.—M.

Sig. Five minims three times daily by hypodermic. (*In
paroxysmal dyspnœa of phthisis.*) RIESS.

1680—℞ Pulv. agarici . . . . 3j.

In pulv. no. xii div.
Sig. One powder every two hours (for three doses) if necessary. (*For night-sweats.*) A. PETER.

1681—℞ Atropinæ sulphatis . . . . gr. j.
Aquæ destillatæ . . . . 3v.—M.

Sig. Twelve minims hypodermically. (*For hæmoptysis.*)
HAUSMANN.

1682—℞ Pyridin . . . . 3j.

Sig. Six to ten drops, increased to twenty-five drops daily, in
three-drop doses. In urgent cases three to five drops may
be inhaled directly from a handkerchief. (*For dyspnœa.*)
DE RENZI.

1683—℞ Codein . . . . gr. iv.
Acid. hydrocyanic. dilut . . . . gtt. xv.
Ammonii chlorid . . . . gr. xv.
Syrup. pruni virginianæ . . . q. s. ad f3ij.—M.

Sig. A teaspoonful every three or four hours. (*For cough.*)
Roosevelt Hospital.

1684—℞ Terpin. hydratis . . . . gr. lxxv.
Spts. vini rectificati (95 per cent.) . . . f3v.
Glycerini . . . . f3x.—M.

Sig. A teaspoonful or two in a little sweetened or aromatized
water two or three times daily. (*Expectorant.*) VIGIER.

1685—℞ Terpinol.,
Sodii benzoatis . . . . āā gr. xv.
Sacchari albi . . . . q. s.—M.

In capsulas no. x div.
Sig. A capsule every hour or two. (*To diminish the expectoration and remove its odor.*) RABOW.

1686—℞ Amyli hydratis . . . . gr. cv.
Ext. glycyrrhizæ . . . . 3iiss.
Aquæ destillatæ . . . . f3xv.—M.

Sig. The half to be taken at bedtime. (*For the insomnia of
phthisis.*) FISCHER.

1687—℞ Amyli hydratis . . . . 3iss.
Morphinæ muriatis . . . . gr. ⅓.
Ext. glycyrrhizæ . . . . 3iiss.
Aquæ destillatæ . . . . f3xv.—M.

Sig. The half to be taken at bedtime. (*Insomnia of phthisis.*)
FISCHER.

PILES. (See Hemorrhoids.)

PITYRIASIS. (See Skin Diseases.)

PLEURISY.

1688—℞ Tincturæ iodi compositæ . . . . f3ij.

Sig. Divide the surface on the affected side into three sections,
and paint one section each day. (*For chronic pleuritic effusion.*) BARTHOLOW.

1689—℞ Hydrarg. chloridi mitis . . . . gr. vj.
Pulv. opii . . . . gr. iij-vj.
Antimonii et potassii tart . . . . gr. iss.—M.

In pulv. no. xii div.
Sig. A powder every three or five hours. (*In acute pleurisy.*)
HARTSHORNE.

1690—℞ Potassii acetatis . . . . 3vss.
Spts. ætheris nitrosi . . . . 3ij.
Aquæ . . . . ad 3viij.—M.

Sig. A tablespoonful every three or four hours. (*In pleuritic
effusion.*) HARTSHORNE.

1691—℞ Magnesii sulphatis . . . . ʒvj–viij.
In pulv. no. viij div.
Sig. A powder in two tablespoonfuls of water before food,
and no fluid for some time afterwards. (*In pleuritic effusion.*)
M. Hay.

1692—℞ Folii jaborandi . . . . f ʒj.
Aquæ bullientis . . . . Oj.—M
Ft. infusum.
Sig. A wineglassful three or four times daily. (*In bad cases
with much effusion.*) Michon.

1693—℞ Potassii acetatis . . . . ʒij.
Infusi digitalis . . . . ʒiij.—M.
Sig. A teaspoonful every three hours to a child of five years.
(*To remove effusion.*) J. Lewis Smith.

1694—℞ Potassii acetatis . . . . gr. xv.
Spiritus ætheris nitrosi . . . . f ʒss.
Vini ipecacuanhæ . . . . gtt. iij.
Syrupi tolutani . . . . f ʒss.—M.
Sig. One dose, four times a day. (*In subacute pleurisy.*)
Da Costa.

1695—℞ Mercuric chloride,
Sodium chloride,
Extract of opium . . . . āā gr xv.
Fresh breadcrumbs . . . . gr. lxxv.
Gluten . . . . gr. xxxviij.
Glycerin . . . . gr. xxx–xlv.
Mix and divide into one hundred pills.
Sig. One, two, or three to be taken daily. (*For pleurisy with
effusion.*) A. Robin.

1696—℞ Potassii iodidi . . . . gr. j.
Ferri et ammonii citratis . . . . . . gr. iij.
Syrupi sarsaparillæ compositi . . . . . f ʒss.
Aquæ destillatæ . . . . f ʒij.—M.
Sig. One dose, three times a day. (*In chronic form with effu-
sion, for children.*) Hazard.

1697—℞ Potassii iodidi . . . . ʒiv.
Aquæ destillatæ . . . . q. s. ad f ʒvj.—M.
Sig. One fluidrachm in milk every four hours. Bartholow.

1698—℞ Tinct. opii deodoratæ . . . . gtt. xx.
Tinct. digitalis . . . . gtt. xvj.
Syr. pruni virginianæ . . . . f ʒj.
Aquæ . . . . f ʒss.—M.
Sig. A teaspoonful every three hours for a child eighteen
months old. (*For first stage.*) J. Lewis Smith.

1699—℞ Tinct. aconiti radicis . . . . f ʒss.
Sig. Half a drop every third hour for a child three years old.
One drop for six years old. If younger, then give—

1700—℞ Tinct. digitalis . . . . f ʒss.
Sig. One drop every three hours for a two-year-old child.
J. Lewis Smith.

1701—℞ Pulv. sinapis . . . . ʒss.
Pulv. lini . . . . ʒviij.
Aquæ bullientis . . . . q. s.—M.
Ft. cataplasma.
Sig. Make the poultice so wet that it moistens the hands in
holding it. Place it between two pieces of muslin, cover
with oiled muslin, and renew when beginning to cool. (*In
pleurisy of children.*) J. Lewis Smith.

1702—℞ Syr. ferri iodidi . . . . f ʒij.
Syr. simplicis . . . . f ʒij.—M.
Sig. A teaspoonful every two hours, with the following:

1703—℞ Iodi . . . . ʒss.
Potassii iodidi . . . . ʒij.
Aquæ destillatæ . . . . f ʒij.—M.
Sig. Apply on the affected side of the chest. Niemeyer.

1704—℞ Tincturæ aconiti radicis . . . . f ʒij.
Tincturæ opii deodoratæ . . . . f ʒvj.—M.
Sig. Eight drops in water every hour or two. (*In acute form
before effusion.*) Bartholow.

1705—℞ Acidi tannici . . . . gr. xxx.
Confectionis rosæ . . . . q. s.

Misce et fiant pilulæ no. xv.
Sig. Four to eight pills daily, one-half in the morning, the
remainder in the evening. (*In purulent pleurisy.*) DEBOUÉ.

1706—℞ Morphinæ acetatis . . . . gr. ss.
Potassii acetatis . . . . 3ss.
Tincturæ veratri viridis . . . . ℳxxiv.
Syrupi tolutani . . . . f3ss.
Liquoris potassii citratis . . . . f3iss.—M.

Sig. Two fluidrachms every three hours. (*In dry pleurisy.*)
DA COSTA.

1707—℞ Morphinæ sulphatis . . . . gr. ¼.
Quininæ sulphatis . . . . gr. xv-xx.

Misce et fiat chartula.
Sig. At once. (*To abort a commencing pleurisy.*) BARTHOLOW.

1708—℞ Collodii cum cantharide . . . . f3ss.

Sig. Apply with a brush over a small area, heal quickly, and
repeat. (*In pleuritic effusion.*) RINGER.

PLEURODYNIA. (See Neuralgia.)

PNEUMONIA.

1709—℞ Pulv. morphinæ comp. (Tully) . . . . 3ss.
In chart. no. xii. div.
Sig. One powder every two hours. J. C. WILSON.

1710—℞ Tinct. aconiti radicis . . . . f3ij.
Tinct. opii . . . . f3iij.—M.

Sig. Thirteen drops at once, followed by five drops every hour
or two. (*In the stage of congestion.*) BARTHOLOW.

1711—℞ Ammonii carbonatis . . . . Əij.
Infusi serpentariæ . . . . f3iv.—M.

Sig. A tablespoonful every three hours. (*About the period of
crisis.*) BARTHOLOW.

1712—℞ Potassii iodidi . . . . 3j.
Ammonii muriatis . . . . 3iss.
Mist. glycyrrhizæ comp. . . . . f3vj.—M.

Sig. A tablespoonful four times daily, to promote absorption,
together with blisters to the chest. DA COSTA.

1713—℞ Pulv. digitalis . . . . gr. vj.
Quininæ sulphatis . . . . gr. xij.
Ext. opii,
Ext. ipecacuanhæ . . . . āā gr. iij.—M.

Ft. massa et in pil. no. xii div.
Sig. One pill thrice daily with the preceding mixture.
DA COSTA.

1714—℞ Tincturæ veratri viridis . . . . f3ij.

Sig. Two or three drops in water until pulse becomes soft and
compressible. (*Only to be given before consolidation has taken
place.*) H. A. HARE.

1715—℞ Liq. trinitrin . . . . f3j.

Sig. One to three drops in water every four hours or oftener.
(*To relieve embarrassed heart.*) J. C. WILSON.

1716—℞ Antimonii et potassii tartratis . . . . . gr. ij.
Morphinæ sulphatis . . . . gr. iij.
Ammonii chloridi . . . . 3ij.
Syrupi glycyrrhizæ . . . . f3iv.—M.
Sig. A tablespoonful every four hours.

And

1717—℞ Pulveris opii . . . . gr. iij.
Pulveris ipecacuanhæ,
Hydrargyri chloridi mitis . . . . āā gr. vj.
Sacchari albi . . . . gr. xxx.

Misce et fiant chartulæ no. vi.
Sig. One powder every four hours, alternately with the preceding prescription: at the end of twenty-four hours omit
powders, and, if typhoid symptoms persist, give the following instead:

1718—℞ Quininæ sulphatis. . . . . gr. ij.
Ammonii carbonatis . . . . gr. iv.

Misce et fiat chartula.
Sig. One dose. If delirium or morbid vigilance is troublesome, add

1719—℞ Chloroformi . . . . ℳx-xij

to each dose of the above. (*In typhoid pneumonia.*)

N. S. DAVIS.

1720—℞ Tinct. ipecac. comp. (Squibb) . . . . . gtt. xxxij.
Tinct. aconiti radicis . . . . gtt. xvj.
Syr. tolutani,
Aquæ . . . . āā f ʒj.—M.

Sig. A teaspoonful every three hours to a child of five years.
(*In the congestive stage.*)

J. LEWIS SMITH.

1721—℞ Morphinæ sulphatis . . . . gr. j.
Syr. ipecacuanhæ . . . . f ʒss.
Syr. tolutani . . . . f ʒiiiss.—M.

Sig. A teaspoonful every three hours to a child of five years.
(*In the stage of hepatization.*)

J. LEWIS SMITH.

1722—℞ Pulv. sinapis . . . . ʒss.
Pulv. seminis lini . . . . ʒviij.—M.

Ft. cataplasma.
Sig. Make as large and thin as a book-cover, and apply to the
chest, covering with oiled silk.

J. LEWIS SMITH.

1723—℞ Morphinæ sulphatis. . . . . gr. ¼ ad ⅓.
Quininæ sulphatis . . . . gr. vi-x.

Misce et fiat chartula.
Sig. One dose. Within twenty-four hours after the chill, to
abort the attack.

A. B. PALMER.

1723bis—℞ Acidi salicylici . . . . gr. xx.

Fiat chartula.
Sig. One every two hours until four or five are taken. (*To
abort an impending attack.*)

L. L. SILVERTHORN.

1724—℞ Potassii iodidi . . . . ʒiss.
Aquæ destillatæ. . . . . f ʒviij.—M.

Sig. A tablespoonful every two hours. (*In double pneumonia,
complicated with pleurisy.*)

M. RIEBE.

1725—℞ Ammonii carbonatis . . . . gr. iv.
Spiritus chloroformi . . . . ℳxx.
Aquæ camphoræ . . . . f ʒx.—M.

Sig. To be given every three or four hours. (*In uncomplicated
cases.*)

A. T. H. WATERS.

1726—℞ Quininæ sulphatis . . . . ʒss.
Acidi sulphurici aromatici . . . . . f ʒiss.
Olei caryophylli. . . . . gtt. iv.
Mucilaginis acaciæ . . . . f ʒj.
Aquæ menthæ pip. . . . . ad f ʒiv.—M.

Sig. A teaspoonful or two every three or four hours. (*In
asthenic pneumonia.*)

HARTSHORNE.

1727—℞ Ext. ergotæ fld. . . . . f ʒiv.
Tinct. digitalis . . . . f ʒj.
Plumbi acetatis . . . . gr. vj.
Aquæ cinnamomi . . . . f ʒij.

Sig. A tablespoonful every two hours till the blood disappears
from the sputa.

WELLS.

1728—℞ Tinct. strophanth. hispid. (1-20,) . . . f ʒj.

Sig. Ten drops in water four or five times daily. (*In the cardiac
lesions of pneumonia.*)

DRASCHE.

1729—℞ Ammonii muriatis . . . . ʒj.
Ext. glycyrrhizæ . . . . ʒj.
Spts. ætheris sulph. . . . . f ʒij.
Aquæ . . . . f ʒiv.—M.

Sig. A tablespoonful every two or three hours. (*In advanced
stages of pneumonia.*)

WARING.

PNEUMONIA (Continued).

1730—℞ Acidi salicylici . . . . f ʒj.
      Ammonii carbonatis . . . . ʒiij.
      Syr. simplicis . . . . f ʒij.
      Aquæ cinnamomi . . . . ad f ʒvj.—M.

Sig. A tablespoonful every hour or two till the fever declines.
                                  FLIESBURG.

1731—℞ Ext. veratri viridis fld. . . . . f ʒj.

Sig. Four to six minims every hour until the pulse falls to
sixty-five or seventy per minute.   STROUD.

1732—℞ Thallin. sulphatis . . . . gr. xxxij.
      Aquæ aurantii flor. . . . . f ʒj.—M.

Sig. A teaspoonful every three hours till the fever declines.
                                  OSLER.

PORRIGO (ECZEMA CAPITIS). (See Skin Diseases.)

PORRIGO DECALVANS (ALOPECIA AREATA). (See Skin Diseases.)

PORRIGO FAVOSA (FAVUS). (See Skin Diseases.)

PRIAPISM. (See Nymphomania.)

PRICKLY HEAT. (See Skin Diseases.)

PROSTATITIS.

1733—℞ Liq. potassæ . . . . f ʒij-iv.
      Ext. hyoscyami . . . . ʒj-iv.
      Syr. aurantii cort.,
      Aquæ cinnamomi . . . . āā f ʒiij.—M.

Sig. A tablespoonful in a wineglassful of water every eight
hours.   VAN BUREN AND KEYES.

1734—℞ Hydrargyri chloridi mitis . . . . . . gr. ij.
      Sodi bicarbonatis . . . . gr. xij.—M.

Fiant chartulæ no. vi.
Sig. One powder on tongue every hour. To be followed by
Seidlitz powder unless free evacuation of bowels. (*Initial
treatment in acute cases.*)

1735—℞ Carbonis animalis . . . . gr. iij.
      Ammonii chloridi . . . . ʒj.
      Extracti conii . . . . gr. ij.
      Pulveris glycyrrhizæ . . . . q. s.

Fiat bolus.
Sig. One three times a day. (*In swelled and scirrhous prostate.*)
                              MAGENDIE.

1736—℞ Iodoform,
      Extract of hyoscyamus . . . . . . āā gr. ss.
      Cocoa butter . . . . gr. xlv.—M.

Sig. Use as a suppository. (*In acute prostatitis.*)
                    Journal des Practiciens.

1737—℞ Extracti glandulæ suprarenalis . . . . ʒiv.

Pone in capsulas no. xlviii.
Sig. One to two capsules after each meal. (*Used in chronic
enlargement of prostate.*)

1738—℞ Argenti nitratis . . . . gr. v.
      Aquæ destillatæ . . . . f ʒj.—M.

Sig. Instil a few drops into deep urethra once daily by means
of a deep urethral syringe. (*Used in chronic prostatitis.*)

1739—℞ Tincturæ cantharidis . . . . ♏xvj.
      Syrupi simplicis . . . . f ʒss.
      Aquæ destillatæ . . . . f ʒiss.—M.

Sig. A teaspoonful every four hours.   RINGER.

PROSTATORRHŒA.

1740—℞ Collodii cum cantharide . . . . f ʒss.

Sig. Paint on one side of the perineum, confining the patient in bed. Paint the other side as soon as the soreness of the first application subsides. VAN BUREN AND KEYES.

1741—℞ Potassii citratis . . . . ʒss-j.
Spts. limonis . . . . f ʒss.
Syr. simplicis . . . . f ʒij.
Aquæ . . . . f ʒj.—M.

Sig. A dessertspoonful, largely diluted with water, three or four times daily. VAN BUREN AND KEYES.

1742—℞ Tinct. ferri muriatis . . . . f ʒvj.
Tinct. cantharidis . . . . f ʒij.—M.

Sig. Fifteen drops in a wineglassful of water three times daily. BARTHOLOW.

1743—℞ Argenti nitratis . . . . gr. v.
Aquæ destillatæ . . . . f ʒij.—M.

Sig. Instil a few drops into deep urethra once daily with deep urethral syringe. (*When resulting from old gonorrhœa.*)

1744—℞ Tincturæ nucis vomicæ . . . . f ʒj.
Tincturæ ferri chloridi . . . . f ʒiij.—M.

Sig. Twenty drops three times a day. (*In debilitated cases.*) GROSS.

PRURIGO, PRURITUS.

1745—℞ Acidi carbolici . . . . ʒj.
Potassæ fusæ . . . . ʒss.
Aquæ . . . . f ʒx.—M.

Sig. Apply locally. J. C. WILSON.

1746—℞ Naphthol . . . . gr. ccxxv.
Saponis viridis . . . . ʒxiiss.
Cretæ præparatæ . . . . ʒiiss.
Adipis . . . . ʒcxxv.—M.

Fiat unguentum.
Sig. Apply to the parts, and then powder them with starch. KAPOSI.

1747—℞ Acidi carbolici . . . . gr. vj.
Aquæ . . . . f ʒj.—M.

Sig. Apply three times daily. (*In pruritus ani.*) CHRISTOPHER HEATH.

1748—℞ Menthol . . . . ʒj.
Alcohol . . . . f ʒss.
Aquæ destillatæ . . . . f ʒj.
Acid. acetic. dilut. . . . . f ʒij.—M.

Sig. Use locally. CUMSTON.

1749—℞ Sodii salicylatis . . . . ʒiij.
Syr. acaciæ . . . . f ʒj.
Aquæ menthæ pip. . . . . ad f ʒiij.—M.

Sig. A dessertspoonful three times daily. (*With rheumatic or diabetic diathesis.*) ICARD.

1750—℞ Chloroform . . . . ℨlxlv.
Vaselin . . . . ʒj.—M.

Sig. Use locally. (*Vulvar pruritus.*)

1751—℞ Sodii hyposulphitis . . . . ʒvliss.
Acidi carbolici . . . . gr. lxxv.
Glycerini . . . . f ʒiv.
Aquæ . . . . f ʒviiss.—M.

Fiat lotio.
Sig. Bathe with cold water and apply the solution every day or two. (*For pruritus ani.*) JOHNSTON.

1752—℞ Resorcin . . . . gr. xxx.
Ichthyol . . . . ʒj.
Lanolin . . . . ʒij.—M.

Sig. Use locally. (*Senile pruritus.*)

1753—℞ Liquoris ammonii acetatis . . . . . . f ʒij.
   Acidi hydrocyanici diluti . . . . . . f ʒj.
   Tincturæ digitalis . . . . f ʒiij.
   Aquæ rosæ . . . . f ʒv.

Fiat lotio.
Sig. Apply to affected part twice daily. (*In senile prurigo.*)
            A. T. THOMPSON.

1754—℞ Olei staphisagriæ . . . . f ʒj.
   Adipis . . . . ʒj.

Fiat unguentum.
Sig. Apply once or twice daily.   BALMANNO SQUIRE.

1755—℞ Aquæ laurocerasi . . . . f ʒj.
   Acidi nitrici diluti . . . . f ʒss.
   Acidi hydrocyanici diluti . . . . . . f ʒiv.
   Glycerini . . . . f ʒj.
   Lactis amygdalæ . . . . ʒxij.

Fiat lotio. (*In pruritus vulvæ.*)   GREENHALGH.

1756—℞ Plumbi iodidi . . . . gr. xlj.
   Unguenti ceræ albæ . . . . ʒj.
   Chloroformi . . . . ꝫ ꟿ viij-xlj.
   Glycerini . . . . f ʒj.

Misce et fiat unguentum. (*In obstinate cases.*)   NELIGAN.

1757—℞ Picric acid . . . . gr. iv.
   Vaselin,
   Lanolin . . . . āā ʒss.—M.

Sig. Use locally.   *Journal de Médecine de Paris.*

1758—℞ Cocainæ muriatis . . . . gr. v.
   Lanolini . . . . ʒj.—M.

Fiat unguentum.
Sig. Apply locally after washing with warm water. (*In pruritus ani.*)
            BESNIER.

1759—℞ Zinci oxidi . . . . ʒiss.
   Potassii bromidi . . . . ʒiiss.
   Ext. cannabis indicæ . . . . ʒss.
   Glyceriti amyli . . . . ʒviiss.—M.

Sig. Wash the parts with very hot lotions of flaxseed, and
then apply the above. (*In vulvar pruritus.*)   MÉNIÈRE.

1760—℞ Hydrargyri chloridi corrosivi . . . . . gr. j.
   Pulv. aluminis . . . . ꝫj.
   Pulv. amyli . . . . ʒiss.
   Aquæ . . . . f ʒvj.—M.

Sig. Apply locally.   GOODELL.

1761—℞ Acidi hydrocyanici diluti . . . . f ʒij.
   Sodii boratis . . . . ʒj.
   Aquæ rosæ . . . . f ʒviij.—M.

Sig. Lotion.   FOX.

1762—℞ Phenazoni . . . . gr. xij.

Fiant chartulæ no. xii.
Sig. A powder to relieve itching of skin.

1763—℞ Argenti nitratis . . . . gr xx.
   Aquæ destillatæ . . . . f ʒj.—M.

Sig. Paint over the affected parts. (*In pruritus vulvæ.*)
            BARTHOLOW.

1764—℞ Iodoformi . . . . ʒj.
   Adipis . . . . ʒj.

Fiat unguentum.
Sig. Apply to affected part once or twice daily.   TANTURRI.

1765—℞ Extracti nucis vomicæ . . . . gr. iij.
   Fellis bovini . . . . gr. vj.
   Extracti taraxaci . . . . gr. xxiv.
   Pulveris myrrhæ . . . . gr. xviij.

Misce et divide in pilulas xxiv.
Sig. One thrice a day.   NELIGAN.

PRURIGO, PRURITUS (Continued).

1766—℞ Morphinæ sulphatis . . . . gr. vj.
    Sodii boratis . . . . ʒiv.
    Aquæ camphoræ . . . . f ʒvj.—M.
Ft. lotio.
Sig. Wash the parts with warm water and castile soap and
apply the lotion twice daily.   BAER.

1767—℞ Chloral. hydratis,
    Pulv. camphoræ . . . . āā ʒj.
    Vaselini . . . . ʒx.—M.
Sig. Use twice daily. (In hemiplegic prurigo.) KOEBNER.

1768—℞ Chloral. hydratis . . . . gr. lxxv-cl.
    Aquæ laurocerasi . . . . f ʒxIiss.
    Aquæ destillatæ . . . . f ʒl.—M.
Ft. solutio.
Sig. Apply locally.   VIDAL.

1769—℞ Iodoformi . . . . ʒj.
    Ceræ flavæ . . . . ʒvj.
    Olei olivæ . . . . q. s. ut ft. ungt.
Ft. unguentum.
Sig. Apply locally.   GREGORY.

PSORIASIS. (See Skin Diseases.)

PTYALISM.

1770—℞ Acidi tannici . . . . ʒj.
    Mellis rosæ . . . . f ʒij.
    Aquæ . . . . f ʒvj.—M.
Sig. Use as a mouth-wash.   BARTHOLOW.

1771—℞ Potassii chloratis . . . . ʒij.
    Infusi rhois glabri radicis . . . . . . Oj.—M.
Sig. Mouth-wash.   FAHNESTOCK.

1772—℞ Phénol sodique . . . . f ʒviij.
Sig. Teaspoonful in half-glass of water as mouth-wash every
two or three hours.

1773—℞ Potassii permanganatis . . . . gr. xxv.
    Sodii biboratis,
    Pulveris aluminis . . . . āā ʒij.
    Potassii chloratis . . . . ʒss.
    Tincturæ capsici . . . . f ʒj.
    Aquæ coloniensis,
    Tincturæ myrrhæ,
    Tincturæ krameriæ . . . . āā f ʒj.
    Tincturæ cinchonæ . . . . f ʒij.
    Aquæ destillatæ . . . . f ʒviij.—M.
Sig. For a mouth-wash.   J. E. GARRETSON.

1774—℞ Sulphuris præcipitati . . . . ʒij-iv.
    Potassii chloratis . . . . ʒij-ʒj.
    Liquoris morphinæ sulphatis . . . . . f ʒj-iss.
    Misturæ amygdalæ . . . . f ʒvij.
Misce bene.
Sig. Two tablespoonfuls every three or four hours.
       STYRAP.

1775—℞ Listerinæ . . . . f ʒiv.
Sig. Teaspoonful in wineglass of water as mouth-wash every
two or three hours.

1776—℞ Potassii permanganatis . . . . gr. ij-x.
    Aquæ destillatæ . . . . f ʒj.—M.
Sig. Use as a mouth-wash. (To correct the fetor.)
       J. E. GARRETSON.

1777—℞ Liquoris plumbi subacetatis . . . . . ʒj.
    Aquæ destillatæ . . . . f ʒviij.—M.
Sig. As a mouth-wash, every hour or two.   GROSS.

1778—℞ Pulv. aluminis . . . . ℨss.
Decocti quercus albæ . . . . Oss.—M.
Sig. Use as a gargle every hour, to remove the fetor of breath of mercurial salivation. KORTÜM.

1779—℞ Acidi hydrochlorici . . . . f℥ij.
Syr. rubi . . . . f℥xv.—M.
Sig. In obstinate salivation, add enough of the above to acidify strongly a portion of sage-tea. Gargle every hour with the mixture. KOPP.

1780—℞ Atropinæ sulphatis . . . . gr. j.
Aquæ destillatæ . . . . f℥ij.—M.
Sig. Four minims three times daily. BARTHOLOW.

1781—℞ Tinct. iodi . . . . f℥ij.
Aquæ rosæ . . . . f℥viij.—M.
Sig. Use as a mouth-wash every hour or two. RINGER.

PUERPERAL CONVULSIONS. (See also Convulsions.)

1782—℞ Naphthol . . . . gr. xxxviij.
Sacchari,
Bismuthi salicylatis . . . . āā gr. xxxj.
Misce et div. in capsulas no. viij.
Sig. One capsule three times a day. (*Preventive.*) RIVIÈRE.

1783—℞ Aquæ destillatæ,
Syrupi pruni virginianæ . . . . . āā f℥ij.
Chloral. hydratis,
Sodii bromidi . . . . āā ℨss-ℨj.—M.
Sig. A tablespoonful in water every hour. RIVIÈRE.

PUERPERAL FEVER. (See Fever.)

PUERPERAL MANIA. (See Mania.)

PUERPERAL PERITONITIS. (See Peritonitis.)

PURPURA.

1784—℞ Sodii sulphatis . . . . ℨij.
Ferri sulphatis . . . . gr. iij.
Acidi sulphurici diluti . . . . ℳxv.
Tinct. hyoscyami . . . . ℳxl.
Infusi calumbæ . . . . f℥ij.—M.
Sig. To be taken in the morning. TANNER.

1785—℞ Quininæ sulphatis . . . . gr. ix.
Acidi phosphorici diluti,
Tincturæ ferri chloridi . . . . . . āā f℥iss.
Liquoris arsenici chloridi . . . . . . ℳxv-xl.
Syrupi zingiberis . . . . f℥vj.
Infusi quassiæ . . . . f℥viij.—M.
Sig. One-sixth part after breakfast, dinner, and supper.
TANNER.

1786—℞ Extracti glandulæ suprarenalis . . . . ℨj.
Pone in capsulas no. xxiv.
Sig. One to four capsules three times a day after meals. (*Used in purpura with vasomotor relaxation.*)

1787—℞ Liq. potassii arsenitis . . . . ℨss.
Sig. Five drops in water, after meals, three times daily. (*When due to iodism.*) PHILLIPS.

1788—℞ Syr. ferri superphosphatis,
Liq. hydrogenii perox. (10 vol.),
Glycerini puri . . . . āā f℥iss.
Aquæ destillatæ . . . . ad f℥vj.—M.
Sig. A tablespoonful thrice daily. GUITÉRAS.

PURPURA (Continued).

1789—℞ Ext. hamamelidis fld. . . . . f 3ij.
Sig. A teaspoonful every one to three hours.
J. V. Shoemaker.

1790—℞ Olei terebinthinæ . . . . f 3iij.
    Extracti digitalis fluidi . . . . f 3j.
    Mucilaginis acacie . . . . f 3ss.
    Aquæ menthæ piperitæ . . . . f 3j.
Misce et fiat emulsio.
Sig. A teaspoonful every three hours. (*In the hemorrhagic form.*)
Bartholow.

1791—℞ Acidi gallici . . . . 3ss.
    Acidi sulphurici diluti . . . . f 3j.
    Tincturæ opii deodoratæ . . . . . . f 3j.
    Infusi rosæ compositi . . . . f 3iv.—M.
Sig. A tablespoonful every four hours or oftener.
Bartholow.

1792—℞ Extracti ergotæ aquosi . . . . ɔj.
    Pulveris ipecacuanhæ . . . . gr. x.
    Acidi gallici . . . . ɔj.
Misce et fiant pilulæ no. xx.
Sig. One pill every hour or two. (*With hemorrhage.*)
Bartholow.

PYÆMIA.

1793—℞ Quininæ sulphatis . . . . gr. v-xx.
Ft. pulv. no. i.
Sig. To be taken every four hours.
Ringer.

1794—℞ Olei eucalypti. . . . . 3j.
Dispensa in capsulas no. xvi.
Sig. One capsule every three hours.
J. C. Wilson.

1795—℞ Salopheni . . . . 3ij.
Fiant chartulæ no. xii.
Sig. One powder three times a day. (*Used as intestinal antiseptic and to neutralize and eliminate toxins.*)

1796—℞ Acidi salicylici . . . . 3ss.
    Sodii biboratis . . . . 3j.
    Glycerini . . . . f 3j.
    Aquæ menthæ piperitæ . . . . f 3v.—M.
Sig. A tablespoonful every two or three hours. Bartholow.

PYROSIS. (See also Acidity.)

1797—℞ Magnesii sulphatis . . . . 3j.
    Tinct. hyoscyami . . . . ℳxv.
    Aquæ . . . . f 3ij.—M.
Ft. haustus.
Sig. To be taken three times daily.
Aitken.

1798—℞ Sodii bicarbonatis . . . . 3iss.
    Olei anisi . . . . : . . . . gtt. j.
    Syrupi aurantii florum,
    Aquæ destillatæ. . . . . ää f 3j.—M.
Sig. One dose.
Piorry.

1799—℞ Quininæ sulphatis . . . . gr. xxij.
    Pepsini . . . . ɔvss.
    Extracti absinthii . . . . q. s.
Misce et fiant pilulæ no. xl.
Sig. Two before each meal.
Piorry.

1800—℞ Tinct. nucis vomicæ . . . . f 3ij-iv.
    Acidi nitrici diluti . . . . f 3vj.
    Syr. zingiberis . . . . ad f 3iij.—M.
Sig. A teaspoonful in a wineglassful of water. Phillips.

1801—℞ Extracti nucis vomicæ . . . . gr. iss.
    Argenti nitratis . . . . gr. ij.
    Extracti lupuli . . . . gr. xij.
Misce et divide in pilulas vi.
Sig. One pill three times a day.
Barlow.

1802—℞ Acidi carbolici . . . . gr. j.
Alcoholis . . . . f ʒj.—M.

Sig. Twenty-five drops in a wineglassful of water before each
meal. PODMORE JONES.

1803—℞ Terebene . . . . gr. ccxxv.
Pulv. acaciæ . . . . ʒiv.
Aquæ . . . . ʒxv.
Pulv. sacchari albi . . . . ʒxlv.
Pulv. tragacanthæ . . . . ʒij.—M.

Ft. trochisci no. c.
Sig. One three times daily. VIGIER.

1804—℞ Sodii bicarbonatis . . . . ʒj.
Aquæ menthæ viridis . . . . . q. s. ad f ʒviij.—M.

Sig. Shake. Tablespoonful two hours after meals.

1805—℞ Acidi sulphurosi . . . . ʒss-j.
Aquæ . . . . f ʒij.—M.

Ft. haustus.
Sig. To be taken shortly before meals. LAWSON.

QUINSY.

1806—℞ Acidi boracici . . . . ʒij.
Eau de Pagliari . . . . f ʒx.
Aquæ . . . . f ʒvij ʒviss.

Misce et fiat gargarisma.
Sig. Use as a gargle several times daily, and each time follow
by an application of—

1807—℞ Iodoformi . . . . ʒj.
Collodii flexilis . . . . ʒvij.—M.

Sig. "Iodoform collodion." LEBRUN.

1808—℞ Tabellas protonucleini no. xxiv . . āā gr. v.

Sig. One tablet dissolved in mouth every hour until flushing
of face ; then one tablet every two or three hours. (*Used at
onset of attack.*)

1809—℞ Tinct. guaiaci ammoniatæ . . . . . . f ʒij.

Sig. A teaspoonful in half a glassful of milk three or four
times daily. (*In the early stage.*) SAJOUS.

1810—℞ Tabellas extracti glandulæ suprarc-
nalis no. xxiv . . . . āā gr. v.

Sig. Dissolve a tablet on the tongue every four hours. (*Used
in formative stage.*)

1811—℞ Tinct. belladonnæ . . . . f ʒss.

Sig. Five drops in a tablespoonful of water every one to
three hours. PHILLIPS.

1811*bis*—℞ Tinct. aconiti radicis . . . . f ʒss.

Sig. Half a drop or a drop every ten minutes or quarter of an
hour for two hours, and afterwards hourly. RINGER.

1812—℞ Quininæ sulphatis . . . . gr. x-xv.

Fiat chartula.
Sig. Take before pus forms. (*To abort an impending attack.*)
BARTHOLOW.

1813—℞ Ichthyoli . . . . f ʒiij.
Unguenti belladonnæ . . . . ʒij.
Olei citronellæ . . . . ℳiiij.
Adipis lanæ hydrosi . . . . ʒij.—M.

Sig. Apply freely externally.

1814—℞ Hydrargyri chloridi corrosivi . . . . . gr. j.
Aquæ destillatæ . . . . f ʒj.—M.

Sig. Five minims every two hours. Or—

1815—℞ Hydrargyri chloridi mitis . . . . gr. ss.
Sacchari lactis . . . . ʒss.

Misce et fiant chartulæ no. x.
Sig. One powder every two hours. Or—

1816—℞ Hydrargyri cum cretâ . . . . ʼ. . . . . gr. ij.
Sacchari albi . . . . ℥ss.

Misce et fiant chartulæ no. x.
Sig. One powder every two hours.   BARTHOLOW.

1817—℞ Hydrargyri cum cretâ . . . . gr. v.
Sacchari lactis . . . . gr. x.—M.

In pulv. no. xv div.
Sig. A powder every hour. (*When the tonsils almost meet.*)
                                                RINGER.

1818—℞ Salinaphthol. . . . . gr. xx–xxv.
Spts. vini rectificati . . . . f℥j.—M.

Sig. One part to twenty parts of water, as an antiseptic gargle.
                                                GEORGI.

1819—℞ Sodii salicylatis . . . . ℥iij–iv.
Syr. acaciæ . . . . f℥ss.
Aquæ cinnamomi . . . . ad f℥iij.—M.

Sig. A dessertspoonful every three hours.   EASBY.

1820—℞ Zinci iodidi . . . . gr. iv.
Aquæ destillatæ . . . . f℥j.—M.

Sig. Apply with a camel's-hair pencil to the hypertrophied
tonsils twice daily.   C. P. W. FISHER.

RACHITIS, RICKETS, SCROFULA, STRUMA.

1821—℞ Phosphori . . . . gr. iij.
Solve in—
  Carbonis sulphureti . . . . ♏lxxv.
  Aquæ destillatæ . . . . f℥v.—M.

Sig. Half a teaspoonful twice daily. The bottle must be kept
tightly corked. No sugar must be combined with the
preparation, but it may be given after taking the dose.
                                                HASTERLIK.

1822—℞ Olei morrhuæ . . . . f℥v.
Phosphori . . . . gr. iij.—M.

Ft. sol.
Sig. One teaspoonful daily.   KASSOWITZ.

1823—℞ Phosphori . . . . gr. ⅛.
Olei amygdalæ dulcis . . . . f℥viiss.
Pulv. acaciæ,
Sacchari albi . . . . āā ℥iv.
Aquæ destillatæ . . . . f℥x.—M.

Ft. emulsio.
Sig. A teaspoonful two or three times daily.   CANALI.

1824—℞ Olei morrhuæ . . . . f℥vj.
Syr. calcis lactophosphatis,
Liq. calcis . . . . āā f℥iij.—M.

Sig. One to two teaspoonfuls three or four times daily. To it
may be added the syrup of the iodide of iron.
                                           J. LEWIS SMITH.

1825—℞ Ferri et quininæ citratis . . . . gr. x.
Olei morrhuæ,
Glycerini . . . . āā f℥ij.—M.

Sig. A tablespoonful thrice daily.   HARTSHORNE.

1826—℞ Olei morrhuæ . . . . f℥iss.
Creasoti . . . . gtt. iv.
Pulv. tragacanthæ comp. . . . . ℈ij.
Aquæ anisi . . . . f℥ivss.—M.

Sig. One-half to two tablespoonfuls thrice daily. THOMPSON.

1827—℞ Morrhuol . . . . f℥j.
Fiant capsulæ no. xx.
Sig. Three to four capsules daily.   LAFARGUE.

1828—℞ Calcii phosphatis . . . . gr. v–x.
Fiat chartula.
Sig. Three times a day, in chalk mixture, or along with cod-
liver oil.   BUDD.

1829—℞ Syrupi calcii lactophosphatis . . . . . f℥iv.

Sig. Adult dose, a teaspoonful three times a day. (*May also be given to the nursing mother.*)   BARTHOLOW.

1830—℞ Calcii phosphatis,

Ferri phosphatis . . . . āā gr. xxxvj.

Misce et fiaut chartulæ no. xii.

Sig. Ouc powder morning and noon.   NELIGAN.

1831—℞ Calcii sulphidi . . . . gr. xv.

Confect. rosæ . . . . q. s. ut ft. massa.—M.

In pil. no. xxx div.

Sig. One to two pills every two to six hours. (*In suppurating scrofulous glands.*)   RINGER.

1832—℞ Syrupi ferri iodidi . . . . f℥j-ij.

Syrupi simplicis . . . . . q. s. ad f℥ij.—M.

Sig. A teaspoonful three times a day.   NIEMEYER.

1833—℞ Syrupi ferri et manganesii iodidi . . . f℥j-ij.

Syrupi simplicis . . . . . . q. s. ad f℥ij.—M.

Sig. A teaspoonful three times a day.   BARTHOLOW.

1834—℞ Potassii iodidi,

Potassii chloratis . . . . āā ʒj.

Potassii bicarbonatis . . . . ʒiij.

Misce et fiaut chartulæ no. xii.

Sig. One three times a day, in warm milk.   ERICHSEN.

1835—℞ Olei delphinidæ (porpoise-oil) . . . . Oss.

Sig. From a teaspoonful to a tablespoonful au hour after meals, thrice daily. Also by inunction.   WEST.

1836—℞ Potassii iodidi . . . . gr. xxx.

Tinct. iodi,

Acidi tannici . . . . āā gr. xv.

Syr. quininæ . . . . f℥viiss.

Syr. acaciæ . . . . f℥iv ʒvss.

Misce.

Sig. A fourth part to be taken every two hours until four doses are taken by an adult. For children, a corresponding fractional dose.   GUIBOUT.

1837—℞ Iodi . . . . gr. x.

Potassii iodidi . . . . gr. xx.

Aquæ . . . . f℥ij.—M.

Sig. Eight to twelve minims in a glassful of water, three or four times daily, for an adult.   SHAPTER.

1838—℞ Iodol. . . . . gr. xxiij.

Olei morrhuæ . . . . f℥viij.

Spts. menthæ pip. . . . . gtt. xx.—M.

Sig. A tablespoonful after each meal. (*In enlarged glands, or strumous skin-diseases.*)   MONIN.

1839—℞ Iodol. . . . . ʒiiss.

Mucil. tragacanthæ . . . . . q. s. ut ft. massa.—M.

In pil. no. xxx div.

Sig. One pill three times daily.   SEIFERT.

1840—℞ Acidi tannici . . . . gr. vj-xij.

Fiant chartulæ no. xii.

Sig. One powder two or three times a day. (*In rickets.*)   ALISON.

1841—℞ Tincturæ nucis vomicæ . . . . f℥j.

Extracti stillingiæ fluidi . . . . . . f℥v.

Syrupi sarsaparillæ compositi . . . . f℥ij.—M.

Sig. Five to fifteen drops three times a day, in water. (*In struma.*)   BARTHOLOW.

1842—℞ Liq. potassii arsenitis . . . . ℳxvj.

Aquæ destillatæ . . . . f℥ij.

Sig. Teaspoonful three times daily after food. (*For a child.*)   HARE.

1843—℞ Calcii chloridi . . . . ℨj.
Extracti conii . . . . gr. xv.
Aquæ cinnamomi . . . . f ℨss.
Solve.
Sig. Shake well. Eight to sixteen drops three times a day,
to a child ten years old. PHOEBUS.

1844—℞ Calcii chloridi . . . . ℨss.
Syr. simplicis . . . . f ℨiv.—M.
Sig. For children, a teaspoonful thrice daily. For adults,
three times the dose is taken. SPILLMANN.

1845—℞ Acidi hydrocyanici dil. . . . . f ℨj.
Glycerini . . . . f ℨij.
Acidi nitrici dil. . . . . f ℨiij.
Infusi quassiæ . . . . ad f ℨxiiss.-M.
Sig. A tablespoonful thrice daily. AITKEN.

1846—℞ Quininæ sulphatis . . . . gr. j.
Acidi sulphurici dil. . . . . ♏j-ij.
Vini ferri . . . . f ℨj-ij.—M.
Sig. To be taken three times daily. WM. JENNER.

1847—℞ Carbonis animalis,
Pulveris glycyrrhizæ . . . . . . āā ℨvj.
Misce et detur in scatula.
Sig. Half or a whole teaspoonful twice a day. RADIUS.

1848—℞ Pulveris glandis quercus torrefactæ . ℨj.
Aquæ bullientis . . . . Oj.
Fiat infusum.
Sig. Three or four teacupfuls during the day, and augmented.
(*In commencing rachitis, glandular swellings, etc. Continue
for a long time.*) HUFELAND.

1849—℞ Ferri bromidi . . . . gr. xij.
Confectionis rosæ . . . . gr. xviij.
Misce et fiant pilulæ no. xx.
Sig. One three times a day. (*In strumous dyspepsia.*)
ROBERT DICK.

RATTLESNAKE-BITE.

1850—℞ Hydrargyri chloridi corrosivi . . . . . gr. j.
Potassii iodidi . . . . gr. ij.
Brominii . . . . ℨiiss.
Alcoholis diluti . . . . ℨxxx.—M.
Ft. sol.
Sig. A teaspoonful in wine or brandy as often as necessary.
BIBRON.

1851—℞ Aquæ ammoniæ . . . . ℨj.
Aquæ . . . . ℨiij.—M.
Sig. Inject thirty minims hypodermically into a superficial
vein above the seat of injury. HALFORD.

1852—℞ Potassii permanganatis . . . . ℨss.
Aquæ destillatæ . . . . ℨiij.—M.
Sig. Apply to the wound, and inject hypodermically above
the seat of injury. At the same time take internally the
following: •

1853—℞ Aquæ ammoniæ . . . . ℨiv.
Sig. A half-teaspoonful in water, repeated every ten or fifteen
minutes. HAWACK AND ARBOC.

REMITTENT FEVER. (See Fever.)

RENAL CALCULI. (See Calculi.)

RENAL DROPSY. (See Dropsy.)

RENAL HEMORRHAGE. (See Hæmaturia.)

1854—℞ Acidi salicylici . . . . ȝiij.
Potassii bicarbonatis . . . . ȝvj.
Aquæ . . . . f ȝij.—M.

Sig. A teaspoonful every three hours. DONNELLY.

1855—℞ Salol . . . . ȝj.
Menthol . . . . gr. xl.
Ether . . . . f ȝj.
Lanolin . . . . ȝviss.—M.

Sig. Locally. LEMOINE.

1856—℞ Acidi salicylici . . . . ȝss.
Ferri pyrophosphatis . . . . ȝj.
Sodii phosphatis. . . . . ȝx.
Aquæ . . . . f ȝvj.—M.

Sig. A tablespoonful every two hours until the improvement
justifies less frequent doses, or unless constitutional effects
are produced. G. L. PEABODY.

1857—℞ Sodii salicylatis . . . . ȝvj.
Glycerini . . . . ȝiv.
Aquæ cinnamomi . . . . ad f ȝvj.—M.

Sig. A tablespoonful every two or three hours until tinnitus
aurium is produced ; then every four to six hours until the
acute symptoms have abated. Then give—

1858—℞ Sodii bicarbonatis . . . . ∴ ȝiv-vj.

In pulv. no. xii div.
Sig. A powder in a half-glassful of water every four hours
until the urine is alkaline to test-paper. If the patient is
anæmic, omit the salicylate and begin on the soda at once,
and give cod-liver oil and iron from the first. (*In robust
cases.*) A. L. LOOMIS.

1859—℞ Ergotinæ . . . . gr. xv.
Sodii salicylatis . . . . ȝiiss.
Aquæ destillatæ . . . . f ȝvj.—M.

Sig. A tablespoonful every hour. (*The ergot obviates thickening
of the tympanum.*) SCHILLING.

1860—℞ Sodii salicylatis . . . . gr. xv.
Sodii bicarbonatis . . . . gr. xxx.
Aquæ menthæ pip. . . . . f ȝss.—M.

Sig. To be taken every third or fourth hour. When the acute
symptoms abate, then give—

1861—℞ Mist. ferri et ammonii acetatis (U.S.P.) ȝiv.

Sig. A dessertspoonful or two in a wineglassful of water,
thrice daily. J. C. WILSON.

1862—℞ Terpinol.
Alcohol (85 per cent.) . . . . āā ȝiiss.
Guaiacol. . . . . ȝj.

Sig. Use locally. LEMOINE.

1863—℞ Liquid vaselin . . . . ȝv.
Methyl salicylate . . . . ȝiij.—M.

Sig. Use locally. LEMOINE.

1864—℞ Sodii bicarbonatis,
Ammonii carbonatis . . . . āā gr. v.
Acidi salicylici . . . . gr. xx.
Aquæ destillatæ . . . . f ȝs.—M.

Sig. One dose. (*This avoids unpleasant cerebral symptoms, sick
stomach, and rapid collapse.*) PRIDEAUX.

1865—℞ Lithii bromidi . . . . ȝij.
Vini cocæ . . . . f ȝiv.—M.

Sig. A dessertspoonful in water every two or three hours.
J. C. WILSON.

1866—℞ Salicinæ . . . . gr. xv.

Fiat chartula.
Sig. This amount every three hours. T. J. McLAGAN.

1867—℞ Olei gaultheriæ . . . . f ℥j.

Sig. Fifteen or twenty minims to be given in capsules or floated on milk or water every two hours until the acute symptoms abate; then gradually diminish to one drachm daily until convalescence; then combine iron. If any joint-stiffness remains, then give—

1868—℞ Lithii salicylatis . . . . ℈ij-iij.

Sig. To be given, dissolved in water, during the twenty-four hours.   KINNICUTT.

1869—℞ Sodii bicarbonatis . . . . ℨiss.
            Potassii acetatis . . . . ℨss.
            Liquoris ammonii acetatis . . . . . . f ℨiij.
            Aquæ destillatæ . . . . f ℥iss.—M.

Sig. One dose. To be taken in a state of effervescence, in combination with—

1870—℞ Acidi citrici . . . . ℨss.
            Aquæ destillatæ . . . . f ℥j.—M.

                                                     FULLER.

1871—℞ Ammonii chloridi,
            Potassii bromidi . . . . āā ℨss.
            Tincturæ cinchonæ compositæ . . . . f ℥ij.
            Syrupi zingiberis,
            Aquæ destillatæ . . . . āā f ℥j.—M.

Sig. One fluidrachm every two hours. With—

1872—℞ Saloli . . . . ℨij.
            Phenacetini . . . . ℨij.—M.

Fiant chartulæ no. xxiv.
Sig. One powder every four to six hours. (Useful in acute and subacute cases with gastric disturbances.)

1873—℞ Tincturæ aconiti (B. P.) . . . . ℳxij.
            Ammonii sulphidi . . . . ℳxvj.
            Aquæ menthæ piperitæ . . . . f ℥vj.—M.

Sig. A fourth part every fourth hour until the fever is abated.
                                      J. MORTIMER GRANVILLE.

1874—℞ Potassii nitratis . . . . gr. xv.
            Pulveris ipecacuanhæ compositii . . . gr. iij.

Misce et fiat chartula.
Sig. One dose. To be taken every fourth hour. (In subacute rheumatism.)   DA COSTA.

1875—℞ Pulveris colchici . . . . gr. iij.
            Potassii sulphatis . . . . gr. iv.
            Potassii bicarbonatis . . . . gr. iij.

Tere simul ut fiat pulvis.
Sig. One every three or four hours. (In subacute rheumatism.)
                                                     HADEN.

1876—℞ Aquæ camphoræ . . . . f ℥iss.
            Liquoris ammonii acetatis . . . . . . f ℥ss.
            Vini antimonii . . . . gtt. xl.
            Tincturæ opii deodoratæ . . . . . . gtt. xx.

Misce et fiat haustus.
Sig. At bedtime.   BLANC.

1877—℞ Hydrochinon . . . . ℨss.
            Aquæ cinnamomi . . . . f ℥iij.—M.

Sig. One-half to three teaspoonfuls two to four times daily until the fever abates.   SYLVESTRINI AND PICCHINI.

1878—℞ Antifebrin . . . . ℨj.

Fiant capsulæ no. xvi.
Sig. One or two capsules three to six times daily.
                                                   EISENHART.

1879—℞ Antipyrin . . . . ℨiij.
            Syr. aurantii cort. . . . . f ℥j.
            Aquæ . . . . ad f ℥iij.—M.

Sig. A dessertspoonful in water thrice daily. (In afebrile cases.)   GERMAIN SÉE.

1880—℞ Propylaminæ . . . . gr. xxiv.
     Aquæ menthæ pip. . . . . f ʒvj.—M.
Sig. A tablespoonful every two or three hours.   JAS. TYSON.

1881—℞ Sodii bicarbonatis . . . . ʒij.
     Acidi salicylici . . . . ʒiij.
     Glycerini,
     Aquæ destillatæ . . . . āā f ʒij.—M.
Sig. One teaspoonful every four hours.   N. B. KENNEDY.

1882—℞ Liq. ammonii ichthyosulphatis (30 per
     cent.) . . . . ʒij.
     Lanolini . . . . ʒj.—M.
Ft. unguentum.
Sig. To be rubbed over the swollen joints. Take internally
the following:

1883—℞ Ichthyol. . . . . ʒj.
Fiant capsulæ no. xx.
Sig. Three to six capsules during the twenty-four hours. (*In
both acute and chronic cases.*)   SCHMIDT.

1884—℞ Sodii salicylatis,
     Potassii citratis . . . . āā gr. xv.
     Aquæ . . . . f ʒss.—M.
Sig. To be given every two hours until the pain and fever
abate. Also the following:

1885—℞ Liq. opii sedativi . . . . ʒj.
     Potassii bicarbonatis . . . . ʒiv.
     Glycerini . . . . f ʒij.
     Aquæ bullientis . . . . f ʒix.—M.
Sig. "Fuller's Lotion." Soak a piece of flannel or spongio-
piline in the above hot solution, and wrap it around the
painful joint.   OSLER.

1886—℞ Pimentæ . . . . ʒvj ʒij.
     Aquæ ammoniæ. . . . . f ʒiij ʒj.
     Ess. thymi,
     Chloral. hydratis . . . . āā ʒiiss.
     Spts. vini rectificati (60°) . . . . . . Oij.—M.
Ft. linimentum.
Sig. "Apone." Use pure or mixed with olive oil. (*For fric-
tion about rheumatic joints.*)   POULET.

RHEUMATISM, CHRONIC.

1887—℞ Lithiæ citratis . . . . ʒij.
     Strychninæ . . . . gr. j.
     Tinct. strophanthi . . . . f ʒiss.
     Aquæ menthæ pip. . . . . . q. s. ad f ʒiv.—M.
Sig. A teaspoonful before each meal, in water.   BROWER.

1888—℞ Aloes . . . . gr. ij.
     Pulv. ipecac. . . . . gr. j.
     Pulv. rhei,
     Ferri sulph. exsiccati,
     Ext. hyoscyami . . . . āā gr. x.—M.
Divide in capsulas no. x.
Sig. One at bedtime.   BROWER.

1889—℞ Lithii salicylatis . . . . ʒiij.
     Syrupi simplicis . . . . f ʒij.
     Aquæ aurantii flor. . . . . ad f ʒvj.—M.
Sig. A tablespoonful thrice daily.   VULPIAN.

1890—℞ Pulveris guaiaci resinæ,
     Potassii iodidi . . . . āā gr. x.
     Tincturæ colchici seminis . . . . . . f ʒss.
     Aquæ cinnamomi,
     Syrupi simplicis . . . . . . āā q. s. ad f ʒj.—M.
Sig. A dessertspoonful to a tablespoonful thrice daily.
                           Philadelphia Hospital.

1891—℞ Sodium iodid.............. ʒiv.
Wine of colchicum .... f ʒiv.
Ammoniated tincture of guaiac.
Fluid extract of erythroxylon .. āā f ʒvij.
Fluid extract of cimicifuga...... f ʒvj.—M.

Sig. One teaspoonful thrice daily.   A. A. ESHNER.

1892—℞ Potassii bicarbonatis .... ʒss.
Vini colchici radicis .... f ʒij.
Tincturæ guaiaci .... f ʒij.
Syrupi aurantii corticis .... f ʒij.—M.

Sig. A dessertspoonful thrice daily in water. (*In rheumatic arthritis.*)   DA COSTA.

1893—℞ Olei terebinthinæ,
Spts. camphoræ,
Aquæ ammoniæ,
Olei olivæ............ āā f ʒj.—M.

Ft. linimentum.
Sig. Use locally.   HARTSHORNE.

1894—℞ Potassii iodidi.............. ʒj-ij.
Aquæ cinnamomi........... f ʒvj.—M.

Sig. A tablespoonful thrice daily.   HARTSHORNE.

1895—℞ Tinct. guaiaci æth. .... f ʒj.
Tinct. cannabis indicæ æth...... f ʒvj.
Tinct. colchici æth........... f ʒij.—M.

Sig. Twenty-five to thirty drops on sugar every four hours.   ATLEE.

1896—℞ Potassii iodidi .... ʒiij.
Vini colchici sem.,
Tinct. opii camph. .... āā f ʒij.
Tinct. stramonii .... f ʒvj.
Tinct. cimicifugæ........... f ʒiij.—M.

Sig. A teaspoonful thrice daily.   *St. Luke's Hospital, N. Y.*

1897—℞ Potassii et sodii tartratis .... ʒss.
Potassii nitratis .... ʒv.
Vini colchici sem............ f ʒij.
Aquæ .. .. q. s. ad f ʒij.—M.

Sig. A teaspoonful thrice daily.   *Bellevue Hospital, N. Y.*

1898—℞ Sulphuris .... ʒj.
Potassii bitartratis .... ʒj.—M.

Pone in cachetas no. xxiv.
Sig. One cachet three times a day after meals.

1899—℞ Sassafras radicis corticis .... ʒiss.
Mezerei .... ʒiv.
Taraxaci radicis .... ʒiij.
Aquæ ferventis .... Oj.

Misce et fiat infusum.
Sig. From one to one and a half fluidounces three times a day, with a plentiful use of diluents.   FULLER.

1900—℞ Iodoformi,
Ferri redacti .... āā gr. xliij.
Extracti glycyrrhizæ .... q. s.

Misce et divide in pilulas no. lx.
Sig. Two to be taken thrice daily.   KNOLL.

1901—℞ Liquoris potassii arsenitis .... f ʒij.
Potassii iodidi............. ʒij.
Syrupi simplicis............ f ʒiij.—M.

Sig. A teaspoonful thrice daily, in water, between meals. (*In rheumatic arthritis.*)   DA COSTA.

1902—℞ Calcii chloridi .... ʒiij.
Syr. simplicis............. f ʒiv.
Olei gaultheriæ .... gtt. iv.—M.

Sig. A tablespoonful thrice daily for adults. One-third dose for children. Also use externally—

1903—℞ Calcii chloridi . . . . ʒj.
Aquæ . . . . f ʒxliss.—M.
Ft. lotio.
Sig. Soak lint in the solution and wrap it about the joints.
DUCKWORTH.

1904—℞ Tinct. aconiti,
Chloroformi,
Aquæ ammoniæ . . . . ãã f ʒij.
Linimenti saponis comp. . . . . . ad f ʒviij.—M.
Ft. linimentum.
Sig. Use locally. *Jefferson Hospital, Phila.*

1905—℞ Linimenti aconiti (B.P.),
Linimenti belladonnæ . . . . . . ãã f ʒij.
Glycerini . . . . ad f ʒij.—M.
Ft. linimentum.
Sig. Apply locally over the seat of pain. FOTHERGILL.

1906—℞ Tincturæ iodi,
Alcoholis . . . . ãã f ʒss.—M.
Sig. Apply morning and evening. DA COSTA.

1907—℞ Aconitinæ . . . . gr. v.
Olei olivæ . . . . f ʒss.
Tere simul et adde—
Adipis . . . . ʒviiss.
Olei bergamii . . . . ℳx.
Olei santali . . . . ℳij.—M.
Ft. unguentum. (*In neuralgic rheumatism.*) FULLER.

1908—℞ Olei cajuputi,
Tincturæ opii . . . . ãã f ʒij.
Olei terebinthinæ . . . . f ʒiv.
Linimenti ammoniæ . . . . f ʒj.—M.
Ft. linimentum. FULLER.

1909—℞ Chloroformi,
Tincturæ aconiti radicis . . . . . ãã f ʒij.
Olei terebinthinæ . . . . f ʒss.
Olei sassafras . . . . ℳxx.
Linimenti saponis camphorati . . . . f ʒiiss.—M.
Ft. linimentum. J. C. WILSON.

1910—℞ Acidi salicylici . . . . ʒj-iss.
Lanolini . . . . ʒiij.
Olei olivæ . . . . q. s. ad f ʒvj.—M.
Sig. Apply as directed. ZEBALD.

1911—℞ Olei monardæ . . . . f ʒss.
Tincturæ opii . . . . f ʒij.
Tincturæ camphoræ . . . . f ʒij.—M.
Ft. linimentum. W. ATLEE.

RHINITIS. (See also Catarrh.)

1912—℞ Menthol . . . . gr. iij.
Caffeæ tostæ,
Sacchari albi . . . . ãã gr. l.—M.
Ft. pulv.
Sig. To be used like ordinary snuff. RABOW.

1913—℞ Cocainæ hydrochloratis . . . . gr. iss.
Caffeæ tostæ,
Sacchari albi . . . . ãã gr. l.—M.
Ft. pulv.
Sig. To be used as snuff. (*Used in rare cases where the preceding is ineffectual.*) RABOW.

1914—℞ Naphthol. (β) . . . . ʒij.
Spts. vini rectificati (90°) . . . . . . f ʒij.—M.
Sig. A teaspoonful in a pint and a half of tepid water. Use as a douche, or with an atomizer. (*In ozæna and purulent rhinitis.*) A. RUAULT.

RICKETS. (See Rachitis.)

RINGWORM. (See Skin Diseases.)

RUBEOLA. (See Fever.)

RUPIA. (See Skin Diseases.)

SALIVATION. (See Ptyalism.)

SARCINÆ ET TORULÆ.

1915—℞ Acidi sulphurosi . . . . fℨj–iss.
      Infusi calumbæ. . . . . fℨxij.—M.
Ft. haustus.
Sig. A wineglassful ten minutes before meals.   LAWSON.

1916—℞ Acidi sulphurosi . . . . fℨss–j.
      Aquæ . . . . fℨij.—M.
Ft. haustus.
Sig. To be taken thrice daily.   TANNER.

1917—℞ Acidi sulphurosi . . . . fℨij.
      Syrupi aurantii corticis . . . . fℨij.
      Aquæ destillatæ . . . . q. s. ad fℨvj.—M.
Sig. One to two tablespoonfuls every four hours.
      RUSSELL REYNOLDS.

1918—℞ Sodii hyposulphitis . . . . ℨij.
      Infusi quassiæ. . . . . fℨvj.
Ft. solutio.
Sig. A tablespoonful three times daily.   R. NEALE.

1919—℞ Sodii sulphitis. . . . . ℨss.
      Aquæ destillatæ. . . . . fℨiss.
Misce et fiat haustus.
Sig. Three times a day. (*The dose may be increased.*)
      JENNER.

SATYRIASIS. (See Nymphomania.)

SCABIES. (See also Lice.)

1920—℞ Oil of sweet almonds . . . . fℨij.
      Salol . . . . ℨj.—M.
Sig. Anoint the body with this mixture every night, and then
rub lightly with flowers of sulphur.
      St. Louis Hospital, Paris.

SCARLATINA. (See also Fever and Diphtheria.)

1921—℞ Ammonii carbonatis . . . . ℨj–iss.
      Syr. simplicis . . . . fℨj.
      Aquæ . . . . ad fℨiss.—M.
Sig. A teaspoonful every hour, or every two or three hours,
according to the severity of the case.   PEART.

1922—℞ Ammonii carbonatis . . . . ℨj.
      Syrupi acaciæ. . . . . fℨvj.
      Liquoris ammonii acetatis . . q. s. ad fℨij.—M.
Sig. A teaspoonful every two hours.   DA COSTA.

1923—℞ Infusi digitalis . . . . fℨiv.

Sig. One-half to one teaspoonful every two, three, or four
hours.   BARTHOLOW.

1924—℞ Tincturæ digitalis . . . . fℨss.
      Syrupi simplicis . . . . fℨss.
      Aquæ destillatæ . . . . q. s. ad fℨij.—M.

Sig. A teaspoonful every hour or two, according to age.
      BARTHOLOW.

1925—℞ Ichthyoli . . . . fℨij.
      Adipis lanæ hydrosi . . . . ℨvj.—M.
Sig. Apply freely in front and to side of neck. (*For anginous
sore throat. To be used in conjunction.*)

—S—

1950—℞ Spiritus glonoini . . . . ꝳij.
Morphinæ sulphatis. . . . . gr. ¼ vel ½.
Aquæ destillatæ . . . . ℳxxx.—M.

Sig. Injected by means of long hypodermic needle deeply inserted into tissues about the nerve.

1951—℞ Antipyrin. . . . . ꝫij.
Syr. aurantii cort. . . . . fꝫss.
Aquæ aurantii flor. . . . . ad fꝫij.—M.

Sig. A dessertspoonful every hour to four hours, until three to six doses are taken.   GERMAIN SÉE.

1952—℞ Methyl. chloridi . . . . fꝫss.

Sig. Apply with an atomizer locally, but with care. DEBOVE.

1953—℞ Saloli . . . . ꝫss.
Olei vaselini . . . . fℨv.—M.

Sig. Inject twenty or thirty minims hypodermically over the course of the nerve.   MEUNIER.

1954—℞ Saloli,
Sacchari lactis . . . . āā ꝫiij.—M.

In pulv. no. xii div.
Sig. A powder every four to six hours.   ASCHENBACH.

1955—℞ Quininæ sulphatis . . . . ꝫss-ꝫj.
Tincturæ ferri chloridi . . . . fꝫij.
Spiritus ætheris nitrosi . . . . fℨiv.
Syrupi simplicis . . . . fꝫij.
Vini xerici . . . . q. s. ad fℨiv.—M.

Sig. A tablespoonful every three or four hours.
H. V. SWERINGEN.

1956—℞ Extracti ergotæ fluidi . . . . fꝫij.
Aquæ cinnamomi . . . . fꝫiij.—M.

Sig. A dessertspoonful in water every three or four hours.
(*Tinct. ferri chloridi may be added if indicated.*)
EDWARD WAAKES.

1957—℞ Emplastri epispastici, 1⅛ × 5 in.

Sig. Apply over affected part for five or six hours, poultice, remove the cuticle, and dress with—

1958—℞ Morphinæ sulphatis . . . . gr. ¼.
Pulveris marantæ . . . . gr. ij.

Misce et fiat chartula.
Sig. Sprinkle over blister. Ten grains of Dover's powder at night.   DA COSTA.

1959—℞ Acidi osmici . . . . gr. ij.
Aquæ destillatæ . . . . ℳcc.—M.

Sig. Sixteen minims hypodermically at the seat of pain, at first daily, then less frequently.   STEKOULIA.

SCIRRHUS. (See Cancer.)

SCLEROSIS (POSTERIOR SPINAL). (See also Locomotor Ataxia.)

1960—℞ Argenti nitratis . . . . : . . . . gr. ¼.
Aquæ . . . . q. s.—M.

Sig. Inject with hypodermic syringe.   ROSENBAUM.

1961—℞ Potassii iodidi . . . . ℨvj-ℨviij.
Ferri et ammonii citratis . . . . ꝫij.
Tincturæ aurantii corticis,
Syrupi simplicis . . . . āā fꝫij.
Aquæ menthæ piperitæ . . . . q. s. ad fℨiv.—M.

Sig. A teaspoonful in water about an hour after each meal.
H. V. SWERINGEN.

1962—℞ Argenti nitratis,
Extracti belladonnæ . . . . āā gr. vj-viij.
Extracti gentianæ . . . . q. s.

Misce et fiant pilulæ no. xxiv.
Sig. One after each meal.   A. McL. HAMILTON.

SCLEROSIS (POSTERIOR SPINAL) (Continued).

1963—℞ Extracti belladonnæ . . . . gr. iv.
　　　Olei terebinthinæ . . . . f ʒij.
　　　Olei theobromæ . . . . q. s.—M.
Fiant capsulæ no. xii.
Sig. One thrice daily.　　　　　　　　A. McL. HAMILTON.

1964—℞ Tincturæ ferri chloridi,
　　　Tincturæ nucis vomicæ,
　　　Acidi phosphorici diluti,
　　　Syrupi simplicis . . . . ãã f ʒj.—M.
Sig. A teaspoonful in water about an hour before each meal.
　　　　　　　　　　　　　　　　H. V. SWERINGEN.

1965—℞ Acidi phosphorici diluti . . . . . . f ʒvj. .
　　　Syrupi simplicis . . . . f ʒiij.—M.
Sig. A teaspoonful in water thrice daily, gradually increased
to a dessertspoonful. (*Along with electricity*.)　W. LAMBERT.

1966—℞ Antipyrin. . . . . ʒij.
　　　Syr. sarsaparillæ comp. . . . . f ʒij.
　　　Aquæ cinnamomi . . . . ad f ʒvj.—M.
Sig. A tablespoonful every hour or two until relieved.
　　　　　　　　　　　　　　　　　　SUCKLING.

1967—℞ Ætheris . . . . f ʒiij.
Sig. Spray over the painful area or nerve-trunk with an
atomizer.　　　　　　　　　　　　　　RAISON.

SCROFULA. (See Rachitis.)

SCURVY.

1968—℞ Succi limonis . . . . f ʒviij.
Sig. Two tablespoonfuls daily. More may be given. With
potatoes and other fresh vegetables.　　　PARKES.

1969—℞ Succi limonis . . . . f ʒvj.
Sig. Use locally and generally *ad libitum*.　　GARROD.

1970—℞ Acidi hydrochlorici . . . . f ʒj.
　　　Mellis,
　　　Aquæ rosæ . . . . ãã f ʒj.
Misce et fiat linctus.
Sig. Apply to affected gums three or four times a day.
　　　　　　　　　　　　　　　　　　BRANDE.

1971—℞ Potassii nitratis . . . . gr. xx.
　　　Acidi citrici . . . . ʒss.
　　　Syrupi aurantii corticis . . . . f ʒvj.
　　　Aquæ destillatæ . . . . f ʒvj.—M.
Sig. The sixth part three or four times a day.　McLACHLAN.

1972—℞ Potassii bitartratis . . . . ʒj.
　　　Olei limonis . . . . ℳxv.
　　　Sacchari albi . . . . ʒij.
　　　Aquæ bullientis . . . . Oij.—M.
Ft. haustus.
Sig. Use when cold as a drink.　　　　　　TANNER.

1973—℞ Sodii chloridi . . . . Ɔx.
　　　Potassii chloratis . . . . ʒss.
　　　Potassii et sodii tartratis . . . . Ɔv.
　　　Sodii phosphatis . . . . Ɔiiss.
　　　Succi limonis recentis . . . . f ʒvj.
　　　Syr. limonis . . . . f ʒxlv.
　　　Aquæ . . . . Ovij.—M.
Sig. To be taken as a drink, iced or not, as agreeable.
　　　　　　　　　　　　　　　　　　TANNER.

SEA-SICKNESS.

1974—℞ Antipyrin. . . . . gr. lxxv.
　　　Cocaïnæ hydrochloratis . . . . gr. iss.
　　　Caffeini . . . . gr. iv.
　　　Strychninæ sulphatis . . . . gr. ⅗.
　　　Spts. vini gallici . . . . f ʒiiss.
　　　Aquæ destillatæ . . . . f ʒxxiiss.-M.
Sig. A tablespoonful before embarking, and two others
during the day, or three during the twenty-four hours.
　　　　　　　　　　　　　　　　　ROUQUETTE.

1975—℞ Amyli nitritis . . . . f ʒij.
Sig. Inhale three to five drops from a handkerchief, with
care. BARTHOLOW.

1976—℞ Cerii oxalatis . . . . gr. ij.
Tincturæ valerianæ ammoniatæ . . . f ʒj.
Aquæ destillatæ . . . . f ʒj.
Misce et fiat haustus.
Sig. Every half-hour. WALSH.

1977—℞ Spiritus chloroformi,
Tincturæ cardamomi compositæ . āā f ʒij.—M.
Sig. A teaspoonful in water every half-hour. BARTHOLOW.

1978—℞ Cocainæ hydrochloratis . . . . 0.15.
Spiritus vini rectificati . . . . q. s. ut fiat solutio.
Dein adde—
Aquæ destillatæ . . . . 150.00.—M.
MANASSEIN.

1979—℞ Acetanilidi . . . . gr. xlviij.
Fiant chartulæ no. xxiv.
Sig. One powder on tongue every two or three hours.

1980—℞ Sodii bromidi . . . . ʒj.
Ammonii bromidi . . . . ʒss.
Aquæ menthæ pip. . . . . f ʒv.—M.
Sig. A tablespoonful before meals and at bedtime. To be
used for three days before embarking. BEDARD.

1981—℞ Chloroformi . . . . f ʒss.
Sig. Two to five minims on sugar every half-hour until relieved. BARTHOLOW.

1982—℞ Chloral. hydratis . . . . ʒss.
Aquæ camphoræ . . . . f ʒj.—M.
Sig. One dose. PRIESTLEY.

1983—℞ Sol. nitro-glycerin. (1 per cent.) . . . . ʒij.
Sig. One or two drops two or three times daily.
TRUSSEWITSCH.

1984—℞ Arseniate of strychnine . . . . gr. ₁⁄₁₀₀.
Hyoscyamine . . . . gr. ₁⁄₃₄₀.
Hydrobromate of morphine . . . . gr. ₁⁄₁₀.—M.
Sig. To be taken every fifteen minutes, for an hour or two.
LE GRIX.

1985—℞ Chloroform . . . . ℳxlv.
Alcohol . . . . f ʒss.
Aromatic elixir . . . . f ʒss.—M.
Sig. Twenty to forty drops as needed.
Journal de Médecine de Paris.

SEPTICÆMIA. (See Pyæmia.)

SHINGLES. (See also Skin Diseases, Herpes Zoster.)

1986—℞ Collodii . . . . f ʒj.
Sig. Paint over the affected parts. WARING.

1987—℞ Collodii flexilis . . . . f ʒj.
Sig. Apply with a brush to the affected area constantly, to
exclude the air. ANSTIE.

1988—℞ Magnesii carbonatis . . . . gr. xx.
Vini colchici radicis,
Tincturæ opii . . . . āā f ʒss.
Aquæ camphoræ . . . . f ʒj.
Misce et fiat haustus. (*To relieve the deep-seated pain in chest.*)
A. T. THOMPSON.

1989—℞ Sulphuris sublimati . . . . ʒj.
Hydrargyri ammoniati . . . . ʒss.
Unguenti simplicis . . . . ʒj.
Misce et fiat unguentum.
Sig. Apply two or three times a day. CORFE.

1990—℞ Zinci phosphidi,
Ext. nucis vomicæ . . . . āā gr. x.—M.
Ft. massa et in pil. no. xxx div.
Sig. One pill every two to four hours.   BULKLEY.

1991—℞ Pulv. amyli . . . . ℥iv.
Sig. Dust over the eruption and on a muslin band sewed tightly around the body, to protect it from the friction of the clothes.   BULKLEY.

1992—℞ Liq. sodæ chlorinatæ . . . . f℥iv.
Aquæ . . . . f℥ij.—M.
Ft. lotio.
Sig. Apply to the ulcerated vesicles.   FOURNIER.

1993—℞ Bismuthi subnitratis . . . . ℥iv.
Hydrarg. chloridi mitis,
Zinci oxidi . . . . āā ℥j.—M.
Ft. pulvis.
Sig. Dust on cotton, and apply to the ulcerated vesicles after washing them with the solution of chlorinated soda.
    FOURNIER.

1994—℞ Veratriæ . . . . ℈j–ij.
Vaselini . . . . ℥j.—M.
Ft. unguentum.
Sig. Apply locally. *(For the neuralgia following shingles.)*
    RINGER.

SICK HEADACHE. (See Headache.)

SINGULTUS. (See Hiccough.)

SKIN DISEASES.

1995—℞ Sulphuris præcip. . . . . ℥iv.
Glycerini . . . . ℥iss.
Spts. camphoræ . . . . f℥j.
Aquæ . . . . f℥iv.—M.
Sig. Apply with a brush to the affected part before retiring at night. *(In acne.)*   LAILLER.

1996—℞ Potassii acetatis . . . . ℥iv.
Tinct. nucis vomicæ . . . . f℥ij.
Ext. rumicis fld. . . . . ad f℥iv.—M.
Sig. One teaspoonful, well diluted, after meals, thrice daily.
(In acne.)   BULKLEY.

1997—℞ Magnesii sulphatis . . . . ℥ss.
Acidi sulphurici aromatici . . . . . ℳxx.
Ferri sulphatis . . . . gr. iij.
Quininæ sulphatis . . . . gr. j.
Vini colchici radicis . . . . ℳx.
Syrupi zingiberis . . . . f℥j.
Aquæ destillatæ . . . . f℥j.
Misce et fiat haustus.
Sig. To be taken twice or thrice a day, with an aperient pill, if necessary. *(In acne.)*   TILBURY FOX.

1998—℞ Hydrargyri oxidi rubri,
Hydrargyri ammoniati . . . . . . āā gr. v.
Adipis . . . . ℥j.—M.
Fiat unguentum. *(In acne.)*   TILBURY FOX.

1999—℞ Creasoti . . . . ℳv–xv.
Adipis . . . . ℥ss.—M.
Fiat unguentum. *(In acne)*   JOY.

2000—℞ Zinci oxidi . . . . ℥ij.
Pulveris amyli . . . . ℥iv.—M.
Fiat pulvis. *(In eczema, acne, impetigo.)*   CAZENAVE.

2001—℞ Sulphuris præcip. . . . . ℨj–iss.
Glycerini . . . . f℥j.
Spts. vini rectificati . . . . f℥ss.
Aquæ rosæ . . . . ad f℥iv.—M.

Ft. lotio.
Sig. To be painted on at night, after steaming the face and washing it with sand-soap. To be washed off in the morning with warm gruel, and the face powdered with—

2002—℞ Zinci oleatis,
Pulv. talci . . . . āā ℨj.—M.
Sig. To be dusted on every morning. (*In acne.*)   JAMIESON.

2003—℞ Acidi chrysophanici . . . . gr. xxiv.
Vaselini . . . . ℨj.—M.

Ft. unguentum.
Sig. Wash the skin with soap and dry it at night. Rub the ointment well in. Repeat every night until a sharp dermatitis is produced. Cease inunction until the dermatitis disappears; then repeat the process. (*In acne.*)
J. T. METCALF.

2004—℞ Saponis mollis . . . . ℨiv.
Aquæ coloniensis . . . . f℥ij.—M.
Sig. Moisten a flannel with hot water, then dip it into the solution, and rub firmly over the skin. Wash well with warm water, dry with friction, and anoint with zinc ointment. (*In acne, with thick, sluggish skin.*)   JAMIESON.

2005—℞ Potassii acetatis . . . . ℨj.
Acidi acetici . . . . ℨss.
Spts. ætheris nitrosi . . . . f℥iss.
Ext. taraxaci fld. . . . . f℥ij.—M.
Sig. A teaspoonful before meals, in water. (*In acne indurata.*)
BULKLEY.

2006—℞ Calcis vivæ . . . . ℨj.
Sulphuris sublimati . . . . ℨij.
Aquæ . . . . f℥x.—M.
Coque ad f℥vi.
Sig. Apply after bathing with hot water at night. Wash off with gruel in the morning, and apply the powder. (*In acne rosacea.*)   VLEMINCKX.

2007—℞ Sulphuris præcip.,
Cretæ præcip.,
Aquæ laurocerasi,
Spts. vini rectificati,
Glycerini . . . . āā ℨij.—M.
Ft. lotio.
Sig. Bathe the face with hot water and dry it with friction, then apply the lotion. (*In acne of the face.*)   LEROY.

2008—℞ β-Naphthol. . . . . 10 gram.
Vaselini flavi,
Saponis viridis . . . . āā 20 gram.
Sulphuris præcip. . . . . 50 gram.
Sig. To be applied by the physician, and to remain fifteen to sixty minutes, then gently removed and replaced by powder or white paste. This is repeated, after the peeled surface is healed, or the following may remain over-night:

2009—℞ Resorcin. . . . . 2.5–5.0 gram.
Zinci oxidi,
Amyli . . . . āā 5 gram.
Vaselini flavi . . . . 12.5 gram.—M.
Ft. pasta. (*In acne vulgaris and rosacea.*)   LASSAR.

2010—℞ Bismuthi oxidi,
Pulv. amyli . . . . āā gr. xxx.
Kaolin. . . . . ℨj.
Glycerini . . . . f℥iss.
Aquæ rosæ . . . . q. s.—M.
Sig. To be painted on the spots and allowed to dry. Wash carefully before making a new application. (*In chloasma.*)
UNNA.

2011—℞ Zinci oxidi . . . . gr. iij.
Hydrargyri ammoniati . . . . gr. iss.
Olei theobromæ,
Olei ricini . . . . āā 3iss.
Ess. rosæ . . . . gtt. x.—M.

Sig. Apply to the face night and morning. (*In the chloasma of pregnancy.*) MONIN.

2012—℞ Ext. opii . . . . gr. x-xx.
Acidi tannici . . . . ǝj.
Unguenti . . . . ʒj.—M.

Sig. Apply after the inflammatory condition has been subdued with lead lotion. (*In idiopathic ecthyma.*)
TILBURY FOX.

2013—℞ Hydrargyri iodidi rubri . . . . gr. xij.
Cerati simplicis . . . . 3viiss.—M.

Ft. unguentum.
Sig. Apply locally. (*In ecthyma syphilitica.*) DIDAY.

2014—℞ Quininæ sulphatis . . . . 3ss.
Acidi sulphurici aromatici . . . . . . fʒss.
Tincturæ cardamomi compositi . . . . fʒiss.
Aquæ destillatæ . . . . q. s. ad fʒiv.—M.

Sig. A dessertspoonful three times a day. (*In ecthyma.*)
RINGER.

2015—℞ Sodii biboratis . . . . ʒij-iij.
Aquæ rosæ . . . . fʒvj.—M.

Fiat lotio.
Sig. Apply two or three times daily. (*In ecthyma.*)
COPLAND.

2016—℞ Chrysarobin. . . . . gr. xx.
Ætheris . . . . fʒj.—M.

Sig. Use as a spray. (*In mycotic eczema.*) HEBRA.

2017—℞ Naphthol . . . . 5 grammes.
Black soap. . . . . 50 "
Powdered chalk . . . . 10 "
Prepared lard . . . . 100 "

Mix.
Sig. Twice daily. (*In eczema.*) KAPOSI.

2018—℞ Calaminæ,
Zinci oxidi . . . . āā ʒij vel ʒiij.
Glycerini,
Alcoholis . . . . āā fʒj.
Liq. calcis,
Aquæ . . . . q. s. ad fʒij.—M.

Sig. Locally. (*In acute eczema.*) STELWAGON.

2019—℞ Acidi hydrocyanici diluti . . . . . . ♏xl.
Olei cadini . . . . fʒj.
Saponis viridis . . . . ʒij.
Olei rosmarini . . . . fʒiss.
Aquæ destillatæ . . . . q. s. ad fʒv.—M.

Fiat linimentum. (*In eczema.*) ANDERSON.

2020—℞ Carbolic acid . . . . gr. x.
Acetanilid . . . . gr. xxx.
Petrolatum . . . . ʒj.

Sig. Locally. Thoroughly cleanse the affected parts with soap and warm water. (*Infantile eczema.*) WELLS.

2021—℞ Citrine ointment,
Chaulmoogra ointment . . . of each ʒss.—M.

Sig. Apply once daily. (*In obstinate chronic eczema, scrofuloderma, lupus, leprosy, and tuberculosis of the skin.*)
SHOEMAKER.

2022—℞ Oil of cade . . . . fʒiss.
Ammoniated mercury . . . . gr. xl.
Chaulmoogra ointment . . . . ʒj.—M.

Sig. Apply thoroughly. (*In chronic eczema, psoriasis, lichen, and scleroderma.*) SHOEMAKER.

2023—℞ Balsam of Peru . . . . ʒj.
Sulphuretted potash ointment . . . . ʒj.—M.

Sig. Apply thoroughly. (*In chronic eczema, psoriasis, and in itch and ringworm.*) SHOEMAKER.

2024—℞ Sodium sozoiodol . . . . ʒij.
Zinc oxid. . . . . ʒiv.
Vaselin . . . . ʒx.—M.

Sig. Apply twice daily. (*Palmar eczema.*)   S. E. Hale.

2025—℞ Cocainæ hydrochloratis . . . . gr. j.
Potassii bromidi . . . . gr. x.
Aquæ destillatæ,
Glycerini . . . . āā fʒiiss.—M.

Sig. Apply to the gums. (*In the eczema of dentition.*) Besnier.

2026—℞ Sodii bromidi . . . . gr. ivss-viiss.
Syr. aurantii flor. . . . . fʒij.—M.

Sig. One teaspoonful every two hours. (*In the eczema of dentition.*) Besnier.

2027—℞ Zinci oxidi . . . . ʒij.
Vaselini . . . . ʒvj.—M.

Sig. Apply locally and cover with a rubber mask. (*In the eczema of dentition.*) Besnier.

2028—℞ Crystallized acetic acid . . . . 2 parts.
Glycerin . . . . 50 "
Cherry-laurel water (dist.) . . . . . . 200 " —M.

Sig.—Paint on the eyelid once a day. (*In palpebral eczema.*)
Lailler.

2029—℞ Liquoris plumbi subacetatis . . . . . . ℥xl.
Vini opii . . . . fʒj.
Aquæ rosæ . . . . fʒviij.

Misce et fiat lotio. (*In eczema.*)   Burgess.

2030—℞ Potassii iodidi . . . . gr. viij.
Decocti dulcamaræ . . . . fʒiv.
Decocti ulmi . . . . fʒxij.—M.

Sig. A wineglassful at bedtime. (*In eczema.*)   Neligan.

2031—℞ Extracti staphisagriæ,
Zinci oxidi . . . . āā ʒss.
Adipis benzoatæ . . . . ʒj.—M.

Fiat unguentum. (*In chronic eczema.*)   Bazin.

2032—℞ Infusi cinchonæ . . . . fʒvj.
Aquæ calcis . . . . fʒixss.
Tincturæ lupulinæ,
Succi conii . . . . āā fʒij.—M.

Sig. A wineglassful three times a day. (*In chronic eczema.*)
Neligan.

2033—℞ Hydrargyri oxidi rubri,
Hydrargyri ammoniati . . . . . . āā gr. vj.
Adipis . . . . ʒj.—M.

Sig. Apply locally. (*In ecthyma syphilitica.*) Startin.

2034—℞ Acidi citrici . . . . gr. xv.
Aquæ laurocerasi . . . . ʒj.
Olei rusci [birch] . . . . gtt. xv.
Ungt. aquæ rosæ . . . . ʒx.—M.

Sig. Use thrice daily. Use starch-powder between the applications. Carefully attend to diet. (*In acute eczema.*) Monin.

2035—℞ Acidi boracici . . . . gr. xv
Pulv. acaciæ . . . . ʒij.
Olei vaselini . . . . ʒviiss.
Aquæ . . . . fʒxv.—M.

Fiat emulsio.
Sig. Apply locally. Bismuth, zinc, sulphur, or other substance may be added. (*In eczema.*) Knaggs.

2036—℞ Pulv. acidi salicylici . . . . gr. xv-xxx.
Pulv. zinci oxidi,
Pulv. amyli . . . . āā ʒiij gr. viij.
Vaselini puri . . . . ʒvj gr. xv.

Misce et fiat unguentum.
Sig. Apply locally, and cover with cotton after rubbing the ointment in. (*In papulous or squamous eczema, or infantile intertrigo.*) Lassar.

2037—℞ Sodii arseniatis . . . . gr. ¾.
Aquæ destillatæ . . . . f ʒiv ʒij.-M.

Sig. A teaspoonful thrice daily. With saline purgative twice weekly. Apply locally the following:

2038—℞ Hydrargyri ammoniati . . . . gr. xv.
Vaselini . . . . ʒv.
Ess. rosæ . . . . ℩lij.—M.

Sig. Apply gently every evening. Every eight or ten days use the following:

2039—℞ Pilocarpinæ nitratis . . . . gr. iss.
Aquæ destillatæ . . . . ℩lxxv.—M.

Sig. Six drops to be injected hypodermically. Contra-indicated in diseases of the heart and great vessels. (*In eczema about the menopause.*)　　　　　　J. CHÉRON.

2040—℞ Olei cadini,
Saponis mollis,
Spiritus rectificati . . . . āā f ʒj.
Olei lavandulæ . . . . f ʒiss.—M.

Sig. After washing, rub in firmly night and morning. (*In eczema.*)　　　　　　ANDERSON.

2041—℞ Zinci oxidi . . . . ʒij.
Glycerini . . . . f ʒij.
Liquoris plumbi subacetatis . . . . . f ʒss.
Aquæ calcis . . . . q. s. ad f ʒvj.—M.

Ft. lotio. (*In eczema.*)　　　　　　TILBURY FOX.

2042—℞ Bismuthi subnitratis . . . . ʒss.

Detur in scatula.
Sig. Dust the affected parts. (*In erythema of the genitals, etc., of infants.*)　　　　　　BARTHOLOW.

2043—℞ Tinct. belladonnæ . . . . f ʒss.

Sig. Five drops thrice daily to a child of two years. The dose should cause dryness of the throat, that it may affect the cutaneous circulation. (*In infantile eczema.*)　　　　　　BARTHOLOW.

2044—℞ Zinci oxidi,
Picis liquidæ . . . . āā partes æquales.

Misce et fiat cataplasma.
Sig. Apply locally. (*In impetiginous eczema after the crusts are removed.*)　　　　　　ELLIOTT.

2045—℞ Pulv. oryzæ . . . . ʒiiss.
Plumbi oxidi,
Glycerini . . . . āā ʒviiss.
Acidi acetici diluti . . . . f ʒxv.—M.

Coque ad ʒxx.
Sig. Use locally. (*In eczema of the hands and fingers. Useful also in painful fissures of the genitals.*) This paste resembles, in color, the skin.　　　　　　UNNA.

2046—℞ Acidi acetici cryst. . . . . gr. iij.
Glycerini . . . . ℩lxxv.
Aquæ laurocerasi . . . . f ʒv.—M.

Sig. Apply daily with a stiff camel's-hair brush. (*In eczema of the eyelids.*)　　　　　　LAILLER.

2047—℞ Olei cadini . . . . ʒss.
Glycerini . . . . ʒj.
Ungt. diachyli. . . . . ʒiiss.—M.

Ft. unguentum.
Sig. Apply locally. (*In squamous eczema with thickened skin.*)　　　　　　TILBURY FOX.

2048—℞ Glyceriti amyli . . . . ʒviiss.
Acidi tannici,
Hydrarg. chloridi mitis . . . . . . āā gr. xv.—M.

Sig. Apply morning and evening. (*In dry eczema with itching.*)　　　　　　VIDAL.

2049—℞ Acidi salicylici . . . . gr. xlv.
Zinci oxidi . . . . ʒij.
Pulv. amyli . . . . ʒv.—M.

Sig. Dust the surface and cover with wadding. (*In acute eczema.*)　　　　　　ELLIOTT.

2050—℞ Menthol . . . . gr. xxx.
Resorcin . . . . gr. xv.
Sulphur. præcipitat. . . . . ʒiiss.
Zinci oxidi,
Vaselin . . . . āā ʒj.—M.
Fiat unguentum. (*Eczema with pruritus.*) THIBIERGE.

2051—℞ Antipyrin . . . . ʒiss.
Aquæ laurocerasi . . . . f ʒiij.—M.
Ft. lotio.
Sig. Apply as a lotion or on compresses. (*In chronic eczema.*)
CHENNEVIÈRE.

2052—℞ Hydrargyri ammoniati . . . . gr. xv.
Unguenti simplicis . . . . ʒv.—M.
Ft. unguentum.
Sig. For local use night and morning. (*In dry eczema, or
chapped lips.*) ROYER.

2053—℞ Resorcin . . . . ʒij.
Vaselini puri . . . . ʒxviij.—M.
Ft. unguentum.
Sig. Rub in three times daily, and dust on rice-powder. (*In
acute eczema of the hands.*) WIFS.

2054—℞ Potassii chloratis . . . . gr. xj.
Vini opii . . . . ♏xx.
Aquæ . . . . Oj.—M.
Sig. Wet compresses with the solution, and apply them to
the affected parts. If the inflammation is very acute, give
first a hot sitz-bath, and use poultices, sprinkled on the
surface with precipitated chalk. (*In eczema.*) MARTIN.

2055—℞ Pulv. camphoræ . . . . ʒss.
Pulv. zinci oxidi . . . . ʒiij.
Glycerini . . . . ♏xl.
Unguenti benzoini . . . . ʒj.—M.
Sig. Apply locally at once, or some isolating powder, as talc,
bismuth, or lycopodium, may be used first. (*In vesiculous
eczema.*) DUHRING.

2056—℞ Pulv. camphoræ . . . . ʒss–j.
Spts. vini rectificati . . . . f ʒj.
Sodii boratis . . . . ϶ij.
Aquæ rosæ . . . . f ʒviij.—M.
Ft. lotio.
Sig. Apply locally several times daily. (*In erythema. Also in
pruritus and eczema.*) TILBURY FOX.

2057—℞ Hydrargyri ammoniati . . . . gr. x.
Acidi carbolici cryst. . . . . gr. viiss.
Ungt. petrolei,
Ungt. zinci oxidi . . . . āā ʒss.
Olei olivæ . . . . ʒss.—M.
Sig. Apply two or three times daily. (*In general infantile
eczema.*) STELWAGON.

2058—℞ Resorcin.,
Zinci oxidi . . . . āā ʒj.
Ungt. aquæ rosæ . . . . ʒx.—M.
Ft. unguentum.
Sig. Apply locally. (*In chronic indurated eczema of infants.*)
FLIESBURG.

2059—℞ Olei morrhuæ . . . . ʒij.
Vitell. ovi . . . . no. j.
Liq. sodii arseniatis . . . . f ʒj.
Syrupi simplicis . . . . f ʒij.
Aquæ . . . . f ʒiv.—M.
Sig. A half-teaspoonful thrice daily. (*In chronic infantile
eczema.*) DOYON.

2060—℞ Ungt. zinci oxidi,
Ungt. plumbi subacetatis . . . . . āā ʒss.
Chloral. hydratis,
Pulv. camphoræ . . . . āā gr. xv.—M. .
Ft. unguentum.
Sig. Use two or three times daily, after bathing with warm
water. (*In general eczema.*) GROSS.

2061—℞ Ferri et ammonii citratis . . . . . . 3j.
 Potassii citratis . . . . 3ij.
 Liq. potassii arsenitis . . . . f3j-ij.
 Tinct. nucis vomicæ . . . . f3j.
 Tinct. cinchonæ comp. . . . . . ad f3iv.—M.
Sig. A teaspoonful in water after meals, as a tonic and alterative. (*In eczema.*) , BULKLEY.

2062—℞ Liq. plumbi subacetatis . . . . f3j.
 Glycerini,
 Aquæ . . . . ââ f3iv.—M.
Sig. To be applied two to four times daily with a camel's-hair pencil. (*In infantile eczema, when the surface is red, angry-looking, and discharging a thin, watery secretion.*)
J. LEWIS SMITH.

2063—℞ Pulv. camphoræ . . . . 3ss-j.
 Zinci oxidi . . . . 3iv.
 Pulv. amyli . . . . 3j.—M.
Sig. Dust on lightly, and do not allow to cake upon the skin. (*In erythema.*) BULKLEY.

2064—℞ Petrolei,
 Balsami peruviani . . . . ââ 3ss.
 Unguenti laurini [bay-leaf] (Ph. P.) . . gr. xvj.—M.
Ft. unguentum.
Sig. Apply with a camel's-hair pencil. Wash off, after remaining three hours, with warm water. (*In erythema following mercurial inunction.*) HEBRA.

2065—℞ Quininæ sulphatis . . . . 3ss.
 Acidi sulphurici aromatici . . . . . . 3ss.
 Ext. taraxaci fld. . . . . 3vj.
 Aquæ . . . . q. s. ad f3iv.—M.
Sig. A dessertspoonful thrice daily. (*In erythema nodosum, with impaired vital forces.*) BARTHOLOW.

2066—℞ Zinci acetatis . . . . gr. ij.
 Aquæ rosæ . . . . f3j.
 Unguenti aquæ rosæ . . . . 3j.—M.
Ft. unguentum. (*In erythema and herpes.*) NEUMANN.

2067—℞ Collodii . . . . f3j.
 Morphinæ . . . . gr. viij.—M.
Sig. Paint the affected surfaces. (*In herpes zoster.*) BOURDON.

2068—℞ Potassii chloratis . . . . Əij.
 Acidi hydrochlorici diluti,
 Spiritus chloroformi,
 Liquoris cinchonæ . . . . ââ f3j.
 Aquæ destillatæ . . . . q. s. ad f3vj.—M.
Sig. Two tablespoonfuls three times a day. (*In herpes zoster.*)
CHARLES STURGES.

2069—℞ Ferri arseniatis . . . . gr. iij.
 Extracti lupulinæ . . . . 3j.
 Pulveris althææ . . . . 3ss.
 Syrupi simplicis . . . . q. s.
Misce et fiant pilulæ no. xlviii.
Sig. One pill daily. (*In herpetic ulcers and cancerous diseases.*)
BIETT.

2070—℞ Ulmi corticis . . . . 3iss.
 Aquæ bullientis. . . . . Oj.—M.
Ft. decoctum.
Sig. Two to four fluidounces thrice daily. (*In ichthyosis.*)
LETTSOM.

2071—℞ Pulveris camphoræ . . . . gr. x.
 Unguenti zinci oxidi . . . . 3j.
Misce et fiat unguentum. (*In ichthyosis.*) ERASMUS WILSON.

2072—℞ Zinci sulphatis . . . . 3j.
 Cerati simplicis . . . . 3j.—M.
Ft. unguentum. (*In ichthyosis.*) ERASMUS WILSON.

2072*bis*—℞ Sodii bicarbonatis . . . . gr. xv-3ss.
 Adipis . . . . 3j.—M.
Ft. unguentum. (*In ichthyosis.*) DEVERGIE.

2073—℞ Potassii carbonatis . . . . ℈j.
Adipis . . . . ℥j.—M.

Ft. unguentum.
Sig. Smear over the eruption at night, and wash off in the morning with the following :

2074—℞ Potassii carbonatis . . . . ℨss.
Aquæ . . . . Oj.—M.

Ft. lotio.
Sig. Use in the morning locally, as directed. (*In herpes.*)
NELIGAN.

2075—℞ Aquæ coloniensis . . . . f ℨij.
Sig. Apply locally with a camel's-hair pencil. (*In herpes labialis.*)
HARTSHORNE.

2076—℞ Magnesii carbonatis . . . . ℨss.
Spiritus ammoniæ aromatici . . . . . f ℨij.
Tincturæ rhei . . . . f ℨij.
Aquæ calcis . . . . f ℨvss.—M.
Sig. One fluidounce twice daily. (*In acute herpes labialis.*)
BURGESS.

2077—℞ Hydrargyri chloridi mitis . . . . . . gr. x.
Adipis . . . . ℥j.—M.

Ft. unguentum.
Sig. Apply three times daily. (*In chronic herpes labialis.*)
NELIGAN.

2078—℞ Hydrargyri chloridi corrosivi . . . . . gr. iij.
Alcoholis . . . . q. s.
Solve et adde—
Extracti conii . . . . ℥j.
Misce et divide in pilulas no. xl.
Sig. Six pills to be taken in the day, and the quantity gradually increased to nine or ten. (*In herpetic eruptions.*)
KOPP.

2079—℞ Resorcin . . . . gr. xlv.
Cocaine . . . . gr. xv.
Alcohol . . . . f ℨiij.—M.
Sig. This is to be applied by means of a swab to the herpetic spot.

2080—℞ Pulv. camphoræ,
Chloral. hydratis . . . . āā ℨiv.—M.
Sig. Apply locally with a camel's-hair brush. (*In herpes labialis and herpes præputialis.*)
JAMIESON.

2081—℞ Hydrargyri chloridi mitis . . . . ℨj.
Unguenti simplicis . . . . ℥j.—M.

Ft. unguentum.
Sig. Apply locally. (*In herpes.*)
PAREIRA.

2082—℞ Glycerini . . . . ℨj.
Pulv. tragacanthæ comp. . . . . . . ℨij.
Mellis . . . . ℨij.
Liq. calcis saccharati . . . . f ℨiss.
Emulsionis amygdalæ . . . . f ℨviij.—M.
Sig. Apply locally. (*In herpes. Also in burns, chapped hands, etc.*)
TILBURY FOX.

2083—℞ Sodii boratis . . . . ℨss.
Morphinæ sulphatis . . . . gr. vj.
Aquæ rosæ . . . . f ℨviij.—M.
Sig. Apply locally. (*In herpes.*)
MEIGS.

2084—℞ Aluminis . . . . ℨj.
Aquæ . . . . f ℨj.—M.

Ft. lotio.
Sig. Wet a piece of lint with the solution, and apply to the glans penis. (*In herpes præputialis.*)
WARING.

2085—℞ Morphinæ acetatis . . . . gr. v.
Chloroformi . . . . ♏xl.
Unguenti simplicis . . . . ℨv.
Olei amygdalæ dulcis . . . . ♏cc.—M.
Sig. Apply two or three times daily. (*In herpes. Also in pruritus pudendi.*)
ELLEAUME.

2086—℞ Creasoti . . . . f3ss.
Aquæ destillatæ . . . . Oj.—M.
Ft. lotio. (*In impetigo.*) DUNGLISON.

2087—℞ Acidi hydrocyanici diluti . . . . f3ij.
Spiritus rectificati . . . . f3ss.
Aquæ destillatæ . . . . f3vij.—M.
Ft. lotio.
Sig. To be applied with lint covered with oiled silk. (*In impetigo, after removal of scabs.*) PLUMBE.

2088—℞ Tincturæ ferri chloridi . . . . f3ss.
Magnesii sulphatis . . . . 3ij.
Tincturæ calumbæ . . . . f3iss.
Infusi quassiæ . . . . f3xviij.—M.
Sig. A wineglassful every morning. (*In impetigo.*) NELIGAN.

2089—℞ Hydrargyri protiodidi . . . . gr. iv.
Hydrargyri cum cretâ,
Sodii carbonatis . . . . ãã gr. xij.
Pulveris myrrhæ . . . . gr. vj.
Mucilaginis acaciæ . . . . q. s.
Misce et fiant pilulæ no. xii.
Sig. One three times a day. (*In chronic impetigo.*) NELIGAN.

2089bis—℞ Syr. hypophosphitum comp. . . . . . f3vj.
Sig. A teaspoonful thrice daily, in water. (*In impetigo of the anæmic.*) JAMIESON.

2090—℞ Plumbi acetatis . . . . gr. viij.
Acidi hydrocyanici diluti . . . . f3ij.
Spiritus rectificati . . . . f3ss.
Aquæ destillatæ . . . . f3viiss.—M.
Ft. lotio.
Sig. Poison. (*In impetigo.*) PARIS.

2091—℞ Sodii carbonatis . . . . 3ij.
Syrupi violæ . . . . f3xij.—M.
Sig. A tablespoonful night and morning. (*Apply at the same time a poultice containing one drachm of sulphur. In impetigo.*) BIETT.

2092—℞ Hydrargyri chloridi corrosivi . . . . . gr. iss.
Olei theobromæ,
Vaselini . . . . ãã gr. ccxxv.
Misce et ft. unguentum.
Sig. Apply in a thin layer over the eruption. (*In impetigo of the scalp.*) JORISSENNE.

2093—℞ Hydrargyri ammoniati . . . . gr. v.
Adipis . . . . 3j.—M.
Sig. Apply to the surface after the scabs have been removed by poulticing or warm fomentations. (*In impetigo contagiosa.*) TILBURY FOX.

2094—℞ Hydrargyri sulphureti rubri . . . . . gr. xxiiss.
Plumbi oxidi rubri . . . . gr. xxxviiss.
Emplastri diachyli . . . . ad 3j.—M.
Ft. emplastrum.
Sig. "Vidal's Emplâtre Rouge." Remove the crusts by poulticing; wash with dilute spirit of camphor, and cover all the points involved with the paste, renewing daily, after washing with dilute spirit of camphor. A sulphur-bath every two days is desirable; also the following:

2095—℞ Syr. ferri iodidi . . . . f3j.
Sig. Ten to fifteen drops thrice daily, with cod-liver oil and other supporting treatment. (*In impetigo.*)
VIDAL ET THURIES.

2096—℞ Glyceriti acidi tannici . . . . 3ij.
Sig. Apply with a hair-pencil during the day. Poultice at night to remove the crusts. (*In impetigo.*) RINGER.

2097—℞ Acidi boracici . . . . ℥j.
Aquæ . . . . f℥x.—M.

Ft. lotio.

Sig. Wet a compress, and apply to the face as a mask. Place three or four of these compresses the one on the other, and cover with a sheet of thin rubber cloth. Renew this dressing every hour. In forty-eight hours cover the secreting surfaces with adhesive plaster. (*In impetigo of the face.*)   E. BESNIER.

2098—℞ Olei terebinthinæ . . . . ℥iv.

Sig. Cut the hair close, and rub the scalp well with the lotion. Let it remain about five minutes, and then wash it off with warm water and carbolic acid soap, and then with clean warm water. Then apply the following:

2099—℞ Iodi . . . . ℈ij.
Olei terebinthinæ . . . . f℥iv.—M.

Sig. Apply once or twice daily. (*In impetigo.*)   SAERDS.

2100—℞ Acidi salicylici . . . . gr. xv.
Pulv. zinci oxidi,
Pulv. amyli . . . . āā ℥ij.
Lanolini . . . . ℥vj gr. xv.

Misce et fiat unguentum.

Sig. Apply locally. (*In impetigo.*)   LIEBREICH.

2101—℞ Acidi carbolici . . . . gr. x.
Glycerini,
Aquæ rosæ . . . . āā f℥j.—M.

Ft. lotio. (*In impetigo.*)   HEADLAND.

2102—℞ Sulphuris . . . . gr. xxv-l.
Unguenti simplicis . . . . ℥j.—M.

Ft. unguentum.

Sig. Rub in nightly. (*In ichthyosis or xeroderma.*)   UNNA.

2103—℞ Resorcin. . . . . gr. xv.
Adipis. . . . . ℥j.—M.

Ft. unguentum.

Sig. Rub in locally in mild cases. In more severe cases, increase the strength of the ointment from two to six times that given above. (*In ichthyosis.*)   ANDEER.

2104—℞ Zinci sulphatis . . . . ℥j.
Adipis . . . . ℥j.—M.

Sig. Use locally. (*In ichthyosis.*)   ERASMUS WILSON.

2105—℞ Acidi salicylici . . . . ℥ij.
Collodii flexilis . . . . ℥j.—M.

Sig. Use locally with a brush. (*In spinous formations in ichthyosis hystrix.*)   LIVELING.

2106—℞ Sodii bicarbonatis . . . . ℥ij-iij.
Aquæ . . . . Oj.—M.

Ft. lotio.

Sig. Use two or three times daily as a wash. (*In ichthyosis or xeroderma.*)   DEVERGIE.

2107—℞ Unguenti zinci oxidi . . . . ℥j.

Sig. Apply locally. (*In indolent impetigo.*)   RINGER.

2108—℞ Ammonii sulpho-ichthyolati . . . . . gr. iij.
Coumarini . . . . gr. viij-xv.
Unguenti petrolei . . . . ℥v.—M.

Ft. unguentum.

Sig. Apply with the finger after bathing and drying the child. (*In intertrigo.*)   LORENS.

2109—℞ Bismuthi subnitratis . . . . ℥j.

Detur in scatula.

Sig. Dust over the inflamed part. (*In intertrigo.*) BARTHOLOW.

2110—℞ Acidi tannici . . . . ℥ss.
Glycerini . . . . f℥ij.—M.

Sig. Apply locally. (*In intertrigo.*)   BARTHOLOW.

2111—℞ Linimenti aquæ calcis . . . . f 3vj.
Sig. Use locally. (*In intertrigo.*)   TILBURY FOX.

2112—℞ Pulv. amyli . . . . 3iv.
        Zinci oxidi . . . . 3j.
        Zinci carbonatis . . . . 3ss.—M.
Sig. Use as a dusting-powder. (*In intertrigo.*) TILBURY FOX.

2113—℞ Hydrargyri chloridi mitis . . . . 3j-ij.
        Adipis . . . . : . . . 3j.—M.
Ft. unguentum. (*In intertrigo, pruritus vulvæ et ani, eczema of the scrotum, etc.*)   TOURNIE.

2113*bis*—℞ Acidi boracici . . . . 3iss.
        Vaselini . . . . 3j.—M.
Ft. unguentum.
Sig. Apply locally, after washing and drying the parts. (*In intertrigo.*)   WARING.

2114—℞ Calcii sulpho-carbolatis . . . . 3j.
        Liquoris potassii arsenitis . . . . ♏xviij.
        Tincturæ aurantii . . . . f 3vj.
        Aquæ destillatæ . . . . q. s. ad f 3vj.—M.
Sig. A sixth part before breakfast and dinner. (*In itching skin diseases.*)   DOBELL.

2115—℞ Plumbi acetatis . . . . gr. xvj.
        Acidi hydrocyanici diluti . . . . f 3iss.
        Spiritus rectificati . . . . f 3ij.
        Aquæ destillatæ . . . . f 3viiss.—M.
Ft. lotio. (*To allay itching in cutaneous diseases.*) A. T. THOMPSON.

2116—℞ Plumbi carbonatis . . . . 3ij.
        Calcis præparatæ . . . . 3ss.
        Unguenti aquæ rosæ . ·. . . . . 3ij.—M.
Ft. unguentum. (*In papular and itching eruptions.*) BURGESS.

2117—℞ Potassii cyanidi . . . . gr. xij.
        Misturæ amygdalæ . . . . f 3vj.—M.
Ft. lotio. (*In itching eruptions.*)   LOUIS.

2118—℞ Acidi arseniosi . . . . gr. x-xxx.
        Adipis . . . . 3j.—M.
Ft. unguentum.
Sig. Over a patch of skin three or four inches square, rub the ointment in well once daily for a fortnight. Then treat a fresh portion. (*In lepra.*)   TILBURY FOX.

2119—℞ Olei anacardii [cashew-nut] . . . . . f 3iv.
Sig. Soap-and-water baths are used twice daily, followed by frictions over the whole body with cocoanut oil or olive oil. After the oil has remained on for three or four hours, the body is thoroughly cleansed by a soap-and-water bath. Then the oil of cashew-nut is applied on a sponge to a small portion of the skin, as large as the hand. A week or ten days later another application of cashew-nut oil may be made. If any herpetic or other eruption is present, then use the following:

2120—℞ Spts. vini rectificati . . . . f 3j.
        Iodi . . . . q. s. ad ft. sat. sol.
Dein adde—
        Liq. sodæ caust. . . . .·- . . . ad excess.
Dein adde—
        Olei olivæ. . . . . f 3xxiv.—M.
Ft. linimentum.
Sig. Use locally on herpetic or other eruptions that occur. Shake well before using. If there be a squamous or scurfy condition of the skin, then use the following:

2121—℞ Vitell. ovi . . . . no. ij.
        Balsami copaibæ . . . . f 3ivss.—M.
Ft. emulsio et adde—
        Olei olivæ. . . . . Oj —M.
Ft. linimentum.
Sig. To be used instead of the oil baths, when the skin is scurfy. For the feet, hot baths (100° F.) of cocoanut oil are used twice daily. (*In lepra*)   BEAUPERTHUY.

2122—℞ Hydrargyri chloridi corrosivi . . . . . gr. ij-iiss.
　　　　Infusi calumbœ . . . . f℥v.—M.

Sig. A teaspoonful twice daily. Fresh meat and fresh vegetable diet, with good hygienic surroundings, are essential to success. (*In lepra.*) BEAUPERTHUY.

2123—℞ Quininæ diarsenitis . . . . gr. iv.
　　　　Micæ panis . . . . q. s.

Fiant pilulæ no. xii.
Sig. Two, three, or four per day. (*In lepra.*) KINGDON.

2124—℞ Acidi arseniosi . . . . gr. j.
　　　　Piperis . . . . gr. xij.
Tere simul in pulverem subtilissimum, et adde—
　　　　Pulveris acaciæ . . . . gr. ij.
　　　　Aquæ destillatæ . . . . q. s.

Misce et fiant pilulæ no. xvi.
Sig. One morning and night. (*In tuberculous lepra.*)
　　　　　　　　　　　　　　　　　　　Paris Codex.

2125—℞ Unguenti hydrargyri nitratis . . . . . ℥j.
Sig. Use twice daily; dilute if necessary. (*In lepra.*)
　　　　　　　　　　　　　　　　　　　WARING.

2126—℞ Unguenti picis liquidæ . . . . ℥j.
Sig. Apply to affected parts. (*In lepra.*) McCALL ANDERSON.

2127—℞ Sodii carbonatis . . . . ℥ss-j.
　　　　Aquæ . . . . f℥vj.—M.

Sig. A dessertspoonful, well diluted, twice daily. (*In lepra where mercurials are contra-indicated.*) BEAUPERTHUY.

2128—℞ Iodoformi . . . . ℥j.
　　　　Unguenti petrolei . . . . ℥j.—M.

Sig. Apply to the affected parts. (*In lepra.*) GLOVER.

2129—℞ Arsenici iodidi . . . . gr. j.
　　　　Extracti conii . . . . ℈ij.

Fiat massa et divide in pilulas no. xvi.
Sig. One pill night and morning. (*In lepra, impetigo, cancer.*)
　　　　　　　　　　　　　　　　　　　ELLIS.

2130—℞ Acidi carbolici . . . . gr. ij.
　　　　Menthol . . . . gr. iij.
　　　　Talci . . . . ℥j.—M.

Sig. Use as a dusting-powder. (*In acute eczema.*) J. C. WILSON.

2131—℞ Menthol . . . . gr. xxxvij.
　　　　Olei olivæ . . . . ℥ij-iij.
　　　　Lanolini . . . . ℥iss.—M.

Sig. Apply frequently. (*In pruritus.*) LASSAR.

2132—℞ Menthol . . . . gr. xxij-xxxvij.
　　　　Spts. vini rectificati . . . . ℥iss.—M.

Sig. Apply at intervals as required. (*In pruritus.*) LASSAR.

2133—℞ Liquoris potassæ . . . . f℥ij.
　　　　Acidi hydrocyanici diluti . . . . f℥j.
　　　　Misturæ amygdalæ . . . . f℥viij.

Misce et fiat lotio. (*In lichen.*) BURGESS.

2134—℞ Cretæ præparatæ . . . . ℥vj.
　　　　Sulphuris sublimati,
　　　　Olei cadini . . . . āā ℥ix.
　　　　Saponis nigris,
　　　　Adipis . . . . āā ℥xxv.

[Melt the lard at a gentle heat. Then add the black soap and other ingredients, stirring until cold.]
Sig. Apply locally. (*In lichen.*) HEBRA.

2135—℞ Sodii arseniatis . . . . gr. iss.
　　　　Aquæ destillatæ . . . . f℥xxv.—M.

Sig. A teaspoonful every morning at meal-time. At the end of a week increase to two teaspoonfuls. If the eruption is dry, add tonics, as cod-liver oil and phosphate of lime. (*In lichen.*) E. VIDAL.

SKIN DISEASES (Continued).

2136—℞ Sodii carbonatis . . . . ϶j.
Aquæ rosæ . . . . f3vj.
Glycerini . . . . f3ij.—M.
Ft. lotio.
Sig. Apply to the eruption. (*In infantile lichen or strophulus.*)
TILBURY FOX.

2137—℞ Glyceriti amyli . . . . 3v.
Pulv. acidi tartarici . . . . gr. xv.—M.
Sig. Apply locally. (*In chronic lichen simplex.*) E. VIDAL.

2138—℞ Bismuthi subnitratis . . . . 3ij.
Pulv. zinci oxidi . . . . 3ij.
Tinct. digitalis . . . . f3ss.
Aquæ . . . . q. s. ad f3vj.—M.
Ft. lotio.
Sig. To be used as a lotion, after an alkaline bath, as bicarbonate of sodium with bran. (*In lichen planus.*)
TILBURY FOX.

2139—℞ Olei cadini . . . . 3ij.
Glyceriti amyli . . . . 3iss.—M.
Sig. Apply locally. Gradually increase the oil of cade to
equal portions. (*In chronic lichen of the genitals.*) E. VIDAL.

2140—℞ Potassii cyanidi . . . . gr. iv.
Chloroformi . . . . ♏viij.
Glycerini . . . . 3j.
Cerati simplicis . . . . 3vj.—M.
Ft. unguentum.
Sig. Apply locally. (*In lichen agrius. Also in pruritus.*)
NELIGAN.

2141—℞ Acidi salicylici . . . . gr. x.
Vaselini . . . . 3ss.
Zinci oxidi,
Pulv. amyli . . . . ãã 3ij.—M.
Ft. pasta.
Sig. Apply locally. (*In lichen marginatus.*) LASSAR.

2142—℞ Hydrarg. chloridi corrosivi . . . . . . gr. viiss.
Cretæ præparatæ . . . . 3iiss.
Acidi carbolici,
Olei olivæ. . . . . ãã 3v.
Ungt. zinci oxidi . . . . 3xv 3v.—M.
Ft. unguentum.
Sig. Rub diligently into the affected skin. (*In lichen planus.*)
UNNA.

2143—℞ Ferri arseniatis . . . . gr. iij.
Pulveris glycyrrhizæ . . . . 3ss.
Syrupi simplicis . . . . q. s.
Misce bene, et fiant pilulæ no. xlviii.
Sig. One to three pills daily. (*In lichen, elephantiasis, lepra,
lupus, herpetic and squamous affections.*) BIETT AND DUPARC.

2144—℞ Potassii cyanidi . . . . gr. xij.
Olei amygdalæ . . . . f3ij.
Unguenti ceræ albæ . . . . 3ij.—M.
Ft. unguentum. (*In lichen.*) BURGESS.

2145—℞ Sodii biboratis . . . . 3ss.
Acidi hydrocyanici diluti . . . . . . f3ij.
Aquæ rosæ. . . . . f3viij.—M.
Ft. lotio. (*In lichen agrius.*) NELIGAN.

2146—℞ Rosæ petalæ . . . . ϶j.
Aquæ ferventis . . . . f3viij.
Acidi nitrici diluti . . . . f3iiss.—M.
Macera, cola, et fiat lotio. (*In lichen.*) HOOPER.

2147—℞ Liquoris ammonii acetatis . . . . f3iij.
Spiritus rectificati . . . . f3iv.
Aquæ rosæ. . . . . f3iv.—M.
Ft. lotio. (*In lichen.*) BURGESS.

2148—℞ Chloroformi . . . . ♏xx.
Olei olivæ . . . . f3j.—M.
Sig. After a tepid bath, and well dried. (*In lichen.*)
NELIGAN.

2149—℞ Liquoris plumbi subacetatis . . . . . . f3j-ij.
Infusi althææ . . . . f3xvj.—M.
Ft. lotio. (*In lichen.*)   BURGESS.

2150—℞ Pulv. lycopodii . . . . 3ss.
Sig.—Use as a dusting-powder after the bullæ are cut. Then use zinc ointment or an astringent solution; and then use the following:

2151—℞ Argenti nitratis . . . . gr. iij-iv.
Adipis . . . . 3j.—M.
Ft. unguentum.
Sig. Apply locally. (*In chronic ulceration following pemphigus.*)
            TILBURY FOX.

2152—℞ Linimenti calcis . . . . 3j.
Sig. Apply after the bullæ have burst or have been punctured. The parts should be fixed, and no motion allowed. (*In pemphigus.*)   CHAMBARD.

2153—℞ Argenti nitratis . . . . gr. ij.
Aquæ destillatæ . . . . f3j.
Misce et fiat solutio. (*In pemphigus after the bullæ have burst.*)
           ERASMUS WILSON.

2154—℞ Unguenti hydrargyri nitratis . . . . . 3ij.
Unguenti simplicis . . . . 3vj.—M.
Sig. Use twice daily. (*In pemphigus.*)   WARING.

2155—℞ Liquoris potassii arsenitis . . . . f3ij.
Aquæ destillatæ . . . . q. s. ad f3iij.—M.
Sig. A teaspoonful after each meal. (*In the more chronic form of pemphigus.*)   McCALL ANDERSON.

2156—℞ Sulphuris loti . . . . 3j.
Vaselini . . . . 3j.—M.
Ft. unguentum.
Sig. Apply to the scalp every morning. Anoint it with sweet almond oil every evening. (*In pityriasis.*)   JACKSON.

2157—℞ Sodii sulphureti,
Sodii carbonatis . . . . āā 3ij.
Unguenti simplicis . . . . 3iiss.—M.
Ft. unguentum. (*In pityriasis*)   BAREGES.

2158—℞ Tinct. ferri chloridi . . . . gtt. xx.
Liq. sodii arseniatis . . . . gtt. v.
Syrupi simplicis,
Aquæ . . . . āā q. s. ad f3j.—M.
Sig. To be taken thrice daily. (*In pityriasis.*)   DA COSTA.

2159—℞ Vitell. ovi . . . . no. iij.
Liq. calcis . . . . Oj.
Ft. emulsio, dein adde—
Spts. vini rectificati . . . . f3ss.—M.
Sig. Use as a shampoo. (*In pityriasis.*)   JACKSON.

2160—℞ Pilulæ hydrargyri . . . . gr. ix.
Sodii carbonatis . . . . gr. vj.
Extracti taraxaci . . . . gr. xlj.
Extracti hyoscyami . . . . gr. iij.
Misce et fiant pilulæ no. vi.
Sig. One pill two or three times a day, half an hour before meals. (*In pityriasis.*)   NELIGAN.

2161—℞ Potassii sulphureti . . . . 3j.
Aquæ destillatæ . . . . f3iij.—M.
Ft. lotio.
Sig. Use once daily. (*In pityriasis capitis.*)   WINZAR.

2162—℞ Sodii hyposulphitis . . . . 3ss.
Aquæ destillatæ . . . . f3j.—M.
Ft. lotio. (*In pityriasis versicolor.*)   HARLEY.

2163—℞ Liquoris potassii arsenitis . . . . . . ℳiv.
　　　Decocti cinchonæ . . . . f℥x.
　　　Syrupi aurantii corticis . . . . f℥ij.
　　　Tincturæ opii . . . . ℳv.—M.
Ft. haustus.
Sig. Twice daily after meals. (*In chronic pityriasis.*) BURGESS.

2164—℞ Hydrargyri sulphatis flavæ . . . . . . gr. xlv.
　　　Vaselini puri . . . . ℥xv.
　　　Ess. bergamii vel limonis . . . . . . gtt. xx.—M.
Sig. Keep in a porcelain jar. Anoint the scalp every evening.
Wash with tepid water every morning. (*In pityriasis capitis.*)
　　　　　　　　　　　　　　　　　　　　　　P. VIGIER.

2165—℞ Sulphuris loti . . . . gr. viiss.
　　　Tinct. benzoini . . . . ℳxlv.
　　　Medullæ ossium bovinum [beef-mar-
　　　　row] . . . . ℥viiss.
　　　Olei amygdalæ dulcis . . . . f℥iiss.—M.
Ft. unguentum.
Sig. Use daily or semi-weekly, according to the severity of
the case. Wash off the next morning. (*In pityriasis capitis.*)
　　　　　　　　　　　　　　　　　　　　　　FOURNIER.

2166—℞ Hydrarg. ammoniat. . . . . ℈j.
　　　Ungt. petrolei . . . . ℥j.—M.
Sig. Apply. (*For pityriasis capitis.*) VAN HARLINGEN.

2167—℞ Liq. arsenici et hydrargyri iodidi . . . gtt. lxxx.
　　　Syrupi zingiberis . . . . f℥ss.
　　　Aquæ destillatæ . . . . f℥viij.—M.
Sig. One fluidounce every third hour. (*In pityriasis.*)
　　　　　　　　　　　　　　　　　　　　　　OSBREY.

2168—℞ Acidi carbolici . . . . ℥ij.
　　　Glycerini . . . . f℥ss.
　　　Aquæ destillatæ . . . . f℥viij.—M.
Ft. lotio.
Sig. Twice daily. (*In pityriasis.*) J. C. WILSON.

2169—℞ Amygdalarum amararum . . . . . . no. xxx.
　　　Aquæ destillatæ . . . . f℥viij.—M.
Ft. emulsio. (*A lotion for prickly heat.*) WARING.

2170—℞ Acidi hydrocyanici diluti . . . . . . ℳx-xl.
　　　Glycerini . . . . f℥j.—M.
Ft. lotio. (*In prickly heat.*) WARING.

2171—℞ Zinci carbonatis præcip. . . . . . . ℥iv.
　　　Zinci oxidi . . . . ℥ij.
　　　Glycerini . . . . f℥ij.
　　　Aquæ rosæ . . . . f℥viij.—M.
Ft. lotio.
Sig. Apply locally. (*In prickly heat. Also in eczema, when
the surface is red and tender.*) TILBURY FOX.

2172—℞ Acidi hydrocyanici diluti . . . . . . f℥j.
　　　Liq. potassæ . . . . f℥ij.
　　　Mist. amygdalæ . . . . f℥viij.—M.
Ft. lotio.
Sig. Use locally. (*In prickly heat [lichen tropicus].*) BURGESS.

2173—℞ Acidi hydrocyanici diluti . . . . . . f℥iss.
　　　Aquæ rosæ . . . . f℥viiss.—M.
Ft. lotio.
Sig. Use locally. (*In prickly heat.*) A. T. THOMPSON.

2174—℞ Sodii arseniatis . . . . gr. ss.
　　　Ext. gentianæ . . . . gr. xlv.—M.
Ft. massa et in pil. no. xxx div.
Sig. Two or three pills after each meal. Also the following:

2175—℞ Acidi pyrogallici . . . . ℥iss-iv.
　　　Adipis . . . . ℥iij.—M.
Ft. unguentum.
Sig. To be rubbed in twice daily. Also, a thorough cleansing
with soap every two days. (*In psoriasis.*) GUIBOUT.

2176—℞ Chrysarobini . . . . gr. xx-xl.
 Lanolini,
 Vaselini . . . . āā ʒss.—M.

Sig. Apply every second day. (*In psoriasis.*) HEBRA.

2177—℞ Ext. gland. thyroid . . . . ʒj.

Fiant in tabellæ compressæ no xxiv.
Sig. One three times daily. (*In psoriasis.*) H. TUCKER.

2178—℞ Hydrargyri biniodidi . . . . gr. j.
 Extracti sarsaparillæ,
 Extracti gentianæ . . . . āā ɔj.

Misce et divide in pilulas no. x.
Sig. One pill three times a day. (*In psoriasis.*) BURGESS.

2179—℞ Hydroxylamine . . . . 1 part.
 Glycerin,
 Alcohol . . . . of each 500 parts.
Mix.
Sig. Apply with a camel's-hair pencil to each spot. (*In psoriasis.*) HEBRA.

2180—℞ Chrysarobin . . . . gr. xx.
 Collodion . . . . f ʒj.
Mix.
Sig. Apply to each spot. (*In psoriasis.*) HEBRA.

2181—℞ Acidi salicylici . . . . ʒss.
 Acidi pyrogallici . . . . ʒiss-ij.
 Collodii . . . . f ʒij.—M.

Ft. collodium.
Sig. Preserve in a dark-colored bottle. After a warm bath to loosen the scales, the collodion is painted on the patches and a half-inch beyond the border. Reapply every day, preceding the application by a warm bath. If the eruption is general, treat successively the different parts. (*In psoriasis.*) ELLIOTT.

2182—℞ Ichthyol . . . . ʒj.
 Acidi salicylici . . . . ℈j.
 Zinci oxidi . . . . ʒij.
 Amyli . . . . ʒiv.
 Petrolati . . . . ʒj.—M.

Sig. Apply locally twice a day. (*In psoriasis.*) SCHMITZ.

2183—℞ Acidi salicylici . . . . ʒiss.
 Olei cadini,
 Glyceriti amyli . . . . āā ʒxxv.
 Ess. caryophylli . . . . . . , ... ʒiiss.—M.

Ft. glyceritum.
Sig. The scales are first removed with hot water and tar soap, and then a weak alkaline bath is given. The glycerole is then rubbed in. If too much irritation follow, diminish the salicylic acid or the oil of cade. (*In psoriasis.*)
 L. BROCQ.

2184—℞ Acidi pyrogallici,
 Acidi chrysophanici . . . . . . āā gr. lxxv.
 Ætheris,
 Alcoholis . . . . āā q. s. ad ft. sol.
 Collodii . . . . f ʒxxv.—M.

Ft. collodium.
Sig. A prolonged (three hours') hot bath, twice weekly. After the bath, rub the surface well to detach the scales; then cover with the collodion, which should remain on until the next bath, if possible. Observe strict diet, and use internally the following:

2185—℞ Liquoris potassii arsenitis . . . . f ʒss.

Sig. Three to ten drops, well diluted, thrice daily after meals. (*In psoriasis circinatus.*) BESNIER.

2186—℞ Olei cadini,
 Ungt. hydrargyri . . . . āā ʒij.
 Vaselini . . . . ʒj.—M.

Ft. unguentum.
Sig. Apply locally. (*In psoriasis palmaris et plantaris syphilitica.*) MAURIAC.

2187—℞ Hydrargyri chloridi corrosivi,
Ammonii muriatis . . . . āā gr. xv.—M.

Ft. pulv. no. 1.
Sig. Dissolve the powder in two quarts of tepid water, and
bathe the parts for fifteen minutes, morning and evening.
(*In psoriasis palmaris et plantaris syphilitica.*)
GILLES DE LA TOURETTE.

2188—℞ Hydrargyri chloridi corrosivi . . . . . 3j.(!)
Alcoholis . . . . f3j.—M.

Fiat lotio.
Sig. Paint the affected spot. (*In psoriasis.*) NIEMEYER.

2189—℞ Tincturæ guaiaci ammoniatæ . . . . . f3j.
Tincturæ serpentariæ . . . . f3ss.
Mucilaginis acaciæ . . . . ℥xx.
Decocti mezerei . . . . f3viss.
Infusi dulcamaræ . . . . f3j.—M.

Fiat haustus.
Sig. Thrice daily. (*In psoriasis guttata.*) NELIGAN.

2190—℞ Liquoris potassii arsenitis . . . . f3ss.
Liquoris potassæ . . . . f3j.
Spiritus ætheris nitrosi . . . . f3ij.
Infusi gentianæ compositi . . . . . . f3vij.—M.

Sig. Two tablespoonfuls three times a day. (*In psoriasis.*)
S. WRIGHT.

2191—℞ Unguenti picis liquidæ,
Unguenti sulphuris . . . . āā 3j.—M.

(*In psoriasis.*) *Guy's Hospital.*

2192—℞ Liquoris potassii arsenitis . . . . ℥v.
Tincturæ ferri chloridi . . . . ℥xx.
Infusi quassiæ . . . . f3j.

Misce et fiat haustus.
Sig. Three times a day. (*In psoriasis inveterata.*) GUY.

2193—℞ Cupri oleatis . . . . 3ss.
Sig. Apply twice daily. (*In ringworm.*) F. LE SIEURE WEIR.

2194—℞ Sodii biboratis . . . . 3j.
Aceti destillatæ . . . . f3ij.—M.
Fiat lotio. (*In ringworm of the scalp.*) ABERCROMBIE.

2195—℞ Hydrargyri protiodidi . . . . gr. xij-xx.
Unguenti simplicis . . . . 3j.—M.
(*In rupia.*) BIETT.

2196—℞ Unguenti hydrargyri oxidi rubri . . . 3j.
(*In rupia, frambœsia, etc.*) WARING.

2197—℞ Hydrargyri chloridi corrosivi . . . . . gr. iv.
Acidi nitrici diluti,
Acidi hydrocyanici diluti . . . . . āā f3j.
Glycerini . . . . f3ij.
Aquæ . . . . f3viij.—M.

Ft. lotio.
Sig. Apply locally. (*In rupia. Also in pityriasis, chloasma,
etc.*)

2198—℞ Hydrargyri oxidi rubri,
Hydrargyri ammoniati . . . . . . āā gr. vj.
Adipis . . . . 3j.—M.

Ft. unguentum.
Sig. Apply locally. (*In rupia.*) STARTIN.

2199—℞ Potassii bitartratis . . . . 3j.
Reducetur in pulverem subtilissimum, et detur in scatula.
Sig. Dust over ulcer. (*In rupia.*) RAYER.

2200—℞ Hydrargyri iodidi rubri . . . . gr. j-ij.
Ext. gentianæ . . . . ℈iij.—M.

Ft. massa et in pil. no. xij div.
Sig. One pill twice daily. (*In rupia and other syphilodermata.*)
TILBURY FOX.

2201—℞ Hydrargyri cyanidi . . . . gr. vj.
    Cerati simplicis . . . . ℨj.—M.

Ft. unguentum.
Sig. Use locally. (*In rupia when the crusts become loosened.*
Also in syphilitic ulcers.) TILBURY FOX.

2202—℞ Hydrargyri iodidi rubri . . . . gr. iij.
    Potassii iodidi . . . . ℨj-ij.
    Alcoholis . . . . f ℨij.
    Syr. zingiberis . . . . f ℨiv.
    Aquæ . . . . ad f ℨiss.—M.

Sig. Thirty drops thrice daily. (*In rupia and other syphilitic eruptions.*) PUCHE.

2203—℞ Hydrargyri chloridi corrosivi . . . . . ℨj.
    Potassii iodidi . . . . ℨvj.
    Tinct. iodi comp. . . . . f ℨij.
    Aquæ . . . . ad f ℨxvj.—M.

Sig. One-half to one teaspoonful thrice daily. (*In rupia and other syphilodermata.*) STARTIN.

2204—℞ Hydrargyri bicyanidi . . . . gr. j.
    Quininæ . . . . ℨj.
    Ext. gentianæ . . . . ℨss.—M.

Ft. massa et in pil. no. xx div.
Sig. One pill twice daily. (*In ordinary syphilitic eruptions.*) TILBURY FOX.

2205—℞ Sulphuris loti . . . . gr. ccxxv.
    Olei ricini . . . . f ℨxliss.
    Olei theobromæ . . . . ℨij.
    Balsami peruviani . . . . ℨss.—M.

Ft. unguentum.
Sig. Apply night and morning. (*In dry seborrhœa of the scalp.*) VIDAL.

2206—℞ Olei amygdalæ dulcis . . . . ℥l.
    Acidi carbolici . . . . gr. v.
    Alcoholis . . . . q. s. ad f ℨj.
    Olei bergamii . . . . q. s.—M.

Ft. unguentum.
Sig. Soak the scalp at night with sweet oil, and shampoo it in the morning with the officinal tincture of green soap, to remove the crusts. Shampoo twice a week, and apply the ointment every night. (*In dry seborrhœa of the scalp.*) HYDE.

2207—℞ Resorcin. . . . . ℨj
    Ol. ricini . . . . ℥xx.
    Alcoholis . . . . f ℨiv.

Sig. Twice daily. (*In seborrhœa capitis.*) STELWAGON.

2208—℞ Zinci sulphatis.
    Potassii sulphureti . . . . āā gr. xxx.
    Alcoholis . . . . ℥c.
    Aquæ rosæ . . . . q. s. ad f ℨij.—M.

Ft. lotio.
Sig. Wet a soft linen rag with ether, rub the nose with it vigorously at night, and then apply the lotion. (*In obstinate seborrhœa of the nose.*) G. H. FOX.

2209—℞ Potassii carbonatis . . . . ℨij.
    Sodii chloridi . . . . ℨij.
    Aquæ aurantii flor. . . . . f ℨij.
    Aquæ rosæ . . . . f ℨvij.—M.

Ft. lotio.
Sig. Face-wash. (*In tan and freckles.*) BARTHOLOW.

2210—℞ Hydrargyri chloridi corrosivi . . . . . gr. j.
    Zinci oxidi . . . . ℨij.
    Zinci carbonatis . . . . ℨss.
    Glycerini . . . . f ℨij.
    Aquæ rosæ . . . . f ℨvij.—M.

Ft. lotio.
Sig. Apply with a sponge. (*In freckles and sunburn.*) TILBURY FOX.

2211—℞ Liq. potassæ . . . . 3j.
Aquæ rosæ . . . . f3ij.—M.
Ft. lotio.
Sig. Face-wash. (*In tan and freckles.*)   TODD.

2212—℞ Plumbi acetatis . . . . gr. xv.
Acidi hydrocyanici diluti . . . . . . ℳxx.
Alcoholis . . . . f3ss.
Aquæ . . . . q. s. ad f3vj.—M.
Ft. lotio.
Sig. Apply with a sponge. (*In freckles and sunburn.*)
    TILBURY FOX.

2213—℞ Lactis recentis. . . . . f3xiiss.
Glycerini . . . . f3viiss.
Acidi hydrochlorici . . . . ℳlxxv.
Ammonii muriatis . . . . 3j.—M.
Ft. lotio.
Sig. Apply morning and evening with a camel's-hair brush.
(*In tan and freckles.*)   MONIN.

2214—℞ Unguenti hydrargyri nitratis . . . . . 3ss.
Unguenti picis liquidæ . . . . 3j.—M.
(*In tinea capitis.*)   ELLIS.

2215—℞ Olei juniperi . . . . f3iss.
Olei anisi . . . . ℳvj.
Axungiæ . . . . 3ij.
Misce bene ut fiat unguentum. (*In tinea capitis.*)   SULLY.

2216—℞ Sodii bicarbonatis . . . . 3ij.
Acidi hydrocyanici diluti . . . . . . f3ss.
Lactis vaccæ . . . . f3viij.
Misce et fiat lotio. (*In milk crust.*)   A. T. THOMPSON.

2217—℞ Pulveris carbonis . . . . 3iij.
Adipis . . . . 3j.—M.
Fiat unguentum. (*In tinea capitis.*)   ALIBERT.

2218—℞ Sodii hyposulphitis . . . . 3iij.
Acidi sulphurosi diluti . . . . f3ss.
Aquæ . . . . q. s. ad Oj.—M.
Ft. lotio.
Sig. Apply thoroughly to the scalp, to loosen the crusts. (*In
linea favosa.*)   STARTIN.

2219—℞ Acidi sulphurosi . . . . f3ij.
Aquæ destillatæ . . . . f3viij.
Sig. Apply constantly. (*In tinea favosa.*)   W. JENNER.

2220—℞ Iodi . . . . gr. x.
Potassii iodidi . . . . gr. xv.
Tinct. iodi comp. . . . . f3j.—M.
Sig. Apply to the scalp after the crusts have been removed
by soaking in oil or poulticing. (*In tinea favosa.*)
    TILBURY FOX.

2221—℞ Sodii hyposulphitis . . . . 3j.
Aquæ destillatæ . . . . f3xij.
Misce et fiat lotio. (*In tinea favosa.*)   TILBURY FOX.

2222—℞ Sulphuris loti . . . . f3j.
Olei cadini,
Hydrarg. chloridi corrosivi . . . . āā gr. v.—M.
Sig. Apply four times daily, on the hairy portion of the skin
and scalp. (*In tinea favosa.*)   BAZIN.

2223—℞ Sulphuris iodidi . . . . 3j.
Unguenti simplicis . . . . : . . 3iss.
Ft. unguentum. (*In tinea favosa.*)   DONAVAN.

2224—℞ Acidi salicylici,
Acidi chrysophanici . . . . āā 3ij gr. viiss.
Cretæ præparatæ . . . . 3ij gr. xlv.
Vaselini . . . . 3xviiss.—M.
Ft. unguentum.
Sig. Remove the crusts, epilate the hairs, and rub in the oint-
ment for fifteen minutes at night. (*In tinea favosa.*) MONOE.

2225—℞ Hydrargyri chloridi corrosivi . . . . . gr. x.
      Aquæ destillatæ . . . . f ℨj.

Solve.
Sig. Apply with a camel's-hair brush, after epilation. (*In tinca sycosa.*)   HARLEY.

2226—℞ Iodi . . . . ℨj-ij.
      Olei picis decoloratæ . . . . f ℨj.—M.

Ft. pasta.
Sig. Apply every fourth or sixth day. When the mass begins to flake off, wash well, and reapply the paste. (*In tinca tonsurans, or ringworm of the scalp. Also in linea circinata.*)   COSTER.

2227—℞ Hydrargyri oleatis (5–10 per cent.) . . ℨj.
Sig. Paint over the affected part. (*In tinea sycosa.*)   LEONARD CANE.

2228—℞ Liquoris arsenici et hydrargyri iodidi . f ℨij.
      Syrupi zingiberis . . . . f ℨj.
      Aquæ destillatæ . . . . q. s. ad f ℨiij.—M.

Sig. A teaspoonful after each meal. (*In linea sycosa.*)   ERASMUS WILSON.

2229—℞ Acidi carbolici . . . . ℨj.
      Glycerini . . . . f ℨss-j.—M.

Ft. lotio.
Sig. Use locally night and morning, rubbing in well. (*In linea tonsurans.*)   TILBURY FOX.

2230—℞ Hydrargyri ammoniati,
      Hydrargyri oxidi rubri . . . . . . āā gr. vj.
      Adipis . . . . ℨj.—M.

Ft. unguentum.
Sig. Use after epilation and washing. (*In linea tonsurans.*)   STARTIN.

2231—℞ Sulphuris loti . . . . ℨij.
      Spts. camphoræ . . . . f ℨss.
      Glycerini . . . . f ℨss.
      Hydrargyri bisulphidi . . . . ℨss.
      Pulv. amyli . . . . ℨij.
      Aquæ . . . . q. s. ad Oj.—M.

Ft. lotio.
Sig. Use locally night and morning. (*In linea tonsurans.*)   STARTIN.

2232—℞ Aceti cantharidis . . . . ℨss.
Sig. Apply lightly with a camel's-hair pencil; epilate around the patch, and use the following:

2233—℞ Hydrargyri chloridi corrosivi . . . . . gr. ij.
      Adipis . . . . ℨj.—M.

Ft. unguentum.
Sig. Rub in well for ten days or a fortnight; then stimulate with cantharidal ointment. (*In linca decalvans.*)   TILBURY FOX.

2234—℞ Naphthol . . . . ℨj-iiss.
      Saponis viridis,
      Cretæ præparatæ,
      Sulphuris loti,
      Lanolini . . . . āā ℨvj gr. xv.

Misce et fiat unguentum.
Sig. Apply locally. (*In linea sycosis.*)   LIEBREICH.

2235—℞ Acidi acetici glacialis . . . . ℨj.
Sig. Use as a paint, once or more, and dry off with blotting-paper if it produces much irritation. (*In tinea circinata.*)   TILBURY FOX.

2236—℞ Cupri carbonatis : . . . . ℨij.
      Adipis . . . . ℨj.—M.

Ft. unguentum.
Sig. Rub in well. (*In linea sycosis.*)   DEVERGIE.

2237—℞ Hydrargyri nitratis . . . . ℨiss.
      Adipis . . . . ℨj.—M.

Ft. unguentum.
Sig. Rub in night and morning, for a day or two. (*In linea circinata.*)   TILBURY FOX.

2238—℞ Ungt. hydrargyri nitratis . . . . ʒiv.
Sulphuris . . . . ʒij.
Creasoti . . . . gtt. x.
Adipis . . . . ʒj-ij.—M.

Ft. unguentum.
Sig. Rub in well. (*In tinea sycosis. See also tinea tonsurans.*)
TILBURY FOX.

2239—℞ Hydrargyri chloridi corrosivi . . . . . gr. ij.
Adipis . . . . ʒj.—M.

Ft. unguentum.
Sig. Use locally, rubbing in well. (*In tinea circinata.*)
TILBURY FOX.

2240—℞ Hydrargyri ammoniati . . . . gr. v.
Adipis . . . . ʒj.—M.

Ft. unguentum. (*In tinea circinata, where the surface is discharging.*) TILBURY FOX.

2241—℞ Acidi sulphurosi . . . . ʒij.
Aquæ . . . . ʒviij.—M.

Ft. lotio.
Sig. Wash the surface with soap and water, and apply the
lotion, night and morning, on compresses of lint covered
with oiled silk for at least one hour. (*In tinea circinata,
where the disease is more or less general.*) TILBURY FOX.

2242—℞ Resorcin. . . . . ʒj-iiss.
Olei ricini . . . . ʒxiss.
Alcoholis . . . . ʒxxxviiiss.
Balsami peruviani. . . . . gr. viiss.—M.

Ft. lotio.
Sig. Apply locally. (*In tinea versicolor. Also in seborrhœa and
atopecia areata.*) IHLE.

2243—℞ Sodii hyposulphitis . . . . ʒiv-vj.
Aquæ . . . . ʒvj.—M.

Ft. lotio.
Sig. Wash the parts well with yellow soap (sapo terebinthinæ),
then sponge with weak vinegar and water, and apply the
lotion freely, even after the disease has vanished. (*In tinea
versicolor.*) TILBURY FOX.

2244—℞ Acidi salicylici . . . . gr. xxx.
Sulphuris loti . . . . ʒiiss.
Lanolini . . . . ʒxxv.—M.

Ft. unguentum.
Sig. Apply with friction. (*In tinea versicolor.*) LIEBREICH.

2245—℞ Acidi salicylici . . . . gr. xlv.
Sulphuris loti . . . . ʒiiss.
Lanolini,
Vaselini . . . . āā ʒxiiss.—M.

Ft. unguentum.
Sig. After rubbing well with tar-soap, rub in the ointment
well every evening. Wash off in the morning. (*In tinea
versicolor.*) E. BESNIER.

2246—℞ Acidi carbolici . . . . ʒj.
Glycerini . . . . f ʒix.—M.

Ft. solutio.
Sig. Cut the eyelashes short. Scrape off all crusts and the
surface of the exposed ulcerations. Paint the raw surface
with the solution. Dress with iodoform. (*In tinea tarsi.*)
TEALE.

2247—℞ Sodii bicarbonatis . . . . ʒij-x.
Aquæ ferventis (90°–95° F.) . . . . cong. xx-xxx.

Misce.
Sig. Alkaline bath. (*In eczema, psoriasis, urticaria, lichen, and
prurigo, where there is much local irritation.*) TILBURY FOX.

2248—℞ Potassii carbonatis . . . . ʒij-vj.
Sodii boratis . . . . ʒij.
Aquæ ferventis (90°–95° F.) . . . . . cong. xx-xxx.

Misce.
Sig. Alkaline bath. Use the same as the preceding.
TILBURY FOX.

2249—℞ Acidi sulphurosi,
    Aquæ destillatæ . . . . āā partes æquales.
Misce et fiat lotio. (*In fungous skin diseases.*)   BIETT.

2250—℞ Hydrargyri chloridi corrosivi . . . . ℈j.
    Hydrargyri oxidi rubri,
    Cupri subacetatis,
    Cupri sulphatis . . . . āā ℈ij.
    Adipis . . . . ℥v.—M.
Ft. unguentum. (*For fungous growths and granulations.*)
                    B. C. BRODIE.

2251—℞ Cupri sulphatis . . . . ℈ss.
    Spiritus rectificati . . . . f℥j.
    Aquæ destillatæ . . . . f℥j.—M.
Ft. lotio. (*In chronic molluscum.*)   NELIGAN.

2252—℞ Acidi nitrici diluti . . . . f℥iss.
    Spiritus lavandulæ compositi . . . . . f℥ss.
    Syrupi aurantii corticis . . . . f℥iss.
    Aquæ destillatæ . . . . ℥iss.—M.
Sig. A wineglassful three or four times a day. (*In chronic, obstinate ulcers and skin diseases.*)   M RYAN.

2253—℞ Amygdalæ dulcis excorticatæ . . . . . ℈j.
    Aquæ florum aurantii . . . . f℥ij.
    Aquæ rosæ . . . . f℥viij.
Fiat emulsio, et adde—
    Ammonii chloridi . . . . ℈j.
    Tincturæ benzoini . . . . f℥ij.—M.
Fiat lotio cosmetica. (*In pimples, freckles, and dryness of the skin.*)   HERMANN.

2254—℞ Sodii arseniatis . . . . gr. ij.
    Aquæ destillatæ . . . . q. s.
Solve et adde—
    Pulveris guaiaci . . . . ℈ss.
    Antimonii sulphurati . . . . ℈j.
    Mucilaginis acaciæ . . . . q. s.
Misce caute et divide in pilulas xxiv.
Sig. Two to three pills daily. (*In chronic skin diseases.*)
                   ERASMUS WILSON.

2255—℞ Phosphori . . . . gr. iij-℈j.(!!)
    Olei caryophylli . . . . ℳx-f℥j.
    Mucilaginis acaciæ . . . . . q. s. ut fiant pilulæ xii.
Sig. One twice a day. (*In obstinate, scaly, tubercular, and syphilitic skin diseases.*)   BURGESS.

2256—℞ Hydrargyri chloridi mitis . . . . ℈j-℈j.
    Adipis benzoatæ . . . . ℥j.—M.
Ft. unguentum. (*In most chronic eruptions.*)   BURGESS.

2257—℞ Hydrargyri biniodidi . . . . gr. j.
    Unguenti simplicis . . . . ℥v.—M.
Sig. Strength may be gradually increased. (*In elephantiasis Arabum.*)   WARING.

2858—℞ Acidi arseniosi . . . . gr. j.
    Piperis nigri . . . . gr. x.
Tere simul per horam dimidiam; dein adde—
    Mucilaginis acaciæ . . . . q. s. ut fiant pilulæ xv.
Sig. One pill once or twice daily. (*In elephantiasis.*)
                   HENRY BEASLEY.

2259—℞ Hydrargyri sulphureti . . . . ℈ss.
    Pulveris olibani . . . . ℈ij.—M.
Sig. To be thrown on a red-hot iron, and the diseased parts *only* exposed to the fumes. (*In chronic skin disease.*) FOY.

2260—℞ Iodi . . . . ℈j-℈j.
    Sulphuris sublimati . . . . ℈ss-℈iss.
Misce et fiat pulvis.
Sig. One-twelfth of a part to be used as a fumigation in *skin-diseases.*   HOOPER.

2261—℞ Menthol . . . . gr. xlviij.
    Balsami peruviani . . . . gr. xcvj.
    Unguenti zinci benzol.,
    Lanolini puri . . . . āā ad ℥ij.—M.
Sig. Apply twice daily. (*In prurigo.*)   SAALFELD.

2262—℞ Potassii sulphureti . . . . ʒij-ʒiv.
　　　　Aquæ calidæ . . . . ℔c-℔cc.
　Solve et adde—
　　　Ichthyocollæ . . . . ℔j-℔ij, in
　　　　　　　　　　　aquæ bullientis solutæ, ℔x.
　Fiat balneum. (*Bath for skin diseases.*)　　DUPUYTREN.

2263—℞ Sodii carbonatis,
　　　　Sodii biboratis . . . . āā ʒv.
　　　　Aquæ pluvialis (caloris grad. 76°-98° F.) cong. xxx.
　Solve ut fiat balneum alkalinum. (*For many skin diseases.*)
　　　　　　　　　　　　　　　　　　NELIGAN.

2264—℞ Acidi nitrici vel muriatici . . . . . . ʒj.
　　　　Aquæ ferventis . . . . cong. xxx.
　Misce. Fiat balneum acidum. (*In chronic lichen and pru-
　rigo.*)　　　　　　　　　　　　　TILBURY FOX.

2265—℞ Sodii hyposulphitis,
　　　　Sulphuris sublimati . . . . āā ʒij.
　　　　Aquæ pluvialis (caloris grad. 80° F.) . cong. xxx.
　Solve. Fiat balneum sulphureum. (*For scaly diseases of the
　skin.*)　　　　　　　　　　　　　NELIGAN.

2266—℞ Furfuris [bran] . . . . ℔ij-vj.
　　　　vel lini seminis . . . . ℔j.
　　　　Aquæ ferventis . . . . cong. xx-xxx.
　Misce.
　Sig. Emollient bath. (*In erythematous, itchy, and scaly diseases.*)
　　　　　　　　　　　　　　　　　TILBURY FOX.

2267—℞ Potassii sulphidi . . . . ʒii-iv.
　　　　Aquæ ferventis . . . . cong. xxx.-M.
　Sig. Sulphuret of potash bath. (*In scabies, chronic eczema,
　lichen, and psoriasis.*)　　　　　　TILBURY FOX.

SLEEPLESSNESS. (See Insomnia.)

SMALL-POX.

2268—℞ Aristol. . . . . ʒj.
　Sig. Use as a dusting-powder from the appearance of the
　pustules.　　　　　　　　　　　J. J. LEVICK.

2269—℞ Acidi salicylici . . . . gr. xx.
　　　　Sodii bicarbonatis,
　　　　Ammonii carbonatis . . . . āā gr. iv.
　Misce et fiat chartula.
　Sig. This amount in water every two to four hours, accord-
　ing to severity. (In the later stage, ferri et ammonii citras
　may be added.)　　　　　　　　　PRIDEAUX.

2270—℞ Acidi carbolici,
　　　　Acidi acetici . . . . āā f ʒj-iss.
　　　　Tincturæ opii,
　　　　Spiritus chloroformi . . . . . . āā f ʒj.
　　　　Aquæ destillatæ . . . . q. s. ad f ʒviij.—M.
　Sig. A tablespoonful every four hours.　　NAPHEYS.

2271—℞ Sodii sulphitis . . . . ʒj.
　　　　Aquæ destillatæ . . . . f ʒj.
　Misce et fiat haustus.
　Sig. To be taken every four hours.　　A. E. SANSOM.

2272—℞ Ichthyol . . . . ʒij.
　　　　Olei amygdalæ dulcis . . . . ʒiiss.
　　　　Lanolin . . . . ʒv.—M.
　Or,
2273—℞ Ichthyol . . . . ʒj.
　　　　Vaselin . . . . ʒj.—M.
　Sig. These allay itching and pain, modify the degree of sup-
　puration, and decrease pitting.　　KOLBASSENKO.

2274—℞ Pulv. folii belladonnæ . . . . gr. vj–xij.
   Sacchari lactis. . . . . Əj.—M.
In pulv. no. xii div.
Sig. A powder every three to six hours, till dilatation of the
 pupils and some stupor follow.   WARING.

2275—℞ Liquoris ammonii acetatis . . . . . . f℥iiss.
   Spiritus ætheris nitrosi . . . . f℥ss.—M.
Sig. A tablespoonful every two or three hours, in a wine-
 glassful of water.   HARTSHORNE.

2276—℞ Sodii salicylatis . . . . ℥ij.
   Glycerini . . . . f℥j.
   Aquæ menthæ pip. . . . . ad f℥iij.—M.
Sig. One or two teaspoonfuls three or four times daily.
             REIMER.

2277—℞ Hydrargyri chloridi corrosivi . . . . . gr. ij–iv.
   Aquæ . . . . f℥vj.—M.
Ft. lotio.
Sig. Wet compresses and apply to the eruption.   SKODA.

2278—℞ Calcis calcinatæ . . . . ℥iv.
   Sulphuris . . . . ℥viij.
   Aquæ . . . . Ov.—M.
[Boil in an earthenware pan, evaporate to three pints, and
 filter.]
Sig. Apply locally as a lotion to the eruption. (*To prevent
 pitting and secondary fever.*)   PETERS.

2279—℞ Collodii flexilis . . . . ℥j.
Sig. Apply every day or two with a brush to the eruption.
 (*To prevent pitting.*)   RINGER.

2280—℞ Argenti nitratis . . . . Əij.
   Aquæ destillatæ . . . . f℥ij.—M.
Sig. Paint the skin that is exposed to the light. (*To prevent
 pitting.*)   RINGER.

2281—℞ Zinci oxidi . . . . ℥j.
   Zinci carbonatis . . . . ℥iij.
   Olei olivæ . . . . q. s. ut fiat unguentum.
             BENNETT.

2282—℞ Atropinæ sulphatis . . . . gr. j.
   Aquæ destillatæ . . . . f℥ss.—M.
Sig. Three to five minims every three or four hours.
          W. HITCHMAN.

2283—℞ Acidi carbolici,
   Gelatinæ. . . . . āā ℥j.
   Glycerini . . . . f℥vj.
   Aquæ . . . . f℥xxvj.—M.
Sig. For local use. (Daily, after bathing, paint over the body.
 After the pustules in the face are filled, prick them, and
 apply the lotion frequently.)   PRIDEAUX.

SPERMATORRHŒA.

2284—℞ Pulv. opii . . . . gr. v.
   Pulv. camphoræ . . . . Əiv.
   Pulv. acaciæ,
   Syr. simplicis . . . . . . āā q. s. ut ft. massa.—M.
In pil. no. xl dividenda.
Sig. Two pills thrice daily.   WARING.

2285—℞ Tinct. cantharidis . . . . ℥ij.
   Tinct. ferri chloridi . . . . ℥vj.—M.

Sig. Twenty drops in water thrice daily. (*In impotence, with
 spermatorrhœa.*)   H. C. WOOD.

2286—℞ Pulv. ergotæ . . . . ℥ss.
   Pulv. nucis vomicæ . . . . gr. vj.
   Sacchari albi . . . . Əj.—M.
In pulv. no. xx div.
Sig. One or two powders at meal-time.   SINÉTY.

2287—℞ Potassii bromidi . . . . ℨj.
Aquæ destillatæ . . . . q. s. ad f ℨij.—M.

Sig. A teaspoonful three times a day. (*In the strong and ple-thoric.*)
BARTHOLOW.

2288—℞ Quininæ sulphatis . . . . gr. vj.
Acidi sulphurici diluti . . . . f ℨj.
Tincturæ cardamomi compositæ . . . f ℨij.
Aquæ cinnamomi . . . . f ℨvss.—M.

Sig. Two tablespoonfuls twice daily.
MILTON.

2289—℞ Tincturæ cimicifugæ . . . . f ℨij.
Sig. A teaspoonful three times a day.
MORSE.

2290—℞ Digitalinæ. . . . . gr. j.
Pulveris acaciæ . . : . . . . Ʒij.
Syrupi simplicis . . . . q. s.

Fiat massa, in pilulas no. xxxv dividenda.
Sig. One pill three times a day.
CORVISART.

2291—℞ Pulveris opii . . . . gr. v.
Camphoræ . . . . Ʒiv.
Pulveris acaciæ,
Syrupi simplicis . . . . āā q. s.

Fiat massa, in pilulas no. xl dividenda.
Sig. Two pills three times a day.
WARING.

2292—℞ Pulveris digitalis . . . . gr. ij.
Lupulinæ . . . . gr. xv.

Misce et fiat chartula.
Sig. Daily at bedtime.
PESCHECK.

2293—℞ Ext. belladonnæ,
Pulv. belladonnæ . . . . āā gr. iij.
Confect. rosæ . . . . q. s. ut ft. massa.—M.

In pulv. no. x div.
Sig. From one to three pills at bedtime, and during the day from fifteen to sixty grains of potassium bromide in divided doses.
SINÉTY.

2294—℞ Antipyrin. . . . . Ʒij.
Syr. acaciæ . . . . Ʒss.
Aquæ cinnamomi . . . . ad f ℨiv.—M.

Sig. A dessertspoonful or two on retiring. (*When due to neurasthenia.*)
THOR.

2295—℞ Hyoscinæ hydrobromatis . . . . gr. ¼.
Sacchari lactis . . . . gr. xxxvj.
Alcohol . . . . q. s.—M.

Fiant tabellæ triturationes no. xxv.
Sig. One tablet at bedtime.

2296—℞ Tinct. gelsemii . . . . Ʒj.
Tinct. belladonnæ . . . . Ʒij.—M.

Sig. Fifteen drops at bedtime.
BARTHOLOW.

2297—℞ Lupulinæ . . . . gr. x.
Pulv. camphoræ . . . . gr. vj.
Ext. belladonnæ . . . . gr. ij.—M.

In pil. no. xii div.
Sig. One pill thrice daily.
BARTHOLOW.

2298—℞ Infusi digitalis . . . . Ʒiv.
Sig. One or two teaspoonfuls twice or thrice daily.
RINGER.

2299—℞ Argenti nitratis . . . . gr. v-x.
Aquæ destillatæ . . . . Ʒj.—M.

Sig. Inject into the prostatic portion of the urethra, using a deep urethral syringe.
VAN BUREN AND KEYES.

2300—℞ Acidi tannici . . . . Ʒj.
Glycerini . . . . q. s.—M.

Ft. pasta.
Sig. Apply to the deep urethra with a cupped sound, placing the paste in the cups.
VAN BUREN AND KEYES.

SPLEEN, ENLARGEMENT OF. (See Fever, Intermittent, and Leucocythæmia.)

STOMATITIS. (See Aphthæ.)

STRANGURY.

2301—℞ Ext. belladonnæ . . . . gr. j-iv.
    Olei theobromæ . . . . 3ss.—M.
Ft. suppositorium no. i.
Sig. Introduce into the bowel, and repeat in four hours, if it
be necessary.   HARTSHORNE.

2302—℞ Pulv. opii . . . . gr. ij-iv.
    Olei theobromæ . . . . 3j.—M.
Fiant suppositoria no. ii.
Sig. Introduce one into the bowel, and repeat, if necessary, in
four hours.   HARTSHORNE.

2303—℞ Pulv. opii . . . . gr. iv.
    Pulv. folli hyoscyami . . . . gr. xx.
    Olei theobromæ . . . . 3j.—M.
Fiant suppositoria no. ii.
Sig. Introduce one into the rectum.   PHILLIPS.

2304—℞ Tincturæ cannabis indicæ . . . . f3j.
Sig. A half-teaspoonful every few hours. (*Especially with
bloody urine, and when due to spinal disease.*)   RINGER.

2305—℞ Aceti scillæ,
    Spiritus ætheris nitrosi . . . . . . ãã f3ss.—M.
Sig. A half-teaspoonful in some demulcent tea every hour or
oftener.   WARING.

2306—℞ Tincturæ veratri viridis . . . . f3ss.
    Morphinæ acetatis . . . . gr. ij.
    Spiritus ætheris nitrosi . . . . f3j.
    Liquoris potassii citratis . . . q. s. ad f3viij.—M.
Sig. Shake. Tablespoonful in water every two hours. (*Used
in acute inflammation of bladder and prostate.*)

2307—℞ Ext. nucis vomicæ . . . . gr. vilj.
    Ext. glycyrrhizæ . . . . q. s.—M.
Ft. massa et in pil. no. l div.
Sig. Two pills on retiring. (*For strangury and dysuria of old
age.*)   FISCHER.

STRUMA. (See Rachitis.)

STYE (HORDEOLUM).

2308—℞ Acidi borncici . . . . ϶iv.
    Aquæ destillatæ . . . . 3v.—M.
Ft. lotio.
Sig. Apply to the eyelids several times daily.   ABADIE.

2309—℞ Hydrarg. oxidi rubri . . . . gr. xv.
    Ungt. aquæ rosæ . . . . 3j.—M.
Sig. Apply night and morning, after bathing with hot water
containing a pinch of salt to the cupful.   J. C. WILSON.

2310—℞ Calcii sulphidi . . . . gr. lx.
In pil. (gelatin-coated) no. xxx. div.
Sig. One pill after each meal and at bedtime.   J. C. WILSON.

SUPPURATION. (See Abscess.)

SWEATING. (See Phthisis.)

SWEATING, LOCAL. (See Bromidrosis.)

SYCOSIS. (See also Tinea, in Skin Diseases.)

2311—℞ Acidi tannici . . . . gr. xlv.
    Sulphuris præcip. . . . . 3iss.
    Zinci oxidi,
    Amyli . . . . ãã 3iv.
    Vaselini . . . . 3j.—M.
Sig. Use twice daily.   ROSENTHAL.

SYNOVITIS.

2312—℞ Vitell. ovi . . . . no. ij.
Pulv. sacchari albi . . . . ℨiv.
Olei amygdalæ amaræ . . . . gtt. ij.
Aquæ aurantii flor. . . . . ƒℨij.
Olei morrhuæ . . . . ƒℨv.—M.

Sig. From a teaspoonful to a tablespoonful thrice daily. (*In
strumous synovitis.*) HEDER.

2313—℞ Liquoris plumbi subacetatis . . . . . ƒℨij.
Tincturæ opii . . . . ƒℨij.
Aquæ bullientis . . . . q. s. ad ƒℨxxxij.—M.
Sig. Apply upon soft cloths saturated with solution, and place
joint at rest. (*Acute synovitis.*)

2314—℞ Tinct. iodi . . . . ƒℨj.
Sig. Apply with a brush every second or third day. · RINGER.

2315—℞ Morphinæ . . . . gr. viij.
Hydrargyri oleatis (5–10 per cent.) . . . ℨj.—M.
Sig. Apply twice daily with a soft brush. (*In the acute form.*)
MARSHALL.

2316—℞ Emplastri cantharidis . . . . 1 in. × 2 in.
Sig. Apply every night until the skin is well reddened. If
this does not avail, leave on until a bleb is formed, which
may be cut, poulticed, and dressed with simple cerate. (*In
the chronic form.*) RINGER.

2317—℞ Argenti nitratis . . . . ℨj.
Aquæ destillatæ . . . . ƒℨj.
Solve.
Sig. Apply almost to vesication. (*In acute synovitis.*)
FURNEAUX JORDAN.

2318—℞ Ichthyoli . . . . ƒℨj.
Adipis lanæ hydrosi . . . . ℨj.—M.
Sig. Apply freely upon cloth, and place joint at rest. (*Used
in acute cases.*)

2319—℞ Iodi . . . . ℨiv.
Potassii iodidi . . . . ℨj.
Aquæ destillatæ . . . . ƒℨvj.— M.
Sig. Apply externally, with a brush. LUGOL.

2320—℞ Unguenti hydrargyri . . . . ℨj.
Sig. As an injunction to the previously blistered surface.
(*In the subacute form.*) W. ADAMS.

SYPHILIS.

2321—℞ Hydrargyri protiodidi,
Lactucarii . . . . āā gr. xv.
Ext. opii . . . . gr. ij¼.
Ext. guaiaci . . . . ℨss.—M.
Ft. massa et in pil. no. xx div.
Sig. One pill at breakfast and after supper, followed by a
draught of water. DIDAY.

2322—℞ Hydrargyri chloridi corrosivi . . . . . gr. viiss.
Amyli . . . . ℨj.
Syrupi acaciæ . . . . q. s.
Misce et fiant pilulæ no. lx.
Sig. One pill three times a day. TROUSSEAU.

2323—℞ Hydrargyri chloridi corrosivi,
Ammonii chloridi . . . . āā gr. iiss.
Aquæ destillatæ . . . . ƒℨiv.--M.
Ft. solutio et adde—
Potassii iodidi . . . . ℨj.
Aquæ destillatæ . . . . ƒℨxvj.—M.
Sig. A tablespoonful before each meal. BESNIER.

2324—℞ Hydrargyri chloridi corrosivi . . . . . gr. ss.(!)
Extracti cinchonæ . . . . gr. x.
Extracti opii aquosi . . . . gr. ss.—M.
Fiant pilulæ ii.
Sig. One or two pills daily, closely watching. DUPUYTREN.

2325—℞ Pilulæ hydrargyri . . . . ₃ss.
Divide in pilulas no. x.
Sig. One pill night and morning. ("One of the best methods
of treatment in the *secondary form*.") ELLIS.

2326—℞ Pil. hydrargyri . . . . ℈ij.
Ferri sulphatis exsiccatæ . . . . ℈j.
Ext. opii aquosi . . . . gr. v.—M.
In pil. no. xx div.
Sig. One pill thrice daily. F. N. OTIS.

2327—℞ Hydrargyri chloridi corrosivi,
Ammonii chloridi . . . . āā gr. iij.
Tinct. cinchonæ comp.,
Aquæ . . . . āā f₃iij.—M.
Sig. A teaspoonful thrice daily. BUMSTEAD.

2328—℞ Hydrargyri cyanidi . . . . gr. iv.
Aquæ destillatæ . . . . f₃viij.—M.
Sig. A teaspoonful three times a day. The *Liqueur Anti-syphi-
litique* of CHAUSSIER.

2329—℞ Mercauro . . . . f₃ss.
Sig. Five to fifteen drops in water thrice daily. H. TUCKER.

2330—℞ Hydrargyri protiodidi . . . . gr. iij.
Potassii iodidi . . . . ₃ij.
Tincturæ gentianæ compositæ,
Syrupi sarsaparillæ compositæ . . āā f₃ij.—M.
Sig. A teaspoonful thrice daily. HORACE GREEN.

2331—℞ Olei hydrargyri (gray oil) . . . . . . f₃ij.
Olei olivæ (sterilized) . . . . f₃j.—M.
Sig. Two to three minims injected deeply into gluteal region
with hypodermic syringe every two or three days until
slight tenderness of gums, then administer every fourth,
sixth, or tenth day to keep patient under the influence of
mercury.

2332—℞ Hydrargyri chloridi corrosivi . . . . . gr. iv.
Ammonii chloridi . . . . gr. iv.
Aquæ destillatæ . . . . f₃iv.—M.
Sig. (Ten minims equal ⅛ grain of corrosive sublimate.) Ten
minims hypodermically into the gluteal muscles used once
every seven days until the patient is impressed with the
mercury, then once in two weeks until all symptoms disappear, and finally once a month. Continue treatment for
eighteen to twenty months in severe cases. (*Used to secure
rapid disappearance of symptoms.*)

2333—℞ Hydrargyri iodidi rubri . . . . gr. j.
Potassii iodidi . . . . ₃iv.
Syr. sarsaparillæ comp.,
Aquæ . . . . āā f₃ij.—M.
Sig. A teaspoonful thrice daily, after meals. (*Mixed treatment.*)
R. W. TAYLOR.

2334—℞ Hydrargyri biniodidi . . . . gr. j.
Potassii iodidi . . . . ₃j.
Aquæ destillatæ . . . . f₃j.
Syrupi simplicis . . . . f₃v.—M.
Sig. A tablespoonful thrice daily. *Hôpital Saint-Louis.*

2335—℞ Hydrargyri chloridi corrosivi . . . . . gr. j.
Tincturæ ferri chloridi . . . . f₃iij.
Aquæ destillatæ . . . . q. s. ad f₃vj.—M.
Sig. A tablespoonful three times a day. ERNEST GOODMAN.

2336—℞ Hydrargyri chloridi corrosivi . . . . . gr. j.
Potassii iodidi . . . . ₃ij.
Tinct. gentianæ comp. . . . . f₃iij.—M.
Sig. A teaspoonful thrice daily, after meals. (*Mixed treat-
ment.*) *Charity Hospital, N. Y.*

2337—℞ Hydrargyri chloridi corrosivi . . . . . gr. iv.
Tinct. benzoini . . . . ₃ss.
Aquæ coloniensis . . . . f₃j.
Aquæ rosæ . . . . f₃ivss.—M.
Ft. lotio.
Sig. Apply locally with a sponge to the skin for twenty
minutes. (*For squamous syphilides.*) S. W. GROSS.

2338—℞ Hydrargyri chloridi mitis,
Lycopodii . . . . āā ℥ij.—M.
Sig. Use as snuff thrice daily. (*In syphilitic lesions of the nose.*)
S. W. GROSS.

2339—℞ Potassii iodidi . . . . ℈ij.
Sacchari albi . . . . ℥j.
Extracti sarsaparillæ fluidi . . . . . . f ℥ss.
Aquæ destillatæ . . . . f ℥iij.—M.
Sig. A tablespoonful three times a day. ELLIS.

2340—℞ Potassii iodidi . . . . gr. iij.
Aquæ destillatæ . . . . f ℥j.
Solve et adde—
Hydrargyri biniodidi . . . . gr. ivss.—M.
Sig. From two to five drops three times a day, much diluted.
CHANNING.

2341—℞ Auri chloridi . . . . gr. j.
Extracti aconiti . . . . ℈ss.
Pulveris glycyrrhizæ . . . . ℈ij.
Syrupi simplicis· . . . . q. s.
Misce intime, et fiant pilulæ no. xx.
Sig. One pill three times a day. NELIGAN.

2342—℞ Potassii iodidi . . . . ℥ij.
Ammonii carbonatis . . . . ℈ss.
Tinct. cinchonæ comp. . . . . f ℥iv.
Syr. aurantii cort. . . . . f ℥iss.
Glycerini . . . . f ℥j.—M.
Sig. A teaspoonful, well diluted, after each meal.
E. L. KEYES.

2343—℞ Auri chloridi .· . . . . gr. j.
Lycopodii præparati . . . . gr. xv.
Misce et fiant chartulæ no. xvi.
Sig. Rub one on the tongue and gums daily. (Afterwards the
same quantity to be divided successively into twelve and
ten powders.) CHRESTIEN.

2344—℞ Acidi nitro-muriatici diluti . . . . . . f ℥iss.
Syrupi stillingiæ compositi . . . . . f ℥xlijss.
Aquæ destillatæ . . . . f ℥ij.—M.
Sig. One to two teaspoonfuls three times a day, with denu-
trition. (*In cases saturated with the approved remedies, but
still presenting patches on the skin and mucous membranes.*)
BARTHOLOW.

2345—℞ Hydrargyri salicylatis . . . . gr. viiss.
Confectionis rosæ . . . . ℈ss.—M.
Ft. massa et in pil. no. lx div.
Sig. One thrice daily, after meals. CHAVES.

2346—℞ Hydrargyri chloridi corrosivi,
Ammonii chloridi . . . . āā gr. iij.
Aquæ destillatæ . . . . f ℥iss.—M.
Ft. solutio et adde—
Albuminis ovi . . . . ℥iss.
Aquæ destillatæ . . . . f ℥v.
Misce, cola, et adde—
Aquæ destillatæ . . . . q. s. ad f ℥x.—M.
Sig. For hypodermic use. Three to ten minims to be used
for each injection. ℳj contains corrosive sublimate, gr. ₂₅₅.
POTTER.

2347—℞ Hydrargyri carbolatis . . . . gr. xviij.
Ext. glycyrrhizæ,
Pulv. glycyrrhizæ . . . . āā q. s. ut ft. massa.—M.
Ft. massa et in pil. no. lx div.
Obduc balsamo tolutano.
Sig. Two to four pills daily. SZADEK.

2348—℞ Hydrargyri oxidi flavi . . . . ℥iss.
Hydrargyri chloridi corrosivi . . . . . gr. ¾.
Glycerini puri . . . . f ℥xxv.—M.
Sig. For hypodermic use. Twelve and a half minims to be
used for each injection. DE SMET.

2349—℞ Hydrargyri chloridi mitis . . . . gr. xij.
      Olei vaselini . . . . ℳccxxv.
Misce.
Sig. For hypodermic injection. Twenty to thirty minims to
be used.   BALZER.

2350—℞ Hydrargyri chloridi mitis . . . . gr. iss.
      Glycerini . . . . ℳxv.—M.
Sig. For hypodermic injection. To be used each time. Two
or three injections required for an average case, before the
symptoms yield.   SCARENZIO.

2351—℞ Hydrargyri chloridi mitis,
      Sodii chloratis . . . . āā gr. xv.
      Aquæ destillatæ . . . . f ʒiss.—M.
Sig. For hypodermic injection. Twenty to thirty minims to
be used.   KRECKE.

2352—℞ Hydrargyri chloridi mitis . . . . . . gr. xv.
      Olei olivæ . . . . f ʒiss.—M.
Sig. For hypodermic injection. Twenty to thirty minims to
be used.   KOPP.

TABES MESENTERICA. (See Marasmus.)

TAPE-WORM. (See Worms.)

TETANUS.

2353—℞ Extracti physostigmatis,
      Pulveris zingiberis . . . . āā gr. j.
Misce et fiat pilula.
Sig. Every hour or two until effects are noted. (Or begin with
one-third of a grain hypodermically.)   E. WATSON.

2354—℞ Extracti physostigmatis . . . . gr. ij.
      Aquæ destillatæ . . . . f ʒj.—M.
Ft. solutio.
Sig. Ten minims every two hours hypodermically, as required.
To be pushed just short of arresting the breathing.
                              FRASER.

2355—℞ Curaris . . . . gr. j-ij.
      Aquæ . . . . gtt. c.—M.
Ft. solutio.
Sig. Ten drops hypodermically, and repeated every four or
five hours, to control the spasm.   DEMME.

2356—℞ Tincturæ cannabis indicæ . . . . . . f ʒss.
      Mucilaginis acaciæ . . . . f ʒij.
      Aquæ cinnamomi . . . . f ʒss.
Ft. haustus.
Sig. At once, and repeat in two hours, or sooner, if permis-
sible.   NÉLIGAN.

2357—℞ Chloral. hydratis . . . . ʒss.
      Syr. aurantii cort. . . . . f ʒiss.
      Aquæ . . . . ad f ʒiij.—M.
Sig. A dessertspoonful as required.   BARTHOLOW.

2358—℞ Pilocarpinæ muriatis . . . . gr. ij.
      Aquæ destillatæ . . . . f ʒj.—M.
Ft. solutio.
Sig. Ten minims hypodermically daily, with chloral hydrate
at night to produce sleep. (*In rheumatismal tetanus.*)
                           BRUNAUER.

2359—℞ Pulveris opii . . . . gr. iiss.
      Moschi optimi,
      Pulveris camphoræ . . . . āā gr. vj.
Misce et fiat pulvis.
Sig. In syrup.   W. AINSLIE.

TETANUS (Continued).

2360—℞ Pulv. opii . . . . ꞔj.
Pulv. camphorœ . . . . gr. xv.
Adipis præp. . . . . ꞔss.—M.
Ft. unguentum.
Sig. To be rubbed on the parts affected with the spasm.
THOMAS.

2361—℞ Extracti belladonnæ . . . . gr. ss-j.
Ft. pilula.
Sig. One every two hours; to be increased *pro re nata*.
HUTCHINSON.

2362—℞ Extracti conii . . . . gr. v.
Divide in pilulas ii.
Sig. One dose. Every three hours. (The *succus* is more reliable.)
CORRY.

2363—℞ Cocainæ muriatis,
Morphinæ muriatis . . . . āā gr. xij.
Aquæ destillatæ . . . . f ꞔj.—M.
Sig. Twenty to sixty minims hypodermically, as required.
LOPEZ.

2364—℞ Liquoris potassii arsenitis . . . . . . f ꞔj.
Sig. Five to eight drops, well diluted, every three hours.
DALTON.

2365—℞ Strychninæ sulphatis . . . . gr. j.
Aquæ bullientis . . . . f ꞔj.—M.
Ft. solutio.
Sig. Eight to sixteen minims hypodermically, as required.
BARTHOLOW.

2366—℞ Potassii bromidi . . . . ꞔiss.
In pulv. no. xii div.
Sig. A powder dissolved in water every three or four hours.
H. C. WOOD.

2367—℞ Nicotinæ . . . . gr. ss.
Aquæ destillatæ . . . . f ꞔj.—M.
Sig. For hypodermic use. (*Ten minims contain ₁/₂₀ of a grain.*)
ERLENMEYER.

2368—℞ Pilocarpinæ hydrochloratis . . . . . . gr. j.
Aquæ . . . . f ꞔj.—M.
Sig. Ten drops hypodermically and repeat at intervals of twenty minutes until profuse sweating, or until three doses have been administered. (*Used to eliminate poison. Patient must be freely stimulated with alcohol.*)

2369—℞ Tincturæ aconiti (Ph. Br.) . . . . . . ℳ xv.
Spiritus vini gallici . . . . f ꞔij-f ꞔss.
Aquæ destillatæ . . . . q. s. ad f ꞔiss.
Misce et fiat haustus.
Sig. Every fourth hour.
H. JONES.

THREAD-WORMS. (See Worms.)

THRUSH. (See Aphthœ.)

TIC DOULOUREUX. (See Neuralgia.)

TINEA. (See Skin Diseases.)

TINNITUS AURIUM.

2370—℞ Arnicæ . . . . ꞔij.
Aquæ bullientis . . . . Oss.
Macera per horas duas et cola. Dein adde—
Tincturæ arnicæ . . . . f ꞔij.
Tincturæ cardamomi . . . . f ꞔvj.—M.
Sig. A tablespoonful three times a day.
WILDE.

2371—℞ Acidi hydrobromici diluti (10 per cent.) f ꞔij.
Sig. One-half to one teaspoonful, in a wineglassful of sweetened water, thrice daily.
FOTHERGILL.

194

2372—℞ Pilocarpinæ hydrochloratis . . . . . . gr. j.
     Sacchari lactis . . . . gr. xviij.
     Alcohol . . . . q. s.—M.
Fiant tabellæ triturationes no. xii.
Sig. One tablet night and morning. (*In rheumatic and gouty subjects with thickening of the ear-drum.*)

2373—℞ Quininæ muriatis . . . . gr. lx.
In pil. no. xxx div.
Sig. One pill four times a day.   J. C. WILSON.

2374—℞ Sodii salicylatis . . . . ℈iij.
     Vini cocæ. . . . . f ℥iv.—M.
Sig. A dessertspoonful in water three or four times a day; gradually reduce the dose.   J. C. WILSON.

TONSILLITIS. (See also Quinsy.)

2375—℞ Potassii bromidi . . . . ℈iv.
     Potassii chloratis . . . . ℈j.
     Tinct. ferri chloridi . . . . f ℈iiss.
     Ext. glycyrrhizæ . . . . ℈j.
     Aquæ . . . . q. s. ad f ℥iv.—M.
Sig. A teaspoonful in water every two hours. Gargle and swallow.   CARL SEILER.

2376—℞ Creolin. . . . . gr. xv–xxx.
     Aquæ destillatæ . . . . Oj.
     Aquæ menthæ pip. . . . . ℈iij.—M.
Sig. Use as a gargle.   SCHNITZLER.

2377—℞ Protonucleini . . . . ℈ij.
Fiant tabellæ compressæ no. xxiv.
Sig. Dissolve a tablet in mouth every two hours until flushing of face and neck, then one every four hours. (*Used to abort inflammation in early stage.*)

2378—℞ Argenti nitratis . . . . gr. xl.
     Aquæ destillatæ . . . . f ℈j.—M.
Sig. Apply to tonsils with swab.

TOOTHACHE.

2379—℞ Pulv. acidi arseniosi,
     Iodoformi. . . . . partes æq.
     Sol. acidi carbolici (5 per cent.) . . . . q. s.—M.
Ft. pasta.
Sig. Carry the paste to the nerve on a piece of cotton the size of a pin's head. Cover with red gutta-percha to retain it. (*In exposed nerve.*)   TRUMAN.

2380—℞ Acidi arseniosi . . . . gr. ij.
     Morphinæ sulphatis . . . . gr. j.
     Creasoti . . . . q. s.—M.
Ft. pasta.
Sig. Apply by a bit of cotton-wool to carious portion.
     BARTHOLOW.

2381—℞ Pulv. acidi arseniosi,
     Cocainæ hydrochloratis . . . . . . āā gr. xxx.
     Menthol. crystal. . . . . gr. viiss.
     Glycerini . . . . q. s.—M.
Ft. pasta.
Sig. Apply to the carious cavity, and retain with a cotton or rubber plug. (*For devitalizing exposed nerves.*)   E. C. KIRK.

2382—℞ Mastiches . . . . gr. x.
     Acidi tannici . . . . ℈j.
     Ætheris sulphurici . . . . f ℈ss.—M.
     DRUITT.

2383—℞ Linimenti aconiti (B.P.),
     Chloroformi . . . . āā ℈iij.
     Tinct. capsici . . . . ℈j.
     Tinct. pyrethri,
     Olei caryophylli,
     Pulv. camphoræ . . . . āā ℈ss.—M.
Sig. A few drops on cotton placed in the cavity.   MASON.

2384—℞ Olei caryophylli,
　　　Olei cajuputi . . . . āā f3j.
　　　Pulveris opii,
　　　Camphoræ. . . . . āā ℈ss.
　　　Spiritus rectificati . . . . q. s.—M.
Ft. solutio.　　　　　　　　　　　　　　　　COPLAND.

2385—℞ Morphinæ sulphatis . . . . gr. iv.
　　　Atropinæ sulphatis . . . . gr. j.
　　　Aquæ destillatæ . . . . f3j.—M.
Sig. A few drops on cotton placed in the cavity.
　　　　　　　　　　　　　　　　　　　BARTHOLOW.

2386—℞ Creasoti . . . . gr. lxxv.
　　　Tincturæ pyrethri . . . . f3iss.—M.
Sig. Put in the hollow tooth by means of a little cotton.
　　　　　　　　　　　　　　TROUSSEAU ET REVEIL.

2387—℞ Olei pimentæ . . . . f3ij.
Sig. Cleanse cavity and pack with cotton saturated with
the oil.

2388—℞ Liq. cocoainæ muriatis (3 per cent.) . . 3vij.
　　　Morphinæ sulphatis . . . . gr. xij.
　　　Gossypii absorbentis . . . . 3vij.—M.
[Saturate the cotton and dry with a gentle heat, and then re-
card the cotton.]
Sig. Moisten a small piece with a few drops of water, and
place it in the cavity of the tooth.　　　　ELLER.

2389—℞ Olei caryophylli . . . . f3ij.
Sig. Moisten a piece of cotton and insert it into the cavity.
　　　　　　　　　　　　　　　　　　　HARTSHORNE.

2390—℞ Collodii flexilis,
　　　Acidi carbolici crystal. . . . . . . āā 3ij.—M.
Sig. Apply to the tooth-cavity by means of a probe wrapped
on the end with cotton.　　　　　　　　　GUILD.

2391—℞ Tinct. iodi . . . . f3iv.
　　　Tinct. aconiti . . . . f3j.—M.
Sig. Paint the gums twice daily around the painful tooth.
(*In dental periostitis.*)　　　　　　　　RODIER.

2392—℞ Pulv. camphoræ,
　　　Chloral. hydratis . . . . āā gr. xxx.
　　　Cocainæ hydrochloratis . . . . gr. vj.—M.
[Heat to the boiling-point of water, and an oily fluid results.]
Sig. Introduce a small quantity of the mixture into the
carious tooth.　　　　　　　　　　　GSELL-FELS.

2393—℞ Ext. opii alcoholici,
　　　Pulv. camphoræ,
　　　Balsami peruviani. . . . . āā gr. viiss.
　　　Mastiches . . . . gr. xv.
　　　Chloroformi . . . . f3iiss.—M.
Sig. Wet a bit of cotton with the solution, and place it in the
carious cavity.　　　　　　　　　*L'Union Médicale.*

TRICHINOSIS.

2394—℞ Sodii sulphocarbolatis . . . . gr. ij-x.
　　　Aquæ . . . . f3ij.—M.
Ft. haustus.
Sig. To be repeated three or four times daily.　　FUREY.

2395—℞ Saloli . . . . 3iss.
　　　Tetramethyli thionin-chloridi . . . . gr. xxx.—M.
Pone in capsulas no. xxx.
Sig. One capsule every four hours. (*Used in intermediate stage.*)

2396—℞ Acidi sclerotinici . . . . gr. vj.
　　　Acidi carbolici . . . . gr. ½.
　　　Aquæ . . . . f3ss.—M.
Sig. Twenty minims, hypodermically, once a day.
　　　　　　　　　　　　　　　　　J. C. WILSON.

2397—℞ Chloral. hydratis . . . . gr. j-ij.
Syrupi simplicis . . . . ʒj.—M.
Sig. To be given every two hours, unless there be profound
sleep. Double the dose if given by the rectum.
WIDERHOFER.

2398—℞ Coniinæ hydrobromatis . . . . gr. ₁/₆.
Aquæ destillatæ . . . . f ʒij.—M.
Sig. Two to four minims hypodermically and repeat fre-
quently to relax spasm. (*For infant several days old.*)

2399—℞ Tincturæ opii . . . . gtt. v.
Tincturæ asafœtidæ . . . . f ʒiss.
Syrupi simplicis . . . . f ʒv.
Aquæ . . . . ad f ʒxv.—M.
Sig. A half-teaspoonful hourly. EBERLE.

2400—℞ Tincturæ opii . . . . f ʒiv.
Sig. One drop every three hours, alternating with the following:

2401—℞ Pulveris ipecacuanhæ comp. . . . . . . gr. xxiv.
Zinci sulphatis . . . . ʒj.—M.
In pulv. no. xii div.
Sig. A powder every three hours. FURLONGE.

2402—℞ Extracti gelsemii fluidi . . . . ℳviij-xvj.
Syrupi simplicis . . . . f ʒj.
Aquæ destillatæ . . . . q. s. ad f ʒss.—M.
Sig. A half-teaspoonful every two to four hours.
BARTHOLOW.

2403—℞ Tincturæ opii . . . . ℳj.
Olei ricini . . . . f ʒj.—M.
Sig. A teaspoonful every four hours, with a warm bath.
DRUITT

TUBERCULOSIS. (See Rachitis and Phthisis.)

TYMPANITES. (See also Fever.)

2404—℞ Olei terebinthinæ . . . . f ʒj.
Olei amygdalæ exprcs. . . . . f ʒss.
Tinct. opii . . . . f ʒij.
Mucil. acaciæ . . . . f ʒv.
Aquæ laurocerasi . . . . f ʒss.—M.
Sig. A teaspoonful every three to six hours. BARTHOLOW.

2405—℞ Olei ricini,
Olei terebinthinæ,
Mucilaginis acaciæ,
Aquæ menthæ piperitæ . . . . . . āā f ʒss.
Misce et fiat haustus. HOOPER.

2406—℞ Olei terebinthinæ . . . . ʒj.
Olei olivæ . . . . ʒiss.
Camphoræ . . . . gr. xx.
Decocti avenæ . . . . f ʒviij.—M.
Ft. enema.
Sig. Inject into the bowel. (*In hysterical tympanites.*)
COPLAND.

2407—℞ Olei terebinthinæ,
Olei ricini . . . . āā f ʒiij.
Olei cajuputi . . . . ℳvj.
Magnesiæ calcinatæ . . . . ʒj.
Aquæ menthæ piperitæ . . . . f ʒiss.
Misce et fiat haustus. JOY.

2408—℞ Guaiacoli carbonatis . . . . ʒj.
Fiant chartulæ no. xxx.
Sig. One powder every four hours. (*Used in tympany of typhoid
fever or in any cases with intestinal fermentation.*)

2409—℞ Pulv. capsici . . . . gr. vj-xxiv.
Sacchari lactis . . . . ʒiss.—M.
In pulv. no. xii div.
Sig. A powder every four hours. PHILLIPS.

2410—℞ Spiritus ætheris compositi,
    Tincturæ cardamomi compositi . . āā f ℨj.—M.
Sig. Teaspoonful every hour or two.

2411—℞ Olei terebinthinæ . . . . f ℨj.
    Olei olivæ . . . . f ℨiss.
    Camphoræ . . . . ℈j.
    Decocti avenæ . . . . f ℨviij.
Misce et fiat enema. (*In hysterical tympanites.*)   COPLAND.

TYPHOID AND TYPHUS FEVER. (See Fever.)

ULCER.

2412—℞ Creasoti . . . . ℳiv.
    Aquæ destillatæ . . . . f ℨvj.—M.
Sig. In tablespoonful doses. (*In chronic gastric ulcer.*)
                             NIEMEYER.

2413—℞ Argenti oxidi,
    Extracti hyoscyami . . . . āā gr. v.
Misce et fiant pilulæ no. x. (*In gastric ulcer.*) BARTHOLOW.

2414—℞ Argenti nitratis . . . . gr. v.
    Pulv. opii . . . . gr. iiss.—M.
Ft. massa et in pil. no. xx div.
Sig. One pill thrice daily. (*In gastric ulcer.*)
                             HARTSHORNE.

2415—℞ Bismuthi subnitratis . . . . ℨij.
    Pulv. opii . . . . gr. iij.—M.
In pulv. no. xii div.
Sig. One powder thrice daily, followed continuously by—

2416—℞ Codein. phosph.,
    Ext. belladonnæ . . . . āā gr. v.
    Bismuthi carb. . . . . gr. l.
    Lactose . . . . ℨj.—M.
Ft. chart. xv.
Sig. Take two or three powders daily. (*Gastric ulcer.*)
                             LEUBE.

2417—℞ Liq. potassii arsenitis . . . . f ℨss.
Sig. One drop, repeated as required, to relieve the pain and
  vomiting. (*In gastric ulcer.*)   BARTHOLOW.

2418—℞ Skimmed milk two parts and liquor calcis one part,
  mixed, as a steady diet. (*In gastric ulcer.*) DA COSTA.

2419—℞ Argenti nitratis fusæ . . . . q. s.
Sig. Apply to the surface and edges, and strap with diachylon
  adhesive plaster. (*In leg-ulcers.*)   T. M. MARKOE.

2420—℞ Balsami copaibæ . . . . ℨij.
    Mucilaginis acaciæ . . . . f ℨss.
Misce et adde—
    Aquæ calcis . . . . f ℨvj.
Fiat injectio. (*In ulceration of the urethra, rectum, or vagina.*)
                           ABERNETHY.

2421—℞ Santonin . . . . gr. j.
    Hydrargyri chloridi mitis . . . . . . gr. iv.
    Sacchari lactis . . . . q. s.—M.
Divid. in chart. iv.
Sig. One every hour, following the last powder with a dose of
  castor oil. (*Corneal ulcer.*)   HANSELL.

2422—℞ Zinci sulpho-carbolatis . . . . ℨvj.
    Aquæ destillatæ . . . . f ℨviij.—M.
Sig. Each portion to be used to be mixed with three parts of
  water. (*A lotion for fetid ulcers.*) H. LEE.

2423—℞ Emplastri plumbi . . . . ℨij.
    Ungt. hydrargyri . . . . ℨss.
    Olei cadini . . . . ℨij.—M.
Ft. unguentum.
Sig. Spread on linen and apply. (*In inflamed syphilitic ulcers.*)
                     BUMSTEAD AND TAYLOR.

2424—℞ Chloral. hydratis . . . . ℈ss-ij.
Aquæ . . . . f ℥vj.—M.

Ft. lotio.
Sig. Use as a wash. (*In sluggish ulcers.*)   KEYES.

2425—℞ Hydrargyri chloridi corrosivi . . . . . gr. xv.
Acidi carbolici . . . . ℳxxx.
Aquæ . . . . q. s. ad ℥iv.—M.

Ft. lotio.
Sig. Pack on cotton and renew daily. (*In syphilitic ulcers.*)
FOX.

2426—℞ Unguenti hydrargyri nitratis,
Unguenti simplicis . . . . āā ℥j.—M.

Ft. unguentum.
Sig. Apply locally. (*In serpiginous ulcers.*)   KEYES.

2427—℞ Tincturæ iodi . . . . f ℥j.
Acidi tannici . . . . . . q. s. ad saturandum.—M.

(*An application to ulcers of the rectum and anus, fissure in ano.*)
BARTHOLOW.

2428—℞ Iodoformi pulverizati . . . . ℥j.

Detur in scatula.
Sig. Use as a dusting-powder.   BARTHOLOW.

2429—℞ Acidi nitrici . . . . ℳxij.
Aquæ destillatæ . . . . f ℥xvj.—M.

Ft. lotio. (*In indolent ulcers.*)   E. HOWE.

2430—℞ Aluminis . . . . ℥ij.
Aquæ destillatæ . . . . f ℥viij.—M.

Ft. lotio. (*In foul ulcers.*)   PENNYPACKER.

2431—℞ Finely powdered chloride of sodium . ℥x.
Powdered menthol . . . . ℥j.

Sig. Mix thoroughly and use as a dusting powder after thoroughly washing the surface of the ulcer clean. (*For leg
ulcer.*)

2432—℞ Acidi pyrogallici,
Pulv. amyli . . . . āā ℥ij.
Vaselini . . . . ℥vj.—M.

Ft. unguentum.
Sig. Preserve in a glass-stoppered jar. Spread on lint and
apply once daily. (*In venereal ulcerations.*)   TERRILLON.

2433—℞ Formaldehydi (40 per cent. sol.) . . . ℳviij.
Aquæ hydrogenii dioxidi . . . . . . f ℥xvj.—M.

Sig. Use locally as wash. (*Used as cleansing and antiseptic
wash for foul ulcers.*)

2434—℞ Piperazini . . . . ℥iv.

Pone in capsulas no. xxiv.
Sig. Dissolve a capsule in about two ounces of water, saturate
a piece of surgeon's lint, and apply to ulcer. The treatment
to be repeated several times a day.

2435—℞ Acidi tannici . . . . gr. lxxv.
Hydrargyri nitratis acid. . . . . . . gtt. xij.
Adipis . . . . ℥viiss.—M.

Ft. unguentum.
Sig. Apply as a dressing. (*For chronic syphilitic ulcers.*)
VENOT.

2436—℞ Bovinine . . . . f ℥vii.

Sig. Apply locally to ulcer. (*In leg ulcer.*)   H. TUCKER.

2437—℞ Ext. colocynth. comp. . . . . gr. xiv.
    Hydrargyri chloridi mitis . . . . gr. vj.—M.

In pil. no. iv div.
Sig. To be taken at once, and in four hours followed by one
ounce of compound infusion of senna.   JOHNSON.

2438—℞ Olei tiglii . . . . gtt. viij.
    Elaterii . . . . gr. ss–j.
    Micæ panis . . . . q. s.—M.

Ft. massa et in pil. no. viii div.
Sig. One or two pills to produce watery stools. Use cautiously.
    BARTHOLOW.

2439—℞ Methyli cærulei (methyl blue) . . . . gr. xij.

Pone in capsulas no. xii.
Sig. One capsule three times a day. (Diuretic.)

2440—℞ Hydrargyri chloridi mitis . . . . gr. vj.
    Pilulæ colocynthidis compositæ. . . . gr. xiv.—M.

Fiant pilulæ ii.
Sig. One dose, to be followed in four hours by a dose of compound liquorice powder.   GEORGE JOHNSON.

2441—℞ Caffeinæ citratæ . . . . gr. xxiv.

Fiant chartulæ no. xii.
Sig. One powder every two hours until three powders have
been taken each day. (Used as diuretic if arterial tension is
low.)

2442—℞ Ext. pilocarpi alc.,
    Ext. scillæ,
    Resinæ jalapæ,
    Resinæ scammonii . . . . āā gr. xv.—M.

Ft. massa et in pil. no. xx div.
Sig. Four or five pills daily for four or five days. Strict milk
diet is requisite.   ROLLAND.

2443—℞ Pilocarpinæ muriatis . . . . gr. ij.
    Aquæ destillatæ . . . . ℥ij.—M.

Ft. solutio.
Sig. Inject hypodermically five minims ; for a child of six
years. Ten minims for an adult.   E. R. STONE.

2444—℞ Acidi benzoici . . . . ℈v.

Divide in chartulas no. v.
Sig. One powder every three hours, largely diluted.
    DA COSTA.

2445—℞ Sodii benzoatis . . . . ℥iij.

In pulv. no. xii div.
Sig. One powder in solution, or in capsules, every three hours.
    PARZEVSKI.

2446—℞ Chloral. hydratis . . . . ℈viij.
    Syr. aurantii cort. . . . . ℥j.
    Aquæ . . . . ad f℥iv.—M.

Sig. A . dessertspoonful as the initial dose, followed by teaspoonful doses, repeated as necessary to relieve the convulsions.   JAS. ANDREW.

2447—℞ Tincturæ scillæ . . . . f℥ii.
    Liquoris ammonii acetatis . . . . . . f℥ij.
    Decocti scoparii . . . . q. s. ad f℥vj.—M.

Sig. Two tablespoonfuls three times daily.   CHARTERIS.

2448—℞ Tincturæ hyoscyami . . . . f℥iij.
    Spiritus ætheris nitrosi . . . . f℥ss.
    Liquoris ammonii acetatis . . . . . . f℥j.
    Aquæ camphoræ . . . . q. s. ad f℥vj.—M.

Sig. A tablespoonful every three hours. (Inhalation of
chloroform during convulsions, or chloral hydrate by the
mouth or hypodermically. In sudden attacks in plethoric
persons, as sometimes in pregnancy, free venesection.)
    CHARTERIS.

URIC ACID DIATHESIS. (See also Gout.)

2449—℞ Lithii carbonatis . . . . ʒiiss.
Ext. gentianæ . . . . gr. lxxv.-M.

Ft. massa et in pil. no. c div.
Sig. One pill after each meal. (*In chronic cases with no complication.*) PIERRE VIGIER.

2450—℞ Lithii carbonatis,
Sodii iodidi . . . . āā ʒiiss.
Ext. gentianæ,
Pulv. acaciæ . . . . āā gr. xxiij.
Ext. glycyrrhizæ . . . . ʒv.—M.

Ft. massa et in pil. no. c div.
Sig. Preserve in a well-stopped bottle. One pill after meals.
(*In chronic cases with tophi in the joints.*) PIERRE VIGIER.

2451—℞ Lithii carbonatis,
Potassii iodidi . . . . āā ʒiiss.
Pulv. acaciæ . . . . gr. xxiij.
Ext. gentianæ . . . . ʒiiiss.—M.

Ft. massa et in pil. no. c. div.
Sig. One pill after each meal. (*In chronic cases with tophi in the joints.*) PIERRE VIGIER.

2452—℞ Lycetoli . . . . ʒj.

Pone in phialus no. xlviii.
Sig. Dissolve the contents of a vial in water and take after each meal. (*Used in subacute and chronic cases.*)

2453—℞ Sodii bicarbonatis . . . . ʒj.
Tincturæ calumbæ . . . . f ʒj.
Infusi quassiæ . . . . f ʒiij.—M.

Sig. A tablespoonful four times a day. HAZARD.

2454—℞ Piperazini . . . . ʒij.

Pone in capsulas no. xxiv.
Sig. Dissolve a capsule in a full glass of water and take after meals.

2455—℞ Sodii boratis . . . . ʒiij.
Sodii bicarbonatis,
Potassii nitratis . . . . āā ʒiss.—M.

In pulv. no. xii div.
Sig. One powder in a full draught of water. DRUITT.

2456—℞ Liq. potassii arsenitis . . . . ℳv.
Potassii bicarbonatis,
Ferri et potassii tartratis . . . . . āā gr. v.
Infusi quassiæ . . . . f ʒj.—M.

Ft. haustus.
Sig. To be taken thrice daily, two hours after meals. (*In asthenic cases.*) FOTHERGILL.

2457—℞ Acidi hydrochlorici diluti . . . . . . f ʒj.
Acidi lactici . . . . f ʒij.
Syrupi simplicis . . . . f ʒss.
Aquæ destillatæ . . . . f ʒj.—M.

Sig. A dessertspoonful after each meal. (*When the excess of acid is due to faulty digestion.*) BARTHOLOW.

URTICARIA. (See also Pruritus.)

2458—℞ Potassii bromidi . . . . ʒss.
Aquæ destillatæ . . . . q. s. ad f ʒiij.—M.

Sig. A dessertspoonful four times a day. McCALL ANDERSON.

2459—℞ Phenazoni . . . . ʒj.

Fiant chartulæ no. xii.
Sig. One powder three times a day. (*Used to relieve itching and abort attack.*)

2460—℞ Quiniæ sulphatis . . . . gr. xij.
Pulveris rhei . . . . gr. xxiv.

Misce et fiant pilulæ no. xii.
Sig. One pill three times a day. (*When intermittent.*)
WARING.

2461—℞ Plumbi acetatis,
Ammonii carbonatis . . . . āā 3j.
Tincturæ opii . . . . f3ss.
Aquæ rosæ . . . . f3viij.—M.

Sig. Apply locally. HAZARD.

2462—℞ Acidi benzoici . . . . gr. x-xx.
Aquæ destillatæ . . . . f3viij.

Misce et fiat lotio. (*To allay itching in chronic cases.*) RINGER.

2463—℞ Chloralis.
Camphoræ . . . . āā 3j.
Amyli pulv. . . . . 3j-ij.—M.

Sig. Keep tightly corked in a wide-mouthed bottle. Rub in
with the hand. BULKLEY.

2464—℞ Sodii biboratis . . . . 3ss.
Aquæ destillatæ . . . . f3viij.—M.

Ft. lotio. (*Also in chloasma, or liver-spots.—PEREIRA.*)
WARING.

2465—℞ Chloroformi . . . . f3j.
Glycerini . . . . f3iv.—M.

Ft. lotio.
Sig. Apply locally with a brush. DUPARC.

2466—℞ Acidi benzoici . . . . gr. viij.
Aquæ . . . . f3iv.—M.

Ft. lotio.
Sig. Apply locally as a wash. SQUIRE.

2467—℞ Hydrargyri chloridi corrosivi. . . . . gr. iss.
Chloroformi . . . . ℳxx.
Glycerini . . . . f3ij.
Aquæ rosæ . . . . f3vj.—M.

Ft. lotio.
Sig. Use locally. (*Also used in pruritus and in papular and
vesicular diseases.*) BURGESS.

2468—℞ Sodii bicarbonatis . . . . 3j.
Glycerini . . . . 3iss.
Aquæ sambuci . . . . f3viss.—M.

Ft. lotio.
Sig. Apply to allay the itching. TILBURY FOX.

2469—℞ Potassii cyanidi . . . . gr. vj.
Pulv. cocci . . . . gr. j.
Ungt. aquæ rosæ . . . . 3j.—M.

Ft. unguentum.
Sig. Apply locally. (*Also used in pruritus.*) ANDERSON.

2470—℞ Salolpheni . . . . 3j.

Fiant chartulæ no. xii.
Sig. One powder before meals. (*Used in lithæmic subjects, and
also in intestinal fermentation.*)

2471—℞ Hydrargyri chloridi corrosivi . . . . . gr. j.
Acidi hydrocyanici diluti . . . . 3j.
Misturæ amygdalæ . . . . f3vj.—M.

Ft. lotio.
Sig. Apply locally, to allay the itching. (*Also used in lichen
and in the syphilodermata.*) TILBURY FOX.

UTERUS, SUBINVOLUTION OF.

2472—℞ Ext. ergotæ fld.,
Ext. viburni fld. . . . . āā f3j.—M.

Sig. A teaspoonful in water three times a day, after meals.
ELLWOOD WILSON.

2473—℞ Strychninæ sulphatis . . . . gr. ⅙.
Quininæ sulphatis . . . . gr. ij.
Ext. ergotæ . . . . gr. j.
Misce et fiat pil. uo. i.
Sig. Oue pill three times a day. B. C. HIRST.

UVULA, RELAXATION OF.

2474—℞ Trochisci acidi tannici . . . . no. xx.
Sig. Let one dissolve slowly in the mouth every two or three
hours. WILLIAM AITKEN.

2475—℞ Zinci chloridi . . . . 3j.
Aquæ . . . . fȝij.—M.
Sig. Apply to the soft palate and uvula. MORELL MACKENZIE.

2476—℞ Pulveris capsici . . . . 3ss.
Potassii nitratis,
Ammonii chloridi . . . . āā 3j.
Misce bene et detur in scatula.
Sig. Apply by meaus of a camel's-hair pencil.
B. GRANVILLE.

2477—℞ Liq. ferri perchloridi . . . . 3ij.
Aquæ . . . . fȝij.—M.
Sig. Apply to the soft palate and uvula. MORELL MACKENZIE.

2478—℞ Argenti nitratis . . . . gr. x.
Aquæ destillatæ . . . . fȝj.—M.
Sig. Apply to uvula on swab night and morniug. (*In acute
cases with pain.*)

2479—℞ Acidi tannici . . . . 3iss.
Aquæ . . . . fȝvj.—M.
Ft. gargarisma.
Sig. Use as a gargle every two or three hours. SAJOUS.

2480—℞ Pulv. aluminis . . . . 3ij.
Aquæ . . . . fȝvj.—M.
Ft. gargarisma.
Sig. Use as a gargle every two or three hours. SAJOUS.

2481—℞ Aluminis . . . . 3j.
Infusi gallæ . . . . fȝvj.—M.
Ft. gargarisma. (*With hypertrophied tonsils.*) WARING.

VAGINISMUS.

$$-\bigvee-$$

2482—℞ Cocainæ (alkaloid) . . . . gr. vj.
Iodoformi . . . . 3j.
Extracti belladonnæ . . . . gr. iij.
Olei theobromatis . . . . 3iij.—M.
Fiant suppositoria no. vi.
Sig. Insert iuto vagina at night.

VAGINITIS.

2483—℞ Tincturæ cubebæ . . . . fȝij.
Sig. A teaspoónful three times a day. PIORRY.

2484—℞ Acidi boracici . . . . 3iiss.
Glycerini . . . . 3xxx.—M.
Sig. Three or four dessertspoonfuls in a quart of water as a
vaginal injection twice daily, or upon a cotton tampou.
CHÉRON.

2485—℞ Cubebæ . . . . 3j.
Aquæ . . . . Oj.—M.
Ft. infusum. (*As a vaginal injection.*) PIORRY.

2486—℞ Hydrastinæ . . . . gr. vj.
Boroglycerini . . . . 3iij.—M.
Fiant suppositoria no. vi.
Sig. Insert a suppository after hot douche twice or thrice daily.

2487—℞ Aluminis . . . . 3j.
Aquæ . . . . Oj.—M.
Ft. lotio. (*In vulvitis of children.*) RINGER.

VAGINITIS (Continued).

2488—℞ Safranin . . . . gr. ⅙.
      ; Salol,
       Chloral,
       Naphthol . . . . āā ʒj.
       Alcohol (90 per cent.) . . . . f ʒvj.
   Sig. A tablespoonful to be added to two quarts of water.
   (*Douche.*)

2489—℞ Glyceriti acidi tannici . . . . ʒj.
   Sig. Apply locally, or diluted, as an injection. (*In chronic
      vaginitis of children.*)   RINGER.

2490—℞ Argenti nitratis . . . . ℈ij.
       Aquæ destillatæ . . . . f ʒj.—M.
   Sig. Apply on a cotton pledget, within the cervical canal and
      over the vaginal mucous membrane.   EMMET.

2491—℞ Potassii permanganitis . . . . ʒiv.
   Sig. Half-teaspoonful in two quarts of water as vaginal douche
      night and morning.

2492—℞ Balsami gurjunæ . . . . ʒij.
       Liquoris calcis . . . . f ʒiv.—M.
   Sig. Saturate a cotton tampon, and leave it in the vagina
      twenty-four hours.   VIDAL.

2493—℞ Glycerini . . . . ʒiv.
       Acidi tannici . . . . ʒss.
       Morphinæ sulphatis . . . . gr. ij.—M.
   Sig. Paint the whole vaginal canal with nitrate of silver solu-
      tion (1 to 8), then saturate a cotton tampon with the above
      solution, and pack it in the vagina to slightly distend it.
      Leave the tampon in for two days. (*In the subacute form.*)
                    T. G. THOMAS.

2494—℞ Acetanilid . . . . gr. v.
       Tannin . . . . gr. j.
       Extract of hyoscyamus . . . . gr. ¼.
       Sugar of milk . . . . gr. xx.—M.
   Sig. This is for one suppository, to be used for vaginal in-
      flammation.

VALVULAR DISEASE. (See Heart-Disease.)

VARICOSE VEINS.

2495—℞ Ext. hamamelidis fld. . . . . f ʒiij.
   Sig. A teaspoonful three or four times daily, with compresses
      applied externally.   MUSSER.

2496—℞ Ext. ergotini aquosi . . . . ʒj.
       Glycerini . . . . f ʒj.
       Aquæ destillatæ . . . . f ʒvij.—M.
   Sig. Fifteen minims hypodermically, near the veins.
                    BARTHOLOW.

2497—℞ Barii chloridi . . . . gr. xxx.
       Aquæ destillatæ . . . . q. s. ut ft. sol.
       Lanolini . . . . gr. ccxxv.
       Olei amygdalæ dulcis . . . . ♏lxxv.—M.
   Ft. unguentum.
   Sig. Use three times daily, with friction, where blue veins
      shine through the skin.   KOBERT.

2498—℞ Liquoris plumbi subacetatis . . . . . f ʒiv.
       Aquæ . . . . q. s. ad f ʒviij.—M.
   Sig. Apply on cotton saturated with lotion.

VARIOLA. (See Small-Pox.)

VENEREAL DISEASE. (See Syphilis, Chancroid, etc.)

2499—℞ Pil. hydrargyri,
Pil. rhei comp.,
Ext. hyoscyami . . . . āā ǝj.—M.
In pil. no. xii div.
Sig. Two pills occasionally at bedtime. (*In plethoric cases.*)
TANNER.

2500—℞ Hydrargyri chloridi corrosivi . . . . gr. j.
Glycerini . . . . ʒj.
Tinct. cinchonæ comp. . . . . . . ad ʒiij.
Olei menthæ pip. . . . . ♏xxv.—M.
Sig. One teaspoonful in a wineglassful of water thrice daily.
(*In vertigo of the aged.*) TANNER.

2501—℞ Pulv. jalapæ . . . . gr. xij.
Hydrargyri chloridi mitis . . . . . . gr. iij.
Potassii sulphatis . . . . gr. vij.—M.
Ft. pulvis.
Sig. To be taken at bedtime. (*In bilious vertigo.*)
A. T. THOMPSON.

2502—℞ Hydrargyri chloridi corrosivi . . . . . gr. j.
Glycerini . . . . f ʒj.
Tincturæ cinchonæ compositæ . . . . f ʒij.
Olei menthæ piperitæ . . . . ♏xxv.—M.
Sig. A teaspoonful in a wineglassful of water three times a
day. (*In the vertigo and dizziness of the aged.*)
C. HANDFIELD JONES.

2503—℞ Pulveris rhei . . . . ʒj.
Sodii bicarbonatis,
Pulveris gentianæ . . . . āā ʒij.
Aquæ menthæ piperitæ,
Aquæ destillatæ . . . . āā f ʒiij.—M.
Sig. A tablespoonful before each meal. (*When due to indiges-
tion.*) E. C. MANN.

2504—℞ Spiritus glonoini . . . . f ʒj.
Sig. One drop in water three times a day, to be gradually increased until temporal headache. (*Used in aural vertigo.*)

2505—℞ Potassii bicarbonatis . . . . ʒij.
Tincturæ nucis vomicæ . . . . f ʒss.
Tincturæ cardamomi compositæ . . . f ʒiij.
Liquoris lacto-peptini . . . . f ʒj.
Syrupi simplicis . . . . f ʒij.
Aquæ menthæ piperitæ . . . . q. s. ad f ʒiv.—M.
Sig. A tablespoonful in water every three or four hours. (*In
gastric vertigo.*) H. V. SWERINGEN.

2506—℞ Tinct. gelsemii . . . . f ʒj.
Sig. Ten minims thrice daily. (*In aural vertigo.*) RINGER.

2507—℞ Tinct. digitalis . . . . f ʒj.
Sig. Twelve drops in water three or four times a day. (*In
weak heart.*) J. C. WILSON.

VOMITING. (See also Morning Sickness and Sea-Sickness.)

2508—℞ Chloralis . . . . gr. xx.
Potassii bromidi . . . . ʒj.
Mucilaginis amyli . . . . f ʒiv.—M.
Sig. Warm gently and use as rectal injection after first using
enema to unload rectum.

2509—℞ Acidi carbolici . . . . gr. iv.
Bismuthi subnitratis . . . . ʒij.
Mucilaginis acaciæ . . . . f ʒj.
Aquæ menthæ piperitæ . . . . f ʒiij.—M.
Sig. A tablespoonful every two, three, or four hours. (*When
due to acute stomachal and intestinal disorder.*) BARTHOLOW.

2510—℞ Creasoti . . . . ♏vj.
Pulveris tragacanthæ . . . . ʒss.
Aquæ camphoræ . . . . f ʒvj.—M.
Sig. A sixth part to be taken for a dose. (*In obstinate vomiting.*)
KESTEVEN.

2511—℞ Menthol . . . . gr. j.
Sodii bicarb. . . . . gr. c.—M.
Ft. in caps. xii.
Sig. One capsule three times a day. (*Nervous vomiting.*)

2512—℞ Liquoris calcis,
Lactis recentis . . . . āā f ʒiv.—M.
Sig. A tablespoonful every half-hour or hour.   WOOD.

2513—℞ Vini ipecacuanhæ . . . . f ʒss.
Sig. One drop every hour to thrice daily. (*Suitable in all
cases.*)   RINGER.

2514—℞ Extracti nucis vomicæ . . . . gr. j.
Extracti conii . . . . gr. xij.
Misce et fiant pilulæ no. vi.
Sig. One three times a day. (*When due to malignant disease of
the stomach.*)   BARLOW.

2515—℞ Sodii bicarbonatis . . . . gr. xv.
Acidi hydrocyanici diluti . . . . . . ℥iss.
Aquæ camphoræ . . . . f ʒx.—M.
Ft. haustus.
Sig. To be taken thrice daily after meals. (*When due to
acidity.*)   CHAMBERS.

2516—℞ Cocalnæ hydrochloratis . . . . gr. vj.
Aquæ destillatæ . . . . f ʒviiss.—M.
Sig. Two tablespoonfuls every hour, until six grains of cocaine have been taken during the twenty-four hours. To
avoid vertigo, the recumbent posture is necessary. (*In
vomiting of pregnancy.*)   DUJARDIN-BEAUMETZ.

2517—℞ Ext. nucis vomicæ . . . . gr. xv.
Ext. belladonnæ,
Ext. opii . . . . āā gr. iij.—M.
Ft. massa et in pil. no. xx div.
Sig. One pill at night. (*In vomiting of uterine catarrh.*)
AUDHOUI.

2518—℞ Bismuthi subnitratis . . . . ʒij.
Acidi hydrocyanici diluti . . . . . . f ʒss.
Mucilaginis acaciæ,
Aquæ menthæ piperitæ . . . . . . āā f ʒij.—M.
Sig. A tablespoonful thrice daily. (*With gastric ulcer.*)
DA COSTA.

2519—℞ Ext. belladonnæ,
Ext. physostigmatis,
Ext. nucis vomicæ,
Aloini . . . . āā gr. xv.
Ferri sulphatis exsiccatæ . . . . ʒj.—M.
Ft. massa et in pil. no. lx div.
Sig. One pill at bedtime. One grain of permanganate of
potash, in distilled water, is also taken thrice daily. (*In
hysterical vomiting.*)   BARTHOLOW.

2520—℞ Tinct. aconiti . . . . gtt. xxx.
Bismuth. subnit. . . . . ʒiij.
Ft. chart. x.
Sig. One powder every half-hour. (*Vomiting due to excita-
bility of gastric mucous membrane.*)   HARE.

2521—℞ Aloini . . . . gr. v.
Strychninæ sulphatis . . . . gr. j.
Ext. colocynth. comp. . . . . gr. v.
Ext. hyoscyami . . . . ʒj.—M.
Ft. massa et in pil. no. lx div.
Sig. One pill after each meal. (*In obstinate vomiting due to
chronic constipation.*)   DA COSTA.

2522—℞ Iodini . . . . ℥ss vel j.
Acidi carbolici . . . . ℥ij.
Aquæ . . . . q. s. ad ʒj.—M.
HARE.

2523—℞ Acidi hydrobromici . . . . f ʒj.
Sig. Thirty minims in a half-wineglassful of water four times
daily. (*In vomiting due to gastric ulcer.*)   RINGER.

VOMITING (Continued).

2524—℞ Potassii iodidi . . . . ℈iv.
   Infusi quassiæ . . . . f℥viij.—M.
Sig. A tablespoonful three times a day. (*In sympathetic vomiting.*)   SELKIRK.

2525—℞ Chloroformi . . . . f℥j.
Sig. Two to five minims, on sugar. (*In non-inflammatory vomiting.*)   RINGER.

2526—℞ Tinct. nucis vomicæ . . . . ℳij.
   Aquæ laurocerasi . . . . f℥j.—M.
Sig. Ten drops night and morning. (*In pregnancy.*) KROYLA.

2527—℞ Hydrargyri cum cretâ . . . . gr. iv.
   Sacchari lactis . . . . gr. x.—M.
In pulv. no. xii div.
Sig. A powder dry on the tongue every two hours. (*In children with clayey stools.*)   RINGER.

2528—℞ Potassii nitratis . . . . ℨj.
   Acidi hydrocyanici diluti . . . . . . gtt. vj.
   Syr. simplicis . . . . f℥ss.
   Aquæ destillatæ . . . . f℥iss.—M.
Sig. A quarter to a half-teaspoonful thrice daily. (*In infantile vomiting.*)   EUSTACE SMITH.

2529—℞ Liq. potassii arsenitis . . . . f℥ss.
Sig. A drop every half-hour, for six or eight doses. (*In vomiting of drunkards and of pregnancy.*) A. A. SMITH.

VULVITIS. (See Vaginitis.)

WAKEFULNESS. (See Insomnia.)

WARTS. (See also Condylomata.)

2530—℞ Acidi salicylici,
   Alcoholis . . . . āā ℨij.
   Æther. sulph. . . . . ℨv.
   Collodii . . . . ℨx.—M.
Sig. Paint the warts with the solution daily. E. VIDAL.

WHITLOW. (See Onychia.)

WHOOPING-COUGH.

2531—℞ Ext. castaneæ fld. . . . . f℥iiiss.
   Glycerini . . . . f℥ss.
   Potassii bromidi . . . . ℨij.—M.
Sig. A teaspoonful in water every two or three hours, for a child six years old.   J. C. WILSON.

2532—℞ Powdered belladonna-root . . . . . . gr. ⅛.
   Dover's powder . . . . gr. ½.
   Sublimed sulphur . . . . gr. iv.
   White sugar . . . . gr. x.—M.
Sig. Take in one dose from two to ten times a day, according to age of patient and effect produced. GERMAIN SÉE.

2533—℞ Quininæ tannatis . . . . gr. xxiv.
   Theobromatis . . . . ℨvj.
Misce et fiant trochisci no. xxiv.
Sig. One lozenge three or four times a day. (*Used as prophylactic if child is exposed to the contagion, and also as tonic during the continuance of the disease.*)

2534—℞ Antipyrin . . . . gr. ij.
   Sacchari albi . . . . ℨj.—M.
In pulv. no. xiv div.
Sig. A powder three times during the day and once during the night for very young children. Dose increased up to fifteen grains for adults. SONNENBERGER.

2535—℞ Acidi nitrici diluti . . . . f 3xij.
    Syrupi simplicis . . . . f 3iiiss.
    Aquæ destillatæ . . . . f 3j.—M.
Sig. A teaspoonful every three hours.   HAZARD.

2536—℞ Tincturæ lobeliæ,
    Syrupi scillæ . . . . āā f 3j.
    Extracti belladonnæ . . . . gr. iv.—M.
Sig. Thirty drops three times a day.   HAZARD.

2537—℞ Sol. cocainæ muriatis (5 per cent.) . . 3ss.
Sig. Paint the throat and fauces repeatedly, with a camel's-hair brush.   LABRIC.

2538—℞ Tincture of belladonna . . . . f 3ij.
    Phenacetin . . . . 3j.
    Brandy . . . . f 3iij.
    Fluid extract of chestnut leaves . . . f 3xij.
Sig. Ten drops from every two to six hours for a child one year of age; a child ten years of age may be given as much as a teaspoonful.   LANCASTER.

2539—℞ Bromoform. . . . . gtt. xlviij.
    Olei amygdal. dulcis . . . . 3iv.
    Acaciæ pulv. . . . . 3ij.
    Aquæ laurocerasi . . . . 3j.
    Aquæ destillatæ . . . . . . q. s. ad f 3iv.—M.
Sig. For children under five years, four drops three times daily; from five to ten years, twenty drops daily.

2540—℞ Liquoris hydrogenii peroxidi (10 vols.) 3vj.
    Glycerini puriss. . . . . 3iv.
    Aquæ destillatæ . . . . ad 3iij.—M.
Sig. A tablespoonful in a wineglassful of water, five or six times daily.   B. W. RICHARDSON.

2541—℞ Guaiacol,
    Eucalyptol . . . . āā 3j.
    Sterilized olive oil . . . . f 3x.—M.
Sig. Thirty-five minims to be injected subcutaneously daily.
    Centralbl. f. d. gesammte Therapie.

2542—℞ Acidi carbolici puri . . . . gtt. xv-xx.
Sig. Drop on cotton or in an inhaler, and inhale for several hours daily. Renew the cotton three times a day.   PICK.

2543—℞ Sodii benzoatis . . . . 3iv.
    Aquæ menthæ pip.,
    Aquæ destillatæ . . . . āā 3x.
    Syr. aurantii . . . . 3ij.—M.
Sig. A dessertspoonful every hour or two.   LETZERICH.

2544—℞ Quininæ sulphatis . . . . gr. c.
    Pulv. benzoini . . . . gr. x.—M.
In pulv. no vij div.
Sig. One powder to be insufflated into the nose during the day.   BACHEN.

2545—℞ Ext. aconiti . . . . gr. j.
    Syr. ipecac. . . . . ℳxlv.
    Aquæ laurocerasi . . . . 3j.
    Mucilaginis acaciæ . . . . 3viss.—M.
Sig. A teaspoonful to a tablespoonful, according to age, every hour.   DERVIEUX.

2546—℞ Pulv. benzoini,
    Bismuthi salicylatis . . . . āā 3iiss.
    Quininæ sulphatis . . . . gr. xxx.—M.
Sig. Insufflate the fauces several times daily.   MOIZARD.

2547—℞ Pulv. acidi boracici . . . . 3j-iss.
In pulv. no. xxx div.
Sig. Insufflate one powder into each nostril three times during the day and once at night.   HOLLOWAY.

2548—℞ Quininæ sulphatis . . . . gr. l.
Acidi sulphurici . . . . gtt. xxx.
Aquæ destillatæ . . . . ℥v ℥v.—M.

Sig. Use as a spray to the fauces every two hours for the first three days, and every three hours for the remainder of the first week, after which it will be unnecessary. KOLOVER.

2549—℞ Olei terebinthinæ . . . . f℥j-iv.
Olei ricini . . . . f℥j.
Mucilaginis acaciæ . . . . f℥ij.—M.

Sig. One dose. (*In tape-worm.*) MCPHAIL.

2550—℞ Olei terebinthinæ,
Oleoresinæ filicis maris . . . . . . āā ℥j.
Mucilaginis acaciæ . . . . f℥ij.—M.

Ft. emulsio.
Sig. Day before treatment, a milk or thin soup diet, and one drachm of compound jalap powder. The emulsion is taken the following morning, fasting, and a half-hour later a dose of castor oil. (*In tape-worm.*) F. A. A. SMITH.

2551—℞ Pelletierinæ tannatis . . . . gr. ij.
Syrupi acaciæ . . . . f℥iv.
Aquæ . . . . q. s. ad f℥j.—M.

Sig. Shake. Give in two doses at intervals of half an hour, and follow in an hour by brisk purge. (*Use for tape-worm in child four to six years old. Children under two years should not be given pelletierine.*)

2552—℞ Olei tiglii . . . . gtt. j.
Chloroformi . . . . f℥j.
Glycerini . . . . f℥viiss.—M.

Sig. At night give a saline purge; the following morning before breakfast the above mixture. (*In tænia.*) B. PERSH.

2553—℞ Peponis decort. . . . . ℥v-x.
Sacchari albi . . . . ℥vj gr. xv.
Lactis recentis . . . . f℥xv.—M.

Ft. emulsio.
Sig. To be given before breakfast. Two hours later to be followed by castor oil. (*In tape-worm.*) DUPONT.

2554—℞ Pelletierine sulphatis . . . . gr. vj-viiss.
Pulv. acidi tannici . . . . gr. viiss.
Syr. simplicis . . . . f℥ij.—M.

Sig. Take a little milk for supper, and a simple enema at bedtime. Take the mixture the following morning before breakfast, and lie down to prevent vertigo. In a quarter- or a half-hour take an ounce of castor oil. (*In tape-worm.*)
LABBÉ.

2555—℞ Pelletierine tannatis . . . . gr. vij.
Syr. simplicis . . . . f℥ss.—M.

Sig. Milk diet the day before. Before breakfast, a dose of infusion of senna. One hour later, half the medicine, and the rest a half-hour later. A half-hour later, an ounce of castor oil. Patient to remain in bed during treatment. A large vessel of warm water should be ready to receive the worm. (*In tape-worm.*) BÉRENGER-FÉRAUD.

2556—℞ Thymoli . . . . ℥ij.

In pulv. no. xii div.
Sig. A powder every fifteen minutes. A dose of castor oil should precede and follow the powders. (*In tape-worm.*)
N. CAMPI.

2557—℞ Chloroformi . . . . f℥j.
Syr. simplicis . . . . f℥j.—M.

Sig. To be given in three doses, at intervals of two hours; taken fasting, and followed by castor oil. (*In tape-worm.*)
THOMPSON.

2558—℞ Oleoresinæ filicis maris,
Tinct. vanillæ . . . . āā ℥xlv.
Syr. terebinthinæ . . . . f℥vij ℥xv.
Pulv. acaciæ . . . . gr. xxx.
Aquæ destillatæ . . . . f℥vj ℥xv.

Misce.
Sig. To be taken at one dose, in an equal quantity of milk. Castor oil should be given a few hours later. (*In tape-worm.*) EILLARD.

2559—℞ Kamalæ,
Confectionis sennæ . . . . āā gr. xx.—M.

Sig. Take at one dose after fasting for twenty-four hours. (*Used for tape-worm in child six to eight years old. Not to be given to younger children. No purge is required.*)

2560—℞ Ext. filicis maris fl. . . . . f℥ss–f℥ij.
Ess. anisi . . . . ℳx.
Aquæ menthæ pip. . . . . f℥ss.
Aquæ anthemidis . . . . f℥j.
Syrupi,
Syrupi aurantii cort. . . . . āā f℥vj.—M.

Sig. (*For children.*)   DUCHENNE.

2561—℞ Olei tiglii . . . . gtt. j.
Chloroformi . . . . ℥j.
Glycerini . . . . ℥x.—M.

Sig. One dose.   KAISER.

2562—℞ Extracti spigeliæ fluidi,
Extracti sennæ fluidi,
Syrupi rosæ . . . . āā f℥ij.—M.

Sig. Teaspoonful night and morning. (*Used to remove round worms in child four or five years old.*)

2563—℞ Santonini . . . . gr. viij.
Extracti sennæ et spigeliæ fluidi . . . f℥j.—M.

Sig. One teaspoonful to a child of five years. (*In lumbrici and ascarides.*)   J. LEWIS SMITH.

2564—℞ Hydrargyri chloridi mitis . . . . gr. ij.
Santonini . . . . gr. iss.
Sacchari lactis . . . . gr. xv.

Misce et fiat pulvis.
Sig. One dose, in honey. (*Infant two years old. In lumbrici.*)   EUGENE BOUCHUT.

2565—℞ Mucunæ . . . . ℈ij–℥j.
Syrupi simplicis . . . . ℥ss.—M.

Sig. A teaspoonful every morning before breakfast for three days, and a dose of castor oil after the last dose. (*Children from two to five years old. In lumbrici.*)   CORREA.

2566—℞ Tinct. rhei . . . . gtt. iij.
Tinct. zingiberis . . . . gtt. j.
Magnesii carbonatis . . . . ℥v.
Aquæ . . . . f℥iij.—M.

Sig. This dose should be taken three or four times daily, according to the effect on the bowels. (*In oxyuris.*)   SYDNEY MARTIN.

2567—℞ Sodii chloridi . . . . ℥x.
Aquæ . . . . f℥vj.—M.

Ft. solutio.
Sig. To be injected by the rectum. (*In oxyuris.*)   EILLARD.

2568—℞ Acidi tannici . . . . gr. xv.
Olei theobromæ . . . . ℥j.—M.

Ft. suppositorium no. i.
Sig. To be introduced into the rectum. (*In thread-worms.*)   EILLARD.

2569—℞ Tinct. ferri chloridi . . . . ℥ss.
Aquæ . . . . Oj.—M.

Sig. One-fourth to one-third, as a rectal enema. (*In seat-worms.*)   RINGER.

2570—℞ Trochisci santonini (U.S.P.) no. xxiv.

Sig. One to six at bedtime for children, with a dose of castor oil the following morning. (*In ascarides.*)   BARTHOLOW.

2571—℞ Infusi quassiæ . . . . ℥vj.

Sig. Use as a rectal injection. (*In seat-worms.*)   RINGER.

2572—℞ Santonini . . . . gr. **xij.**
   Olei theobromæ . . . . 3j.—M.

Fiant suppositoria no. iv.
Sig. One at bedtime, introduced into the bowel. (*For seat-worms.*)   HARTSHORNE.

2573—℞ Tincturæ ferri chloridi . . . . f 3ss.
   Aquæ . . . . f 3viij.—M.

Ft. enema. (*In ascarides.*)   DARWALL.

2574—℞ Fuliginis ligni . . . . 3j.
   Aquæ . . . . f 3v.—M.

Coque per quartam partem horæ et cola.
Ft. enema. (*In ascarides.*)   TROUSSEAU.

2575—℞ Sodii chloridi . . . . 3ij.
   Infusi quassiæ . . . . Oj.—M.

Ft. enema.
Sig. Use once a day. If this fails to dislodge them com-pletely, give—

2576—℞ Ferri sulphatis,
   Quininæ sulphatis,
   Pilulæ aloës cum myrrhâ,
   Pilulæ galbani compositæ . . . . . āā gr. l.

Misce et fiant pilulæ no. l.
Sig. Take one pill three times a day. Keep up for a fortnight.
Adult dose. (*In oxyuris vermicularis.*)   W. DATE.

WOUNDS.

2577—℞ Acidi carbolici,
   Olei ricini . . . . āā f 3ss.
   Collodii . . . . f 3j.—M.

Sig. "Carbolized collodion."

2578—℞ Acidi tannici . . . . 3iiss.
   Alcoholis absoluti . . . . f 3ss.
   Ætheris . . . . f 3iiss.
   Collodii . . . . f 3xij.—M.

Sig. "Styptic colloid."

2579—℞ Iodoformi . . . . 3j.
   Collodii flexilis . . . . 3vij.—M.

Sig. Hold or stitch the edges of the wound together, and
apply with a brush. (*In superficial wounds.*)   BRUNS.

2580—℞ Saloli,
   Ætheris . . . . āā 3j.
Solve et adde—
   Collodii flexilis . . . . f 3viiss.—M.

Sig. Apply with a camel's-hair brush.   NICOT.

2581—℞ Hydrargyri chloridi corrosivi . . . . . gr. viiss.
   Aquæ ferventis . . . . Oij.—M.

Sig. "Sublimate solution (1 to 2000)." (*For washing wounds,
irrigating cavities, or saturating dressings.*)

2582—℞ Pulv. acidi salicylici . . . . 3j.
Sig. Use as a dusting-powder.   THIERSCH.

2583—℞ Formaldehydi (40 per cent. sol.) . . . f 3j.
Sig. Ten drops in a pint of water and apply as wash. This
solution is much too strong to be used about the eyes.

2584—℞ Aristolis,
   Acidi borici . . . . āā 3ij.—M.

Sig. Used as dusting powder.

2585—℞ Acidi boracici . . . . 3iss.
   Glycerini . . . . f 3iij.
   Infusi caryophylli (3iv ad Oj) . . . . Oij.
   Olei menthæ pip. . . . . ♏vj.—M.

Sig. "Aseptin."   MAGNUS TROILIUS.

2586—℞ Pulv. saloli,
　　　　Pulv. amyli . . . . āā Ꝝss.—M.
　　Sig. Use as a dusting-powder. 　　　　CREYX ET JARRY.

2587—℞ Pulv. naphthol. . . . . ꝛj.
　　Sig. Use as a dusting-powder. 　　　　BOUCHARD.

2588—℞ Iodoformi . . . . gr. c.
　　　　Thymoli . . . . gr. cc.
　　　　Sacchari lactis . . . . gr. j.—M.
　　Ft. pulvis.
　　Sig. Apply as a powder thrice daily. 　　R. G. REYNOLDS.

2589—℞ Europheni . . . . Ꝝij.
　　Sig. Used as dusting powder.

2590—℞ Phenol sodique . . . . fꝜvj.
　　Sig. In all wounds and surgical operations. J. E. GARRETSON.

2591—℞ Acidi carbolici . . . . ꝛj.
　　　　Glycerini . . . . fꝜj.—M.
　　　　　　　　　　　　　　　　　　HAZARD.

2592—℞ Tincturæ eucalypti . . . . fꝜlj.
　　　　Aquæ destillatæ . . . . fꝜiv.—M.
　　　　　　　　　　　　　　　　　　GIMBERT.

2593—℞ Acetanilidi . . . . Ꝝij.
　　Sig. Used as dusting powder.

2594—℞ Iodol. . . . . ꝛj.
　　　　Glycerini . . . . fꝜj.
　　　　Vaselini . . . . Ꝝvij.—M.
　　Ft. unguentum.
　　Sig. Use locally. 　　　　　　　WOLFENDEN.

2595—℞ Acidi boracici . . . . Ꝝiiss.
　　　　Ess. eucalypti . . . . fꝜiiss.
　　　　Vaselini . . . . Ꝝxxv.—M.
　　Ft. unguentum.
　　Sig. To be used as a dressing. (*The boracic acid may be re-
　　placed by mercuric chloride corr., gr. iss., if desired.*) BRONDEL.

XERODERMA. (See Ichthyosis.)

YELLOW FEVER. (See Fever.)

II

Special List of New Remedies, with their Dosage, Solubilities, and Therapeutic Applications.

Acetophenone.

Syn. Hypnone; Phenyl-Methyl Ketone.
Dose, 1½ to 5 minims, in almond emulsion or with mucilage or syrup, in peppermint water, or in capsules with oil.
Insoluble in water, but soluble in alcohol, ether, and oil.
As a hypnotic; useful in nervous affections and insomnia without pain; action uncertain.

Acid Felicic—Felicinic Acid.

Amorphous, sticky powder; odorless, tasteless; anthelmintic.
Dose, 5 to 15 grains.

Acidum Phenylaceticum—Phenylacetic Acid.

Syn. Alphatoluic Acid.
Dose, 1 to 3 grains, in alcoholic or oily solution.
Soluble 1 in 1 of spirit, 1 in 20 of oils.
Phthisis, in doses of 10 to 20 minims of a 1 in 6 alcoholic solution, freely diluted, three times a day.

Acidum Phenylpropionicum — Phenylpropionic Acid.

Syn. Hydrocinnamic Acid; Homotoluic Acid.
Dose, 1 to 3 grains, in alcoholic or oily solution.
Soluble 1 in 1 of spirit, 1 in 6 of oils.
In phthisis, same dose as preceding, but less useful.

Adonis Vernalis.

Dose, in powder, 3 to 6 grains; of the infusion, 1 in 40, 4 drachms.

Adonidin.

Dose, ¼ to ½ grain daily.
Cardiac tonic and diuretic.
Useful in the præcordial pains of cardiac disease.

Agaricin.

Dose, $\frac{1}{12}$ to ⅛ grain.
In night-sweats.

Airol—Bismuth Oxyiodogallate.

Grayish-green, odorless, tasteless powder.
Insoluble in water, alcohol, etc.
Antiseptic, local, intestinal, and antigonorrhœic.
Dose, 2 to 5 grains.

Alantol.

Amber liquid; odor like peppermint.
Soluble in alcohol, chloroform, and ether.
Internal antiseptic, anticatarrhal.
Dose, ⅙ minim ten times daily.

Aldehyde, Diluted.

A mixture of spirit and aldehyde, containing 15 per cent. of the latter.
Dose for inhalation, 10 minims in a pint of hot water.
In catarrhal congestion and ozæna.

Metaldehyde.

Dose, 2 to 8 grains, in cachets or pills.
Insoluble in water, slightly soluble in alcohol and ether.
Sedative and hypnotic.

Paraldehydum—Paraldehyde.

Dose, 30 to 60 minims, in diluted syrup or almond mixture.
Soluble 1 in 10 of water.
Hypnotic; resembling chloral in its effects. but without its depressing influence upon the heart. Is sedative rather than anodyne.

Aletris Cordial. (Proprietary.)

Stated, from aletris farinosa (or true unicorn) with aromatics.
Uterine tonic and restorative.
Dose, 1 to 4 fluidrachms daily.

Ammonol. (Not completely defined.)

Stated, ammoniated phenylacetamide.
Yellow, alkaline powder.
Antipyretic, analgesic.
Dose, 5 to 20 grains three to six times daily.

Amyl Nitrite.

Dose, by inhalation, the vapor of 2 to 5 minims; by the mouth, $\frac{1}{2}$ to 1 minim.
Soluble in spirit, insoluble in water.
In angina pectoris, sea-sickness, ague, spasmodic asthma, migraine, neuralgic dysmenorrhœa, post-partum hemorrhage, as an antidote to chloroform, to ward off epileptic attacks, and for the spasm of false croup and whooping-cough.
Sold in the shops in glass capsules, 1, 2, 3, or 5 minims.

Isobutyl Nitrite.

When pure, has effects analogous to the above, for which it may be used as a substitute.

Amylene, Hydrate of.

Syn. Dimethyl-Ethyl Carbinol.
Dose, 30 to 80 minims, flavored with extract of liquorice.
Soluble in 12 parts of water, and in spirit.
Hypnotic; intermediate in its effects between chloral and paraldehyde.

Anacardium Occidentale—Cashew-Nut.

Best given in the form of a 10-per-cent. tincture, of which the dose is 2 to 10 minims.
In leprosy; also as a vermifuge. Locally in ringworm and obstinate ulcers.

Aniline.

Syn. Phenylamine, Mono-Phenylamine.
In phthisis, by inhalations from a specially-designed inhaler, 1 part of aniline to 7 parts of oil of eucalyptus, anise, peppermint, or gaultheria.

Anthrarobin.

Five to ten per cent. ointment, or as a tincture.
Sparingly soluble in chloroform and ether, but readily so in alcohol or weak alkaline solutions.
In psoriasis.

Antifebrin. (Patented under this name.)

Syn. Acetanilide; Phenylacetamide.
Dose, 4 to 15 grains, in cachets, or suspended by means of mucilage of tragacanth or acacia in an aqueous vehicle.
Almost insoluble in cold water, but freely soluble in spirit; neutral in reaction.
As a febrifuge and antipyretic, hypnotic, sedative, anti-epileptic, anti-arthritic, and nervine.
Useful in alcoholic delirium and in the hectic of phthisis; also for the relief of the pains of locomotor ataxia and in sciatica.
Applied locally in psoriasis, erysipelas, and eczema.

Antikamnia. (Not completely defined.)

Stated, coal-tar derivative.
White, odorless powder.
Antipyretic, analgesic.
Dose, 5 to 15 grains.

Antinosine—Sodium Salt of Nosophene.

Greenish-blue powder, faint iodine odor.
Soluble in water.
Antiseptic.
Use, chiefly vesical catarrh.
$\frac{1}{10}$ to $\frac{1}{2}$ per cent. solution.

Antipyrin. (Patented.)

Syn. Analgesine; Dimethyloxychinizin (?); Phenyldimethylpyrazolon.
Dose, 4 to 30 grains, in cachets or aqueous solution.
Readily soluble in water.
An analgesic, febrifuge, hæmostatic; especially useful in various forms of neuralgia; may be employed hypodermically.
A measly rash has been observed after its use.
Incompatible with spirit of nitrous ether and other nitrites in the presence of free acid, a brilliant bluish-green compound being formed, which appears to be inert.
Also incompatible with the cinchona alkaloids
Liquefactions occur on trituration with butyl-chloral hydrate or sodium salicylate or with β-naphthol.

Antithermin.

Syn. Phenyl-Hydrazin-Levulinic Acid.
Dose, 8 grains.
Allied to antipyrin; apt to cause gastric irritation.

Antitoxine, Diphtheria.

From serum of blood that has been subjected to diphtheria.
Liquid, limpid.
Dose (children), severe cases, 1500 to 3000 units; ordinary, 500 to 1000 units; prophylactic, 200 to 300 units. Adults, twice dose to a child.
Given hypodermically, and repeat if necessary.

Apiol.

Greenish, oily liquid.
Soluble in alcohol and ether.
Emmenagogue, antiperiodic.
Dysmenorrhœa, malaria.
Dose, 5 to 10 minims three times daily..

Arbutin.

Dose, 15 to 60 grains.
In chronic cystitis and vesical catarrh.

Argonin—Silver Casein Compound, 4.25 per cent. Silver.

White powder.
Soluble in hot water.
Antiseptic.
Used in gonorrhœa, 1 to 2 per cent. solution injection.

Aristol.

Syn. Di-Thymol Iodide.
Insoluble in water, soluble in ether and oils. Useful in psoriasis, mycosis, and lupus, and as a dusting powder for wounds and burns.

Arsenauro. (Not completely defined.)

Stated, 10 minims contain $\frac{1}{32}$ each of gold and arsenic bromides.
Alterative, tonic.
Dose, 5 to 15 minims in water three times daily.

Arsen-Hæmol—Hæmol with 1 per cent. Arsenous Acid.

Brown powder.
Alterative, hæmatinic.
Dose, 1½ grains three times daily, increasing 1 daily until 10 are taken.

Asaprol—Calcium β-Naphtol-α-Monosulphonate.

White or reddish-gray powder.
Soluble in water and alcohol.
Analgesic, antiseptic, antirheumatic, antipyretic.
Dose, 8 to 15 grains.
Externally, 2 to 5 per cent. solution.
Incompatibles, antipyrin and quinine.

Aseptol—Sozolic Acid, 33⅓ per cent. solution of Ortho-phenolsulphonic Acid.

Yellow-brown liquid, odor of carbolic acid.
Soluble in alcohol, glycerin, water.
Antiseptic, disinfectant.
Use externally.
1 to 10 per cent solution.
Keep from light.

Auri Bromidum—Bromide of Gold—Auric Bromide.

Dose, ₁/₃₀ to ₁/₆ grain, increased to ¼ grain, well diluted.
In epilepsy and migraine.

Beberine, Sulphate of.

Dose, 1 to 10 grains, in pills with glycerin of tragacanth, or in aqueous solution.
Soluble 1 in 80 of water, slightly in spirit.
In neuralgia and as an antiperiodic.

Benzanilide.

Syn. Phenyl Benzamide.
Dose, 3 to 12 grains.
Insoluble in water, soluble 1 in 60 of spirit.
Chemically and therapeutically allied to acetanilide.
Especially useful in the treatment of diseases of children.

Benzosol—Benzoyl-Guaiacol; Guaiacol Benzoate.

White, odorless, almost tasteless powder.
Soluble in alcohol, insoluble in water.
Antitubercular, intestinal antiseptic.
Dose, 3 to 15 grains.

Bismal—Bismuth Methylene-Digallate.

Grayish powder.
Soluble in alkalies; insoluble in water or gastric juice.
Intestinal astringent.
Dose, 3 to 15 grains.

Blatta Orientalis—Cockroach.

Dose, 2 to 8 grains, in powder.
A Russian domestic remedy for dropsy; it has recently attracted some attention.

Boldoa Fragrans.

Tincture of Boldo, 1 in 5 of rectified spirit.
Dose, 10 to 20 minims.
In dyspepsia, liver-affections, rheumatism, and as a diuretic.

Boldin.

A glucoside.
Hypnotic properties; local anæsthetic like cocaine.

Borolyptol. (Not completely defined.)

Stated, 5 per cent. aceto-boro-glyceride, 0.1 per cent. formaldehyde, with pinus pumilio, eucalyptus, myrrh, storax, and benzoin.
Antiseptic and disinfectant.
Dose, ½ to 1 fluidrachm, diluted.
Externally, 5 to 50 per cent. solution.

Bromal, Hydrate of.

Dose, 2 to 5 grains—3 grains to relieve pain or produce sleep.
Less soluble in water than chloral hydrate.
Physiologically more active than chloral; not suitable for internal administration, by reason of producing vomiting and diarrhœa.

Bromoform.

Dose, 5 to 20 drops per diem.
A limpid, sweet liquid, with an agreeable odor.
Soluble in alcohol and ether, slightly soluble in water.
Useful in whooping-cough.

Bromo-Hæmol—Hæmol with 2.7 per cent. Bromine.

Brown powder.
Nerve tonic and sedative.
Dose, 15 to 30 grains three times daily.

Cactus Grandiflorus.

Tincture, 1 to 20.
Dose, 1 to 5 minims.
In cardiac asthenia with dropsy.

Cadmium Iodide.

Lustrous tablet.
Soluble in water and alcohol.
Resolvent, antiseptic, scrofulous gland, chronic joint-inflammation.
Applied in ointment, 1 to 8 per cent. lard.

Caffeinæ Sodio-Salicylas.

Dose, 1 to 4 grains, hypodermically.

Caffeinæ Tri-Iodidum.

Dose, 2 to 4 grains.

Caffeinæ Valerianas.

Dose, ½ to 3 grains.
The above three preparations are tonic and stimulant, useful in cardiac failure with dropsy.
In unilateral headache and in bronchial asthma.

Carbon, Tetrachloride of.

By inhalation.
Anæsthetic, hay fever, dysmenorrhœa, and tic-douloureux.
Locally for neuralgia.

Carnogen. (Not completely defined.)

Stated, unaltered fibrin of ox-blood with medullary glyceride.
Hæmatinic.
Dose, 2 to 4 fluidrachms in water three times daily.

Caulophyllin.

Dose, 1 to 4 grains, in a pill with glycerin of tragacanth.
An emmenagogue, parturient, and antispasmodic.

Celerina. (Not completely defined.)

Stated, each drachm equals 5 grains each of celery, coca, kola, viburnum, and aromatics.
Sedative, nerve tonic, vomiting of pregnancy, sea-sickness, etc.
Dose, 1 to 2 fluidrachms.

Chaulmoogra Oil.

Dose, 2 to 15 grains, filled into empty capsules, or in cod-liver oil or milk.
Used externally and internally in leprosy, phthisis, scrofula, marasmus, psoriasis, and lupus; also locally in chronic rheumatism and rheumatic gout.

Chekan.

Dose of the fluid extract, ½ to 3 drachms.
In chronic coughs and bronchitis.

Chinolinum—Chinoline.

Dose, 3 to 10 minims.
Soluble in alcohol, insoluble in water.
Locally in diphtheria, 5 per cent. in solution of equal parts of spirit and water.

Chinolini Tartras.

Dose, 5 to 15 grains, in chloroform water with syrup of orange, or in wafer paper.
Soluble 1 in 40 of water.
Chinolini salicylas is less soluble than the above.
Antipyretic, anti-neuralgic, local antiseptic.

Chloral, Hydrate of.

Dose, 5 to 30 grains, in aqueous solution or in chloroform water well diluted.
Soluble 3 in 1 of water, freely soluble in rectified spirit, and in ether, 1 in 4 of chloroform, also in oils and fats.
A pure hypnotic. Contra-indicated in heart-affections, feeble circulation, Bright's disease, and asthenic conditions.
An antidote to strychnine-poison; useful in tetanus, chorea, and hysteria. There is danger of formation of the chloral habit.
As a vesicant.
Toxic effects best treated, after emesis, by hypodermic injection of sulphate of strychnine and inhalations of amyl nitrite. Picrotoxin is also an antidote.

Chloralamide.

Syn. Chloral Formamide.
Dose, 20 to 50 grains, in weak spirituous or acidulated solution. Incompatible with alkalies.
Soluble 1 in 9 of water, 1 in 2 of spirit; decomposed at a temperature of 120° F.
Hypnotic without analgesic effects.

Chloral cum Camphora, B.P.C.—Pigmentum Chloral et Camphoræ.

Locally in neuralgia and rheumatism.

Hydrate of Butyl-Chloral.

Syn. Croton-Chloral Hydrate,—wrongly so called.
Dose, 2 to 15 grains or more.
Soluble 1 in 100 of cold water, freely soluble in rectified spirit, and about 1 in 4 of glycerin.
Facial neuralgia, toothache, neuralgic toothache; hypnotic.

Chrysarobin.

Syn. Araroba Powder, Goa Powder, Pó di Bahia.
Dose, ⅛ to ½ grain.

Pure Chrysarobin.

Dose, ⅛ to ½ grain.
Freely soluble in hot benzene, hot chloroform, hot oil of turpentine, and certain volatile oils.
Insoluble in water, rectified spirit, and ether.
Parasiticide in many skin-affections.

Cocaina—Cocaine.

Dose, $\frac{1}{8}$ to 1 grain, in a pill or tablet.
The alkaloid soluble 1 in 700 of water, 1 in 20 of alcohol, freely in chloroform, ether, oil of cloves, etc., 1 in 10 of vaseline and castor oil, 1 in 3 of benzol, toluol, and amylic alcohol. The salts are soluble in water.
A powerful local anæsthetic on mucous surfaces. Mydriatic, and paralyzes the accommodation. Irritability of inflamed mucous surfaces much relieved by applications of solutions of the cocaine salts. Useful in hay fever, influenza, coryza, bronchitis, spasmodic asthma, laryngitis, and pharyngitis. Much employed as a local anæsthetic in minor gynæcological operations. In dentistry it deadens the sensibility of exposed pulp. Acts as a cardiac stimulant. Morphine and cocaine appear to be mutually antagonistic. A valuable stomachic.

Colchi-Sal. (Not completely defined.)

Stated, each capsule contains $\frac{1}{50}$ grain of colchicine in 3 minims of methylsalicylat.
Antirheumatic, antipodagric.
Dose, 2 to 4 capsules three times daily.

Colocynthin—Glucoside.

Yellow powder.
Soluble in water and alcohol.
Cathartic.
Dose, ⅙ to ⅔ grain.

Condurango.

Dose of the fluid extract, 20 to 40 drops.
Alterative. Has been unsuccessfully used in the treatment of cancer and syphilis. Said to be a useful stomachic tonic.

Convallaria Majalis—Lily of the Valley.

Convallarin.

Dose, 2 to 4 grains.
Soluble in alcohol, insoluble in water.
No effect other than purgative.

Convallamarin.

Dose, ½ to 2 grains.
Soluble in water and alcohol.
Said to contain the active principles of the drug.

Extractum Convallariæ.

Dose, 2 to 8 grains.

Extractum Convallariæ Fluidum.

Dose, 2 to 10 minims.

Tinctura Convallariæ.

Dose, 5 to 20 minims.

The physiological action of convallaria approaches that of digitalis; its action is cumulative; it is a powerful diuretic.

In mitral and aortic regurgitation, dilatation of the heart, senile hypertrophy, chronic pericarditis, anæmia, and diabetes.

Coumarinum.

A neutral crystalline principle obtained from the Tonka bean, also synthetically from salicylic aldehyde.

Readily soluble in hot water, dilute acids, and alcohol.

It has an agreeable aromatic odor, and is employed to disguise the odor of iodoform.

Creolin.

A dark alkaline liquid prepared from coal tar, forming a white emulsion with water.

Dose, 1 to 5 grains.

Used in the form of lotion, strength of 1 to 100 or more of water.

An antiseptic and sedative.

Crotalus.

A solution of the pure venom of the rattlesnake, 1 to 1000.

Dose, 3 drops every three hours.

Has been used in malignant scarlet fever.

Cupro-Hæmol.

Substitute for copper compounds.

Dose, 1 to 3 grains three times daily.

Dermatol—Bismuth Subgallate. Merck.

Siccative, antiseptic. Substitute for bismuth subnitrate.

Externally on wounds, ulcers, eczema, etc.

Internally, gastro-intestinal affections.

Dose, 4 to 8 grains several times daily.

Diabetin—Levulose.

White powder. Substitute for sugar.

Diuretin.

A sodio-salicylic compound of theobromine, about 50 per cent.

Dose, 90 grains, daily, in divided doses.

Diuretic.

Emblic Myrobalan Fruit.

Dose, 1, 2, or more, as required.

Stomachic and purgative.

Ergotole.

Liquid preparation of ergot, 2½ times strength of fluid extract.

Inject 5 to 20 minims.

Ethidene, Dichloride of.

Syn. Monochlorethyl Chloride—Chlorinated Chloride of Ethyl.

An anæsthetic.

Ethyl Chloride.

Gas. When compressed, colorless liquid.

Soluble in alcohol.

Local anæsthetic for minor surgery, as a spray.

Eucaine, Alpha-Hydrochlorate.

White powder. Soluble in 10 parts of water.

Local anæsthetic.

1 to 5 per cent. solution on mucous surfaces.

15 to 60 minims of 6 per cent. subcutaneously.

Eucalyptol. U. S. P., C. P.

    Dose, 5 to 16 minims three times daily, in capsules.

Eudoxine—Bismuth Salt of Nosophene.

    Odorless, tasteless, insoluble powder; 52.9 per cent. iodine.
Intestinal antiseptic and astringent.
Dose, 4 to 10 grains three times a day.

Eugenol.

    Syn. Eugenic Acid.
An oxidation product of oil of cloves.
Antiseptic and antiputrescent.
Lowers sensibility of the mucous membranes; does not
produce anæsthesia.

Europhen.

    Yellow powder; 27.6 per cent. iodine.
Soluble in alcohol, ether, chloroform, and fixed oils.
Insoluble in water and glycerin.
Antisyphilitic and antiseptic.
Dose (by injection), ½ to 1½ grains once daily.
Externally, like iodoform.

Exalgin.

    Syn. Methylacetanilide.
Dose, 2 to 6 grains, in cachets or aqueous or weak alcoholic
solutions.
Soluble 1 in 60 of water, freely soluble in spirit.
An analgesic, antipyretic, and antiseptic.
Toxic effects, with cyanosis, have followed its employment.

Ferri Albuminati Liquor—Solution of Albumi-
        nated Iron.

    Dose, 1 to 4 drachms.

Ferri Peptonati Liquor—Solution of Peptonated
        Iron.

    Dose, 1 to 4 drachms.

Ferri Pomati Tinctura.

    Dose, 15 to 30 minims.

Formaldehyde—Aqueous solution of **Gas,** about 35 per cent.

    Colorless, volatile liquid.
Surgical and general antiseptic.
Applied in vapor or solution.
In surgery, ½ to 1 per cent. solution.
General antisepsis, ½ to 2 per cent. solution.
Also use to preserve anatomical specimens, $\frac{1}{10}$ per cent. so-
lution.

Fuchsine—Rosaniline Mono-Hydrochlorate.

    Syn. Magenta; Roseine.
Dose, ½ to 4 grains, in a pill with glycerin of tragacanth.
Freely soluble in water.
In albuminuria.
Apt to contain arsenic in variable quantities.

Globon—Chemically pure **Albumin.**

    Yellowish, dry, tasteless, odorless powder.
Nutritive and reconstructive.
Dose, ½ to 1 drachm several times daily.

Glycozone. (Not completely defined.)

    Stated, chemical result of glycerin treated by 15 volumes
of ozone under normal pressure at 0° C.
Colorless viscid liquid. Specific gravity, 1.26.
Disinfectant and antizymotic.
Dose, 1 to 2 fluidrachms.

Guaiacol.

    Dose, ½ to 2 minims.
Soluble in alcohol, ether, fats, oils, and glycerin, slightly
soluble in water.
In phthisis.
Capsules containing 1 minim sold in the shops.

Gurjun Balsam—Wood Oil.

Dose, ½ to 2 drachms.
Not fully soluble in ether or alcohol.
In leprosy, and, in an emulsion of acacia, in gonorrhœa.

Gynocardic Acid.

Dose, ½ to 3 grains.
Supposed to be the active principle of Chaulmoogra oil.

Hamamelin.

Syn. Hamamelidin.
Dose, ½ to 2 grains, in a pill with mucilage of acacia.
Hæmostatic.
In hæmoptysis, hemorrhoids, menorrhagia, and all passive hemorrhages.

Hæmoglobin—Hæmoglobin reduced by Pyrogallol.

Brownish-red powder or scales.
Soluble in water.
Hæmatinic, anæmia, chlorosis.
Dose, 75 to 150 grains daily.

Hæmol—Hæmoglobin reduced by Zinc.

Dark brown powder, containing iron and trace of zinc.
Anæmia, chlorosis, neurasthenia.
Dose, 2 to 8 grains before meals.

Hydracetin.

Syn. Acetyl-Phenyl-Hydrazin.
Dose, ½ to 3 grains daily, in one or two doses.
Soluble 1 in 50 of water, freely in alcohol.
Administration requires caution; must not be continuous.
An impure preparation sold under the name of pyrodin.
A somewhat uncertain antipyretic.
Ten-per-cent. ointment in psoriasis. Its absorption apt to be followed by toxic effects.

Hydrargyri Naphtholacetas—Mercur-β-Naphthol Acetate.

Dose, ½ to 1 grain.
A mild antisyphilitic.

Hydrargyri Succinimidum — Succinimide or Imido-Succinate of Mercury.

Used hypodermically in 2-per-cent. solution in the treatment of syphilis.

Hydrargyri Thymolacetas—Mercury Thymolacetate.

Dose, ¾ to 1½ grains, in pill, also hypodermically.
Antisyphilitic.

Hydrogen, Peroxide of.

Syn. Hydroxyl, in aqueous solution.
Dose, ½ to 2 drachms.
As made for medical purposes, the solution contains ten times its volume of active oxygen.
It possesses disinfecting and bleaching properties.
Readily decomposed.

Ozonic Ether.

Dose, ½ to 1 drachm.
Ether containing in solution peroxide of hydrogen in 30-volume strength with the addition of alcohol.
In diabetes, whooping-cough, scarlet fever, diphtheria, rheumatism, albuminuria, etc.

Hydroleine. (Not completely defined.)

Stated, 2 drachms contain 80 minims cod-liver oil, 35 minims distilled water, 5 grains pancreatin, ⅕ grain soda, ¼ grain salicylic acid.
Dose, ¼ to 1 fluidounce after meals.

Hydroquinone.

Syn. Quinol; Hydrochinon (German).
Dose, ½ to 5 grains.
Soluble 1 in 20 of water, also in alcohol and ether; slightly soluble in olive oil.
Antiseptic and antipyretic.

Hydroxylamine.

Results from the action of nascent hydrogen on nitric acid.
Aqueous solution odorless and colorless.
Has powerful reducing properties.
The hydrochlorate is freely soluble in water.
Used in solution 1 in 1000 in the treatment of lupus and parasitic skin-diseases.

Ichthyol.

Syn. Sulpho-Ichthyolate of Ammonium.
Dose, 10 to 30 grains per diem.

Lithii Sulpho-Ichthyolas.

Dose, 10 to 30 grains per diem.

Sodii Sulpho-Ichthyolas.

Dose, 10 to 30 grains per diem.

Zinci Sulpho-Ichthyolas.

These preparations are miscible with water, glycerin, fats, oils, vaseline, and lanolin, and may be combined with preparations of lead and mercury, without the formation of sulphide.
Used locally in chronic skin-diseases, such as eczema, psoriasis, acne, and favus. Also used in chronic rheumatism.

Ingluvin—Digestive Ferment from Gizzard of Chicken.

Dose, 5 to 20 grains.

Iodoform.

Dose, ½ to 3 grains.
Soluble 1 in 8 of ether, 1 in 12 of chloroform, 1 in 80 of rectified spirit, 1 in 11 of oil of eucalyptus, 1 in 10 of collodium, 1 in 60 of vaseline and oil of almond; insoluble in water.

Iodoformi Pulvis.

Minute crystals.

Iodoformum Præcipitatum.

A primrose-yellow-colored impalpable powder.

Iodoformum Aromaticum.

Is scented with coumarin, 1 in 50.
Powerful antiseptic, sedative, and alterative.
Especially useful in the treatment of surgical and other wounds, the ulcerative processes of chronic infectious diseases, etc.

Iodol.

Syn. Tetra-Iodo-Pyrrol.
Dose, 1 to 3 grains.
Insoluble in water; soluble 1 in 34 of glycerin, 1 in 6 of alcohol, and freely in ether.
Useful for the same purposes as the preceding.

Sozoiodol.

Dose, 20 grains 3 times a day.
Soluble 1 in 14 of water.

Iodo-Salicylic Acid and Di-Iodo-Salicylic Acid.

Dose, 20 to 60 grains in the course of twenty-four hours.
Slightly soluble in water; soluble in alcohol, ether, and fixed oils.
Antiseptic, analgesic, and antithermic.

Syrupus Acidi Hydriodici.

Dose, 20 to 40 minims.
A mild preparation of iodine.

Iodide of Ethyl.

Syn. Hydriodic Ether.
Soluble in alcohol and ether, not readily soluble in water.
By inhalation in asthma and laryngitis; also in nervous dyspnœa and certain forms of bronchial catarrh.
Dispensed in the shops in glass capsules containing 5 minims each.

Iodothyrine—Thyroidine.

Dry preparation of thyroid gland.
Alterative, discutient.
Use in goitre, corpulency, myxœdema, etc.
Dose, 15 to 40 grains per day.

Jambul.

Dose, 5 to 10 grains.
Said to check the diastasic conversion of starch into sugar.
In diabetes.

Kava-Kava.

Fluid extract dose, 15 to 60 minims; extract, 3 grains.
A bitter tonic.

Kairine. (Patented.)

Syn. Oxychinoline-Ethyl Hydrochloride.
Dose, 5 to 8 increased to 15 grains, in pills with glycerin of tragacanth, or in cachets.
Freely soluble in water, less soluble in alcohol; insoluble in ether.
Taste saline, bitter, and nauseous.
Powerful antipyretic.

Kyrofine—Methoxy. Acet. Phenetidine.

Colorless, odorless powder; pungent taste.
Soluble in water, 600 parts; freely in alcohol and ether.
Analgesic, antipyretic.
Dose, 8 to 15 grains.

Lactopeptine. (Not completely defined.)

Stated, pepsin-pancreatin, ptyalin, lactic and hydrochloric acid; grayish powder.
Digestant.
Dose, 10 to 20 grains.

Lanolin.

Syn. Adeps Lanæ—Wool Fat.

Lanolinum Anhydricum—Anhydrous Lanolin.

Sapolanolin.

Lanolin 5 parts, soft soap 4 parts.
In acne, eczema.

Agnine.

These preparations consist of a purified fat from sheep's wool.
Used as a basis for ointments, and readily absorbed by the integument.

Lipanin.

A mixture of olive oil with 6 per cent. of oleic acid.
Has been used as a substitute for cod-liver oil.

Listerine. (Not completely defined.)

Stated, thyme, eucalyptus, baptisia, gaultheria, and mentha arvensis, with 2 grains benzo boric acid in each drachm.
Clear yellow, aromatic.
Antiseptic, deodorant, disinfectant.
Dose, 1 drachm, diluted.
Externally, in solution, to 40 per cent.

Losophan—Tri-Iodo-Cresol.

Colorless needles; peculiar odor; 80 per cent. iodine.
Soluble in ether and chloroform.
Insoluble in water.
Antiseptic.
Externally, 1 per cent. solution.

Lycetol—Dimethyl-Piperazine Tartrate.

White powder; soluble in water.
Diuretic and uric acid solvent.
Dose, 4 to 10 grains.

Maidis Stigmata.

Dose of the fluid extract, 1 drachm.
Demulcent and diuretic.
In acute and chronic affections of the kidney and bladder;
also in cardiac dropsy.

Maidis Ustilago.

Dose, 15 to 60 grains; of the fluid extract, ½ to 1 drachm.
Used in parturition instead of ergot.

Maltzyme—Concentrated, unfermented, diastasic Extract of Malt.

Uses, malnutrition, starchy indigestion.
Dose, ½ to 1 fluidounce.

Manganesii Hypophosphis—Hypophosphite of Manganese.

Dose, 1 to 10 grains.

Manganesii Oxidum Præcipitatum.

Dose, 3 to 10 grains or more, in pills with syrup.

Manganesii Phosphas—Phosphate of Manganese—Manganous Phosphate.

Dose, 1 to 5 grains.
In gastrodynia and amenorrhœa, chlorosis, jaundice.

Mandragorine.

A crystallized alkaloid from mandrake root.
A solution of the sulphate acts as a mydriatic.

Menthol.

Dose, ½ to 2 grains or more, in a pill with powdered soap,
or in solution in olive oil.
Insoluble in glycerin, soluble 2 in 3 of rectified spirit,
also freely in ether, chloroform, and fixed and volatile oils;
sparingly soluble in water.
Internally a diffusible stimulant; externally sedative and
anæsthetic.

Mercauro. (Not completely defined.)

Stated, 10 minims contain $\frac{1}{32}$ grain each gold, arsenic, and
mercury bromides.
Alterative, antisyphilitic.
Dose, 5 to 15 minims, in water, three times daily.

Methacetin.

Syn. Para-Acetanisidin; Oxymethylacetanilide.
Dose, 2 to 6 grains, in cachets or mucilaginous fluid.
Soluble 1 in 260 of water, freely soluble in alcohol, chloro-
form, and glycerin.
Resembles phenacetin in its action.

Methelene Blue. C. P.

Bluish crystal or powder.
Soluble in 40 parts of water.
Uses, gonorrhœa, nephritis, malaria, cystitis, rheumatism.
Dose, 2 to 5 grains three times daily, in capsules.

Methyl Chloride.

This gas is used as a local anæsthetic. Applied as a jet, it
produces intense cold and freezes the part.
Useful in various small operations, such as opening ab-
scesses and in scraping lupus; also in neuralgia, lumbago,
muscular pains.
Employed in microscopical work to freeze specimens for
section-cutting.

Methylal.

Dose, 15 to 30 minims, in aqueous mixture.
Topically as an anæsthetic.
Used internally in angina pectoris, delirium tremens.

Methylene.

Syn. Methylene Dichloride; Dichlormethane; formerly
called Bichloride of Methylene.
Used as an anæsthetic.

Mollin.

A white, inodorous, superfatted soap, containing about 17
per cent. excess of fat.
A basis for ointments, readily washed off with water, with
which it forms a lather.

Monobromacetanilide.

Syn. Monobromphenylacetamide.
A bromine substitution compound of acetanilide.
Dose, 3 to 15 grains.
Facial neuralgia, neuritis, and rheumatism.
Its employment has been followed by cyanosis.

Morrhuol.

Dose, in capsules containing 0.20 gramme, 1 or 2, each
equivalent to 5 grammes of cod-liver oil.

Nitrate of Muscarine.

Dose, (?) ½ to ¾ grain hypodermically, etc.
Muscarine and its alkaloid, the nitrate of muscarine, are
uncrystallizable. The latter is a viscid, yellowish-brown
liquid, hygroscopic, soluble in water. Applied topically to
the eye it dilates the pupil, but given internally it contracts
it. Causes salivation, perspiration, flow of tears, and purgation.
Useful in checking night-sweats.

Myrtol.

Dose, 2 to 4 minims, in capsules.
In putrid affections of the lungs and air-passages.

β-Naphthol.

Syn. Naphthyl Alcohol.
Dose, 2 to 15 grains.
Soluble in alcohol, ether, and benzene; sparingly soluble
in hot water; soluble 1 in 8 of olive oil and lard, and 1 in 80
of vaseline.
Powerfully antiseptic and germicide.
In scabies, psoriasis, and hyperidrosis of palms, soles, and
axillæ; has been administered in enteric fever, in various
gastric and intestinal disorders, and by inhalation in pharyngitis, catarrh, and bronchitis.

α-Naphthol.

Powerfully antiseptic, and less poisonous than β-naphthol.

Acidum α-Oxynaphthoicum — α-Oxynaphthoic Acid.

Syn. α-Naphthol-Carbonic Acid : α-Carbonaphtholic Acid.
Powerfully antizymotic; said to possess this property to
five times the degree of salicylic acid.

Naphthol cum Camphora—Naphthol Camphor.

β-Naphthol 1, Camphor 2, mixed to form a viscid liquid.
A powerful non-toxic antiseptic; has been used to protect
surgical instruments.

Hydronaphthol.

A commercial preparation in the form of a grayish-white
crystalline powder, with a faint odor of iodine.
A non-toxic antiseptic in solution or dusting-powder.

Naphthalene.

Dose, 2 to 15 grains or more, in cachets or pills with mucilage and syrup.
Insoluble in water; soluble in ether, in hot alcohol, and in
fats, also in fixed and volatile oils.

Naphthalene Tetrachloride.

Syn. Naphthalon Hydrochlorate.
Dose, 3 to 12 grains, in cachets or pills.

α-Dichloronaphthalene.

Naphthalene, not being absorbed by the system, acts only on the mucous membrane of the bowel.

In dysentery and the catarrhal diarrhœa of enteric fever and phthisis.

Used locally in foul ulcers, etc.; also very useful in fetid urine.

Nitroglycerin.

Syn. Glonoine; Trinitrate of Glycerol; Nitric Ether of Glycerin (formerly considered as the Trinitrite of Glycerol or Nitrous Ether of Glycerin); Trinitrine.

Dose, $\frac{1}{200}$ to $\frac{1}{50}$ grain, increased to $\frac{1}{10}$ grain.

Slightly soluble in water, freely in ether and in absolute alcohol, 1 in 6 of almond oil, 1 in 15 of rectified spirit.

Nervous sedative and muscular depressant; an active depressant of the inhibitory apparatus of the heart and of the vaso-motor centres and muscular coats of the blood-vessels.

In angina pectoris, and in spastic neuralgias, asthma, headaches, sea-sickness, and Bright's disease.

Less fugacious in its effects than nitrite of amyl, and more powerful than the other nitrites.

Has been used in myxœdema, puerperal convulsions, epileptic vertigo, epilepsy, and specially in *petit mal.*

Acidum Oleicum—Oleic Acid.

Dissolves many of the metallic oxides, with the resulting formation of oleic solutions of the oleates in an excess of oleic acid. Also dissolves alkaloids, but not their salts.

The following are used in medicine:

Oleatum Cocainæ.

Cupri Oleas.

Oleatum Hydrargyri.

5 per cent., 10 per cent., and 20 per cent.

Quininæ Oleatum.

Oleatum Zinci.

Chartazinc.

Tissue-paper saturated with oleate of zinc.

In chronic ulcers.

The metallic oleates are made by the double decomposition of soluble metallic salts and castile soap; they contain no free oleic acid.

Pulvis Zinci Oleatis.

An example of the above.

A fine white powder, resembling chalk.

Used in moist eczema and for the relief of excessive perspiration; especially useful in hyperidrosis and osmidrosis.

Oleanodyne.

A preparation of oleic acid holding in solution the alkaloids aconite, atropine, morphine, and veratrine.

Rapidly absorbed.

Powerfully anodyne.

It can be diluted with chloroform, rectified spirit, or oils.

Nosophene—Tetraiodido-Phenolphtalein.

Yellow, odorless, tasteless, insoluble powder; 60 per cent. iodine.

Surgical antiseptic, like iodoform.

Orexine.

Syn. Orexine Hydrochloride; Hydrochloride of Phenyldihydrochinazolin.

Dose, in coated pills, 3 grains each, 1 to 3 once or twice daily, with a cup of broth or hot fluid.

Freely soluble in water and alcohol.

In failure of appetite.

Acts as a stomachic and appetizer, stimulating the gastric secretion.

Orthoform—Methyl Ester of Para-amido-meta-Oxybenzoic Acid.

White, odorless powder.
Slightly soluble in water.
Local and internal anodyne, antiseptic.
Dose, 8 to 15 grains.

Osmic Acid.

Syn. Tetroxide of Osmium; Perosmic Acid; Hyerposmic Acid.
Soluble slowly, 1 to 5 of water.
Hypodermically for neuralgia, especially obstinate sciatica, enlarged glands, sarcoma, and cancer; also in muscular rheumatism.

Ovariin—Dried Ovaries of Cow.

Coarse powder.
Use in molimena, climacterica, and other ovarian conditions.
Dose, 8 to 24 grains.

Pancreatin.

Dose, 5 to 15 grains.

Paraldehyde—Paraform; Trioxy-Methelene.

White crystal powder.
Soluble in water.
Internally for cholera nostras, diarrhœa, etc.
Externally, antiseptic and disinfectant.
Dose, 30 to 90 minims, well diluted with whiskey.

Pepsin.

Dose, 5 to 15 grains.

Peptenzyme. (Not completely defined.)

Stated, digestive principles of stomach, pancreas, liver, spleen, salivary and Brunner's glands, and Lieberkühn's follicles.
Digestant.
Dose, 3 to 10 grains three times daily.

Pepto-Mangan. (Gude.) (Not completely defined.)

Stated, aromatic solution of peptonized iron and manganese.
Hæmatinic.
Dose, 1 to 4 fluidrachms before meals.

Phenacetin.

Syn. Para Acet-Phenetidin.
Dose, 4 to 8 increased to 15 grains, in cachets, or suspended in mucilaginous fluids.
Inodorless and tasteless.
Insoluble in water or glycerin; freely soluble in hot alcohol. Insoluble in both acid and alkaline solutions.
Antipyretic and anodyne.
Rheumatism, neuralgia, migraine, hysteria, pertussis.
Causes neither rashes nor cyanosis.

Phenalgin. (Not completely defined.)

Stated, ammonio-phenylacetamide.
White powder, ammoniacal odor.
Antipyretic, analgesic.
Dose, 5 to 15 grains.

Picric Acid.

Syn. Carbazotic Acid; Trinitrophenic Acid.
Dose, ¼ to 2 grains.
Soluble 1 in 90 of water, 1 in 16 of rectified spirit.
In ague, albuminuria, and certain forms of headache; also locally in erysipelas and dermatitis.

Ammonium Picrate.

Dose, ⅛ to 1½ grains four or five times a day.
In ague and malarial fevers.

Piperazin—Diethylene Diamine.

Colorless crystals.
Soluble in water.
Antipodagric, antirheumatic.
Dose, 5 to 10 grains three times daily well diluted.

Potassii Cobalto-Nitris—Cobalto-Nitrite of Potassium.

Dose, ½ grain every two or four hours.
Slightly soluble in water.
Relieves arterial tension.
In dyspnœa of uræmia and asthma ; also in arterial capillary fibrosis.

Priodate, Crystals and Powder.

Dose. 1 to 15 grains.
Slightly soluble in water.
Antiseptic and deodorant.
A weak germicide.

Prostaden—Standardized Dried Extract of Prostate Gland.

Use, hypertrophy of prostate.
Dose, up to 40 grains daily.

Protargol—Proteid Compound of Silver, 8 per cent. Silver.

Yellow powder.
Soluble in water.
Antigonorrhœic.
Dose, ¼ to 2 per cent. solution, injection.

Protonuclein. (Not defined.)

Stated, obtained from lymphoid structures.
Brownish powder.
Antitoxic invigorator, cicatrizant.
Dose, 3 to 10 grains three times daily.

Ptyalin—Amylolytic Ferment of Saliva.

Yellowish powder.
Soluble in glycerin, partly in water.
Use, amylaceous dyspepsia.
Dose, 10 to 30 grains.

Pyridine.

Dose, 5 to 10 increased to 25 minims daily.
Miscible with water, alcohol, ether, and oils.
Used by inhalation in a closet or small room.
In asthma ; also as a heart-stimulant, and in angina pectoris.

Pyrogallic Acid.

Syn. Pyrogallol.
Dose, ½ to 1½ grains, in aqueous solution, or in a pill with syrup.
Soluble in 2½ parts of water and in 10 parts of melted lard.
In hæmoptysis, and locally in psoriasis; also used in the preparation of hair-dyes.

Quinalgen—Analgen.

Derivative of quinoline.
White, tasteless, insoluble powder.
Anodyne, antirheumatic.
Dose, 5 to 15 grains.

Resorcin.

Dose, 5 to 15 or 30 grains.
Soluble in 2 parts of water, in 20 of olive oil.
A powerful antiseptic.
Internally, action analogous to that of quinine, but with excessive diaphoresis.
Used locally in diphtheria, gonorrhœa, vesical catarrh, cancer, eczema, psoriasis, condylomata and mucous patches, and internally, well diluted with water and flavored with syrup of orange, or in infusion of chamomile, in whooping-cough, sea-sickness.

Rubidium-Ammonium Bromide.

Dose, 30 grains three times daily.
In epilepsy.

Saccharin.

A harmless drug, valuable as a substitute for sugar in cases of diabetes.

Syn. Benzoyl-Sulphonic-Imide; Benzoic Sulphinide; Anhydro-Ortho-Sulphamine-Benzoic Acid.

Dose, $\frac{1}{2}$ to 2 grains, or more,—*ad libitum* is recommended.

Soluble 1 in 500 volumes of cold and 1 in 160 of hot water, 1 in 35 of rectified spirit, 1 in 80 of proof spirit, 1 in 100 of ether, 1 in 50 of chloroform, 1 in 50 of glycerin.

Sweetening power variously estimated as from 100 to 300 times that of sugar. 1 part in 10,000 parts of distilled water is perceptibly sweet, and it is possible to detect 1 part in 70,000,—about a grain in a gallon.

Saccharinum Solubile.

Dose, $\frac{1}{2}$ to 2 grains or more.

This substance consists of saccharin, 90 per cent., in combination with soda.

Safrol.

Dose, 20 to 30 minims.

In subacute rheumatism.

Salicylic Acid.

Dose, 5 to 30 grains, in cachets.

Soluble in 760 parts of water, 4 of spirit, 2 of ether, 120 of olive oil, 100 of castor oil, 200 of glycerin; also in melted fats and vaseline. Solubility in water much increased by the addition of borax.

Internally its effects are analogous to those of quinine.

Used in rheumatism, sciatica, Ménière's disease; is a powerful antiseptic.

Bismuthi Salicylas.

Dose, 5 to 20 grains.

Insoluble in water, alcohol, and glycerin.

In diarrhœa, typhoid fever, etc.; also in gastric catarrh.

Cresol Salicylas.

Syn. Para-Cresol Salicylate; Cresalol.

Dose, (?)

Insoluble in water; freely soluble in spirit.

Has been used in acute rheumatism.

Ferri Salicylas.

Dose, 3 to 10 grains, in pills.

Slightly soluble in water.

In certain forms of diarrhœa of infancy.

Quininæ Salicylas.

Dose, 2 to 6 grains.

Soluble in water 1 to 900.

Best administered in pills.

In rheumatic gout.

Sodii Salicylas.

Dose, 10 to 30 grains, in water.

Soluble in its own weight of water, also in rectified spirit.

Antipyretic; chiefly useful in acute rheumatism. Used also in enteric fever, tonsillitis, vesical catarrh, neuralgia, gouty headaches, diarrhœa, influenza, and in vertigo with auditory-nerve symptoms.

Over-doses produce headache, suffusion of the eyes, deafness, flushed face, muscular trembling and weakness.

Sodii Di-Thio-Salicylas.

Dose, 3 grains, morning and evening.

Soluble 1 in 1 of water.

In articular and gonorrhœal rheumatism.

Salicinum—Salicin.

Dose, 5 to 30 grains, in aqueous solution.

Soluble 1 in 20 parts of water, 1 in 50 of spirit; insoluble in ether.

In rheumatism and ague.

Salol.

Syn. Phenyl Ether of Salicylic Acid. (Patented.)

Dose, 4 to 30 grains, in cachets or suspended in milk.

Insoluble in water, faintly soluble in glycerin, soluble in alcohol, ether, and fixed oils.

Antiseptic and antipyretic.

Useful in sciatica; chiefly valuable in acute rheumatism; also employed in the treatment of summer diarrhœas.

Salol cum Camphora—Salol Camphor.

3 parts of salol heated with 2 parts of camphor combine to form a viscid liquid which has been used as an antiseptic.

Betol.

The salicylate of β-naphthol-ether.
Dose, 3 to 8 grains, in cachets or pills, or suspended in almond emulsion or milk.
Insoluble in water, soluble in alcohol.
Rheumatism, cystitis, and intestinal catarrh.

Salophen—Acetyl-Para-Amidophenol-Salicylate.

White, odorless, tasteless powder, 51 per cent. salicylic acid.
Soluble in alcohol and ether, insoluble in water.
Antirheumatic.
Dose, 15 to 20 grains.

Seng. (Not completely defined.)

Stated, active constituent of panax schinseng in aromatic essence.
Stomachic.
Dose, 1 drachm.

Serum, Antituberculous—Maragliano (only in 1 cc. [16 min.] tubes).

Antitoxin against pulmonary tuberculosis.
Dose (subcutaneous) in apyretic cases, 16𝗆 (1 cc.) every other day for ten days, then daily for ten days, and 30𝗆 twice a day thereafter until sweats have ceased, when 16𝗆 are injected for a month every other day, and finally once a week for a year.
In febrile cases, if slight and intermittent, dosage same as given above; if continuous and intense, inject 160𝗆, and, if temperature falls markedly, repeat in one week, and so continue until fever is gone, then inject 16 to 32𝗆 daily.

Simulo.

Used in the treatment of nervous diseases, especially hysteria and epilepsy.

Somnal.

A liquid preparation believed to be a combination of chloral alcoholate and urethane.
Dose, ½ drachm.
Hypnotic.

Sparteine Sulphate.

Dose, ¼ to 1 grain, increased.
Soluble 2 in 3 of water.
Cardiac tonic, non-cumulative; valuable diuretic.

Spermine, Poehl—Essence.

Four per cent. aromatized alcoholic solution of double-salt spermine hydrochlorate-sodium chloride.
Use internally, nervous diseases with anæmia, hystero-epilepsy, angina pectoris, locomotor ataxia, asthma, etc.
Dose, 10 to 30𝗆 in alkaline mineral water every morning.

Strophanthus Hispidus.

Two crystalline substances have been isolated, strophanthin and incin.
The dose of strophanthin, hypodermically, is from 1-120th to 1-160th of a grain; it has been used as a cardiac tonic and diuretic. Its chemical nature has not been fully determined, and it is not a safe therapeutic.
The preparations of strophanthus most available for therapeutic purposes are

Tincture of Strophanthus,

Dose, 2 to 10 minims, and

Pills of Strophanthus

Contain 2 to 4 minims of the tincture combined with sugar of milk.
Dose, 1 to 2.

Sulphonal.

Syn. Diethyl-Sulphon-Dimethyl-Methane.
Dose, 15 to 30 grains (?), in cachets or suspended in water with mucilage.
Soluble 1 in 500 of water, freely soluble in boiling water and in alcohol and ether.
A pure hypnotic, not affecting the digestion, pulse, or temperature.
Especially useful in insomnia of nervous subjects, in mania, delirium tremens, and meningitis, and in the control of night-sweats.

Taka-Diastase—Diastase Takamine.

Brownish powder, almost tasteless.
Soluble in water, insoluble in alcohol.
Starch digestant.
Used in amylaceous dyspepsia.
Dose, 1 to 5 grains.

Terebene, Pure.

Dose, 5 to 30 minims.
Not miscible with water.
Powerful antiseptic, disinfectant, deodorizer.
In phthisis, dysentery, and winter cough.
Used by inhalation and internally.

Terpin Hydrate.

Syn. Terpene Hydrate ; Hydrate of Oil of Turpentine.
Dose, 2 to 6 grains or more.
Soluble 1 in 200 of water, 1 in 20 of alcohol, 1 in 6 of oils.
In chronic and subacute bronchitis.
Also diuretic.

Terpinol.

An aromatic liquid resulting from the action of dilute hydrochloric or sulphuric acid on terpene.

Testadin—Standardized Dried Extract of Testicular Substances—Knoll.

One part represents two parts of fresh gland.
Uses, spinal and nervous diseases, impotence, etc.
Dose, 30 grains three or four times daily.

Tetronal.

Syn. Diethyl-Sulphon-Diethyl-Methane.
Dose, 10 to 20 grains, in cachet.
Soluble 1 in 450 of water, 1 in 15 of spirit.

Thalline—Tetrahydroparamethyloxychinoline, or Tetrahydroparachinanisol. (Patented.)

Syn. Thallinæ Sulphas—Sulphate of Thalline.
Dose, 3 to 8 grains.
Soluble 1 in 5 of cold water.
An irregular and dangerous antipyretic.

Thiol.

Dose, (dry) 2 to 10 grains, in pills.

Thiol Liquidum.

A syrupy liquid containing about 40 per cent. of thiol.

Thiol is soluble in water, alcohol, and ether. It is precipitated by acids; analogous to ichthyol, and used for the same purposes.

Thio-Resorcin.

Insoluble in water, slightly soluble in ether and alcohol.
Used as a substitute for iodoform as a dusting-powder, or in 10 per cent. ointment.

Thymol.

Dose, $\frac{1}{2}$ to 2 grains or more, in pills with powdered soap, or in oily or aqueous solution.
Soluble 1 in 800 of water, 1 in 200 of glycerin, 1 in 8 of equal parts of alcohol and glycerin mixed; also in fats and oils; freely soluble in alcohol and ether.
Powerfully antiseptic and antiputrefactive.
Used in surgical dressings, and as an intestinal antiseptic.

Thyraden—Standardized Dried Extract of Thyroid Gland—Knoll.

One part represents two parts of fresh gland.
Brownish, sweet powder.
Alterative.
Uses, diseases due to altered function of thyroid gland.
(Myxœdema, cretinism, struma, certain skin diseases.)
Dose, 15 to 25 grains daily, gradually increased if necessary.

Tongaline. (Not completely defined.)

Stated, 1 drachm equals tonga, 30 grains; extract cimicifuga, 2 grains; sodium salicylate, 10 grains; pilocarpine salicylate, $\frac{1}{6}$ grain; colchicine, $\frac{1}{600}$ grain.
Antirheumatic, diaphoretic.
Dose, 1 to 2 drachms.

Trimethylamine.

Syn. Secalin; Propylamine (?).
Dose of the solution, 20 to 50 minims every two to four hours.
Commercial preparation miscible with water.
In acute articular rheumatism.
Propylamine is isomeric with trimethylamine.

Trimethylamine Hydrochloras.

Dose, 2 to 3 grains three to five times daily.
Very soluble in water.
In acute articular rheumatism.

Trional. (?)

Intermediate in hypnotic effect between sulphonal and tetronal.

Ulexine.

Ulexine Hydrobromate.

Dose of each, $\frac{1}{20}$ to $\frac{1}{5}$ grain.
Powerful diuretic.

Uralium.

Syn. Ural.
A compound of chloral and urethane.
Dose, 15 to 45 grains.
Hypnotic.

Uranium, Nitrate of.

Dose, $\frac{1}{2}$ to 5 grains.
Soluble in half its weight of water.
Used in solution, 10 grains to the ounce, as a spray for the throat. Has been used in the treatment of diabetes. Not a safe remedy.

Urea—Carbamide.

White crystal, soluble in alcohol, ether, water.
Diuretic, renal calculi.
Dose, 150 to 300 grains a day in water.

Urethane.

Syn. Ethyl Carbamate.
Dose, 10 to 20 grains.
Soluble in water.
A pure hypnotic.
Very useful in diseases of children, in delirium tremens, and in acute mania.

Urotropin—Formin.

Syn. Hexamethylene Tetramine.
Alkaline crystals, powdered.
Soluble in water.
Uric acid solvent and genito-urinary antiseptic.
Use, gout, cystitis, etc.
Dose, 15 to 30 grains daily in lithia water.

Vitogen. (Not defined.)

White, odorless, insoluble powder.
Surgical antiseptic, deodorant.
Used externally only, pure.

Yerba Santa.

Dose of the fluid extract, 10 to 40 minims; aromatic and expectorant.
In bronchitis, phthisis, and pulmonary catarrh.

III

A Table of Formulæ for Suppositories.

A.—RECTAL.

The quantity given is to be thoroughly incorporated with a sufficient quantity of cacao butter—gr. xxx., U.S.P.—to form one suppository.

1. Anodyne.

Pulv. opii . . . . . gr. ⅛-iv.	Ext. hyoscyami. . . gr. iij.
Ext. opii aq. . . . . gr. ¼-ij.	Ext. hyoscyami. . . gr. v.
Morphinæ sulph. . . gr. ₁₂-j.	{ Ext. hyoscyami . . . gr. ij.
Morphinæ acetatis . gr. ₁₂-j.	{ Ext. opii aq. . . . . gr. j.
Ext. belladonnæ . . gr. ¼-j.	{ Morphinæ sulph. . . gr. ⅛.
{ Pulv. opii . . . . . gr. ½.	{ Atropinæ sulph. . . gr. ₁₆₀.
{ Ext. belladonnæ . . gr. ½.	{ Morphinæ sulph. . . gr. ¼.
{ Pulv. opii . . . . . gr. j.	{ Atropinæ sulph. . . gr. ₁₆₀.
{ Ext. belladonnæ . . gr. ¼.	{ Cocain. hydrochlor. gr. ⅛.
{ Pulv. opii . . . . . gr. ij.	{ Morphinæ sulph. . . gr. ½.
{ Ext. belladonnæ . . gr. ½.	{ Atropinæ sulph. . . gr. ₁₆₀.
{ Pulv. opii . . . . . gr. iij.	{ Cocain. hydrochlor. gr. ⅛.
{ Ext. belladonnæ . . gr. ½.	{ Morphinæ sulph. . . gr. ½.
{ Ext. opii aq. . . . . gr. ½.	{ Atropinæ sulph. . . gr. ½.
{ Ext. belladonnæ . . gr. ¼.	{ Cocain. hydrochlor. gr. ½.
{ Ext. opii aq. . . . . gr. i.	{ Ext. cannabis ind. . gr. ½.
{ Ext. belladonnæ . . gr. ½.	{ Codeinæ . . . . . . gr. j.
{ Ext. opii aq. . . . . gr. iss.	{ Ext. hyoscyami . . gr. j.
{ Ext. belladonnæ . . gr. ½.	{ Ext. cannabis ind. . gr. j.
{ Ext. opii aq. . . . . gr. ij.	{ Codeinæ . . . . . . gr. ij.
{ Ext. belladonnæ . . gr. j.	{ Ext. hyoscyami . . gr. ij.
{ Pulv. opii . . . . . gr. ¼.	{ Ext. cannabis ind. . gr. ij.
{ Pulv. ipecacuanhæ . gr. j.	{ Ext. cannabis ind. . gr. ½.
{ Pulv. opii . . . . . gr. j.	{ Ext. hyoscyami . . gr. j.
{ Pulv. ipecacuanhæ . gr. ij.	{ Ext. cocæ . . . . . . gr. ij.

2. Anodyne and Hypnotic.

{ Chloral. hydrat. . . gr. x.	{ Chloral. hydrat. . . gr. xxx.
{ Atropinæ sulph. . . gr. ₁₆₀.	{ Atropinæ sulph. . . gr. ₁₆₀.
{ Morphinæ sulph. . . gr. ¼.	{ Morphinæ sulph. . . gr. ½.
{ Chloral. hydrat. . . gr. xv.	{ Ext. opii . . . . . gr. ½.
{ Morphinæ sulph. . . gr. ¼.	{ Ext. cannabis ind. . gr. j.
{ Atropinæ sulph. . . gr. ₁₂₀.	{ Lupulini . . . . . . gr. v.
{ Chloral. hydrat. . . gr. xx.	{ Ext. hyoscyami . . gr. j.
{ Morphinæ sulph. . . gr. ½.	{ Ext. opii . . . . . gr. j.
{ Atropinæ sulph. . . gr. ₁₀₀.	{ Ext. cannabis ind. . gr. ij.
	{ Lupulini . . . . . gr. xv.
	{ Ext. hyoscyami . . . gr. ij.

3. Hypnotic.

{ Chloral. hydrat. . . gr. xv.	{ Ext. cannabis ind. . gr. j.
{ Camph. monobrom. gr. v.	{ Lupulini . . . . . . gr. xv.
{ Hyoscyam. hydroch. gr. ₁₀₀.	{ Ext. hyoscyami . . gr. ij.
{ Chloral. hydrat. . . gr. xx.	{ Camph. monobrom. gr. v.
{ Camph. monobrom. gr. x.	{ Hyoscinæ hydro-
{ Hyoscyam hydroch. gr. ₈₀.	{ brom. . . . . . . gr. ₁₀₀.
Urethane . . . . . . gr. x.	{ Codeinæ . . . . . gr. j.
Urethane . . . . . . gr. xv.	{ Lupulini . . . . . gr. v.
{ Ext. cannabis ind. . gr. ½.	{ Hyoscinæ hydro-
{ Lupulini . . . . . . gr. v.	{ brom. . . . . . . gr. ₅₀.
{ Ext. hyoscyami . . gr. j.	{ Codeinæ . . . . . gr. ij.
{ Camph. monobrom. gr. ij.	{ Lupulini . . . . . gr. x.

4. Antiseptic.

Iodoformi . . . . . gr. ij.		Acidi borici . . . gr. x.
Thymol. . . . . . . gr. j.		Thymol. . . . . . . gr. j.
Resorcin. . . . . . gr. v.		Ol. eucalypti . . . . ℥iij.

Iodoformi . . . . gr. v.	Acidi benzoici . . . gr. v.
Thymol. . . . . . gr. j.	Hydrarg. chlor. cor. gr. $\frac{1}{20}$.
Resorcin. . . . . . gr. x.	Resorcin. . . . . . gr. x.

Iodoformi . . . . gr. v.	Acidi benzoici . . . gr. x.
Acidi tannici . . . gr. x.	Hydrarg. chlor. cor. gr. $\frac{1}{20}$.
	Resorcin. . . . . . gr. x.

Iodoformi . . . . gr. v.	Naphthalini . . . . gr. ij.
Acidi tannici . . . gr. xx.	Sodii biborat. . . . . gr. x.
	Hydrarg. chlor. cor. gr. $\frac{1}{20}$.
Acidi borici . . . gr. v.	Ol. eucalypti . . . . ℥ij.
Thymol. . . . . . gr. ij.	
Ol. eucalypti . . . ℥j.	Acidi salicylici . . . gr. x.
	Acidi borici . . . gr. x.
Naphthalini . . . gr. v.	Thymol. . . . . . . gr. x.
Sodii biborat. . . . gr. x.	
Hydrarg. chlor. cor. gr. $\frac{1}{20}$.	Iodoformi . . . . . gr. ij.
Ol. eucalypti . . . . ℥ij.	
	Iodoformi . . . . . gr. iij.
Acidi salicylici . . . gr. v.	
Acidi borici . . . gr. v.	Acidi borici . . . . gr. vj.
Thymol. . . . . . . gr. ij.	

5. Astringent.

Pulv. opii . . . . . gr. j.	Ext. krameriæ . . . gr. iij.
Acidi tannici . . . gr. ij.	Ext. krameriæ . . . gr. v.
Pulv. opii . . . . . gr. ij.	Ext. krameriæ . . . gr. x.
Acidi tannici . . . gr. ij.	Acidi tannici . . . . gr. v.
Pulv. opii . . . . . gr. j.	Acidi gallici . . . . gr. ij.
Acidi tannici . . . gr. v.	Ext. krameriæ . . . gr. j.
Pulv. opii . . . . . gr. ij.	Acidi tannici . . . . gr. x.
Acidi tannici . . . gr. v.	Ext. krameriæ . . . gr. v.
Pulv. opii . . . . . gr. j.	Acidi gallici . . . . gr. iv.
Plumbi acetat. . . . gr. ij.	Acidi gallici . . . . gr. ij.
Pulv. opii . . . . . gr. ij.	Ext. ergotæ . . . . gr. v.
Plumbi acetat. . . . gr. ij.	Digitalis . . . . . . gr. j.
Pulv. opii . . . . . gr. j.	Acidi gallici . . . . gr. v.
Plumbi acetat. . . . gr. v.	Ext. ergotæ . . . . gr. x.
Pulv. opii . . . . . gr. ij.	Digitalis . . . . . . gr. ij.
Plumbi acetat. . . . gr. v.	Bismuthi subnitrat.. gr. x.
Ext. belladonnæ . . gr. ¼.	Acidi tannici . . . . gr. v.
Plumbi acetat. . . . gr. iss.	Bismuthi subnitrat. gr. xx.
Ext. belladonnæ . gr. ½.	Acidi tannici . . . . gr. x.
Plumbi acetat. . gr. iij.	Bismuthi subnitrat. gr. x.
Acidi tannici . . . gr. ij.	Thymol. . . . . . . gr. ij.
Acidi tannici . . . gr. v.	Bismuthi subnitrat. gr. xx.
Acidi tannici . . . gr. x.	Thymol. . . . . . . gr. j.
Ext. stramonii . . gr. j.	Acidi tannici . . . . gr. v.
Plumbi acetat. . . gr. ij.	Eucalyptol. . . . . . ℥j.
Ext. stramonii . . gr. ½.	Iodoformi . . . . . gr. ij.
Acidi tannici . . . gr. ½.	Acidi tannici . . . . gr. xx.
Plumbi carbonat. . gr. j.	Eucalyptol. . . . . . ℥ij.
Liquor plumbi sub-acetat. . . . . . . ℥ij.	Iodoformi . . . . . gr. v.
Creasoti. . . . . . . ℥½.	Acidi tannici . . . . gr. x.
Plumbi iodidi . . . gr. iij.	Bismuthi subnitrat. . gr. x.
Ext. belladonnæ . gr. ½.	Hydrarg. chlor. cor.. gr. $\frac{1}{20}$.
Morphinæ sulph. . . gr. ¼.	Acidi tannici . . . . gr. x.
Acidi tannici . . . gr. v.	Bismuthi subnitrat. gr. x.
Ext. stramonii . . gr. j.	Hydrarg. chlor. cor. gr. $\frac{1}{20}$.
Acidi tannici . . . gr. v.	

6. Laxative.

Glycerin. Containing 95 per cent. of glycerin.

7. Antiperiodic.

Quininæ bisulphatis . . . . gr. j-vj.

B.—VAGINAL.

{ Iodoformi . . . . . . gr. v.
{ Hydrarg. chlor. cor. . gr. 1/20.

{ Iodoformi . . . . . gr. x.
{ Hydrarg. chlor. cor. . gr. 1/10.

{ Iodoformi . . . . . gr. v.
{ Acidi tannici . . . gr. xv.

{ Iodoformi . . . . . gr. v.
{ Acidi tannici . . . gr. xxx.

{ Acidi tannici . . . gr. xx.
{ Acidi borici . . . . gr. v.

{ Acidi tannici . . . gr. xl.
{ Acidi borici . . . . gr. x.

{ Acidi salicylici . . gr. x.
{ Acidi borici . . . . gr. v.
{ Acidi tannici . . . gr. xx.

{ Acidi salicylici . . gr. xv.
{ Acidi borici . . . . gr. v.
{ Acidi tannici . . . gr. xx.

{ Bismuthi subnitrat. . gr. xx.
{ Acidi tannici . . . gr. xx.

{ Bismuthi subnitrat. . gr. xl.
{ Acidi tannici . . . gr. xx.

{ Plumbi nitrat. . . . gr. ij.
{ Plumbi acetat. . . . gr. v.

{ Plumbi nitrat. . . . gr. v.
{ Plumbi acetat. . . . gr. x.

{ Bismuthi subcarb. . gr. x.
{ Plumbi carbonat. . . gr. v.
{ Eucalyptol. . . . . mij.

{ Bismuthi subcarb. . gr. xx.
{ Plumbi carbonat. . . gr. v.
{ Eucalyptol. . . . . mij.

{ Zinci oxidi . . . . gr. v.
{ Zinci sulphocarbolat. gr. x.
{ Thymol. . . . . gr. ij.

{ Zinci oxidi . . . . gr. x.'
{ Zinci sulphocarbolat. gr. xx.
{ Thymol. . . . . gr. x.

{ Resorcin. . . . . . gr. v.
{ Bismuthi subnitrat. . gr. xx.
{ Salicini . . . . . gr. v.

{ Resorcin. . . . . . gr. x.
{ Bismuthi subnitrat. . gr. xxx.
{ Salicini . . . . . gr. v.

{ Cocain. hydrochlor. gr. 1/2.
{ Salicini . . . . . gr. xx.

{ Cocain. hydrochlor. gr. j.
{ Salicini . . . . . gr. xxx.

C.—URETHRAL.

Zinci sulph. . . . gr. 1/4.

Zinci chlor. . . . gr. 1/4.

Iodoformi . . . . gr. j.

Hydrastis canad. . gr. v.

{ Zinci sulph. . . . gr. j.
{ Ext. opii aq. . . . gr. j.

{ Zinci sulph. . . . gr. j.
{ Ext. belladonnæ . gr. j.

{ Zinci sulph. . . . gr. j.
{ Ext. opii aq. . . . gr. j.
{ Ext. belladonnæ . gr. j.

{ Zinci sulph. . . . gr. j.
{ Morphinæ sulph. . gr. 1/4.

{ Zinci chlor. . . . gr. 1/4.
{ Ext. opii aq. . . . gr. j.

{ Zinci chlor. . . . gr. 1/4.
{ Ext. belladonnæ . gr. j.

{ Plumbi acetat. . . gr. j.
{ Ext. opii aq. . . . gr. j.

{ Sol. plumbi subacet. gr. v.
{ Ext. opii aq. . . . gr. j.

{ Zinci sulph. . . . gr. j.
{ Acidi carbolici . . gr. 1/2.

{ Iodoformi . . . . gr. iij.
{ Ext. belladonnæ . gr. 1/2.

Iodoformi . . . . gr. v.

{ Zinci sulph. . . . gr. 1/2.
{ Plumbi acetat. . . gr. 1/2.
{ Ext. opii aq. . . . gr. j.

{ Iodoformi . . . . gr. v.
{ Ol. eucalypti . . . gr. x.

{ Zinci sulph. . . . gr. 1/4.
{ Zinci oxidi . . . . gr. ij.

{ Iodoformi . . . . gr. iij.
{ Ext. opii aq. . . . gr. j.

{ Zinci sulph. . . . gr. 1/4.
{ Zinci oxidi . . . . gr. ij.
{ Hydrastis canad. . gr. v.

{ Bismuthi subnitrat. gr. iij.
{ Hydrastis canad. . gr. v.

{ Zinci acetat. . . . gr. 1/2.
{ Iodoformi . . . . gr. ij.
{ Ext. belladonnæ . gr. 1/2.

{ Ext. belladonnæ . gr. 1/2.
{ Ext. opii aq. . . . gr. j.
{ Ext. hyoscyami . gr. ij.

{ Ext. gelsemii fld. . gr. v.
{ Ext. belladonnæ . gr. 1/4.
{ Ext. aconiti rad. fld. gr. j.
{ Ext. opii aq. . . . gr. j.

Boroglyceridi . . . gr. v.

{ Iodoformi . . . . gr. v.
{ Boroglyceridi . . . gr. v.

{ Zinci sulph. . . . gr. 1/4.
{ Boroglyceridi . . . gr. v.
{ Iodoformi . . . . gr. v.

Iodoformi . . . . gr. ij.

Iodoformi . . . . gr. iij.

Cocain. hydrochlor. gr. 1/4.

Zinci sulph. . . . gr. 1/2.

Zinci sulph. . . . gr. j.

Zinci sulphocarb. . gr. 1/2.

{ Cocain. hydrochlor. gr. 1/4.
{ Morph. sulph. . . . gr. 1/2.

{ Cocain. hydrochlor. gr. 1/4.
{ Morph. sulph. . . . gr. 1/2.
{ Atropinæ sulph. . . gr. 1/100.

{ Cocain. hydrochlor. gr. 1/4.
{ Morph. sulph. . . . gr. 1/2.
{ Iodoformi . . . . gr. iij.
{ Thymol. . . . . gr. 1/2.

{ Iodoformi . . . . gr. iij.
{ Morph. sulph. . . . gr. 1/4.

{ Bismuthi subcarb. . gr. ij.
{ Plumbi carb. . . . gr. ij.

{ Bismuthi subcarb. . gr. ij.
{ Plumbi carb. . . . gr. j.

{ Bismuthi subcarb. . gr. iij.
{ Plumbi carb. . . . gr. j.

Hydrastin. muriat. . gr. j.

{ Hydrastin. muriat. . gr. j.
{ Iodoformi . . . . gr. ij.

{ Zinci sulph. . . . gr. j.
{ Plumbi acetat. . . gr. 1/2.
{ Ext. opii aq. . . . gr. j.
{ Ext. belladonnæ . gr. 1/4.

Zinci oxidi . . . . . gr. ij.
Morph. sulph. . . . gr. 1/4.
Iodoformi . . . . . gr. iij.

Hydrarg. chlor. cor. gr. 1/20.
Hydrarg. chlor. mit. gr. ij.
Ol. eucalypti . . . . gr. v.

Hydrarg. chlor. cor. gr. 1/20.
Hydrarg. chlor. mit. gr. v.
Ol. eucalypti . . . . ♏j.

Iodol . . . . gr. ij.

Iodoformi . . . . . gr. iij.
Ergotini . . . . . . gr. v.
Ext. belladonnæ . . gr. 1/4.

Bismuthi subiodidi . gr. iij.

Thallin. sulph. . . . gr. j.
Iodoformi . . . . . gr. j.
Ext. opii aq. . . . gr. 1/2.
Ext. belladonnæ . . gr. 1/4.

Copaibæ . . . . . . ♏ij.
Acidi tannici . . . . gr. ij.

Copaibæ . . . . . . ♏ij.
Acidi tannici . . . . gr. v.

Copaibæ . . . . . . ♏ij.
Bismuthi subnitrat. gr. iij.

Copaibæ . . . . . . ♏iij.
Bismuthi subnitrat. gr. v.

Hydrarg. chlor. mit. gr. j.
Potassii chlorat. . . gr. j.

Hydrarg. chlor. mit. gr. ij.
Potassii chlorat. . . gr. iij.

Hydrastini . . . . . gr. 1/2.
Salicini . . . . gr. ij.

Hydrastini . . . . . gr. j.
Salicini . . . . gr. iij.

Salicini . . . . gr. ij.
Copaibæ . . . . . . ♏ij.
Ol. cubebæ . . . . . ♏j.

Salicini . . . . gr. iij.
Copaibæ . . . . . . ♏ij.
Ol. cubebæ . . . . . ♏j.

Zinci sulph. . . . . gr. j.
Cupri sulph. . . . . gr. j.

Zinci sulph. . . . . gr. iij.
Cupri sulph. . . . . gr. j.

Iodoformi . . . . . gr. ij.
Acidi tannici . . . gr. j.
Thymol. . . . . . . gr. 1/2.

Iodoformi . . . . . gr. ij.
Acidi tannici . . . . gr. ij.
Thymol. . . . . . . gr. 1/2.

D.—AURAL.

Bismuthi subnitrat. gr. j.
Acidi benzoici . . . gr. j.

Bismuthi subnitrat. gr. ij.
Acidi benzoici . . . gr. j.

Iodoformi . . . . . gr. j.
Acidi tannici . . . . gr. ij.

Iodoformi . . . . . gr. j.
Acidi tannici . . . . gr. iij.

Acidi borici . . . . . gr. 1/2.
Acidi tannici . . . . gr. j.

Acidi borici . . . . . gr. j.
Acidi tannici . . . . gr. iij.

Acidi salicylici . . . gr. j.
Acidi borici . . . . gr. 1/2.
Acidi tannici . . . . gr. ij.

Acidi salicylici . . . gr. ij.
Acidi borici . . . . gr. j.
Acidi tannici . . . . gr. iij.

Zinci sulphocarbol. . gr. ij.
Zinci sulph. . . . . gr. j.

Zinci sulphocarbol. . gr. iij.
Zinci sulph. . . . . gr. j.

Hydrarg. oxidi flav. gr. j.

Hydrarg. oxidi flav. gr. iij.

Hydrarg. chlor. cor. gr. 1/10.
Hydrarg. chlor. mit. gr. ij.

Hydrarg. chlor. cor. gr. 1/10.
Hydrarg. chlor. mit. gr. iij.

Thymol. . . . . . . gr. 1/2.
Eucalyptol. . . . . ♏j.
Chloral. hydrat. . . gr. ij.

Thymol. . . . . . . gr. j.
Eucalyptol. . . . . . ♏ij.
Chloral. hydrat. . . gr. iij.

Morphinæ sulph. . . gr. 1/8.
Atropinæ sulph. . . gr. 1/200.

Morphinæ sulph. . . gr. 1/2.
Atropinæ sulph. . . gr. 1/100.

Cocain. hydrochlor. gr. 1/8.
Morphinæ sulph. . . gr. 1/8.

Cocain. hydrochlor. gr. j.
Morphinæ sulph. . . gr. 1/2.

Cocain. hydrochlor. gr. 1/8.
Potassii chlorat. . . gr. j.

Cocain. hydrochlor. gr. j.
Potassii chlorat. . . gr. iij.

Morphinæ sulph. . . gr. 1/8.
Acidi tannici . . . . gr. ij.

Morphinæ sulph. . . gr. 1/2.
Acidi tannici . . . . gr. iij.

Morphinæ sulph. . . gr. 1/2.
Atropinæ sulph. . . gr. 1/100.
Cocain. hydrochlor. gr. 1/2.

E.—NASAL.

Hydrastis canad. . . gr. v.

Zinci sulph. . . . . . gr. j.
Acidi carbolici . . . gr. 1/4.
Hydrastis canad. . . gr. v.

Iodoformi . . . . . . gr. iij.

Iodoformi . . . . . . gr. v.

Zinci sulph. . . . . . gr. j.
Ex. opii aq. . . . . . gr. ij.

Iodoformi . . . . . . gr. ij.
Ext. belladonnæ . . gr. 1/4.

Acidi carbolici . . . gr. 1/4.
Liq. iodi comp. . . . ♏ij.

Ergotin. . . . . gr. v.

Iodoformi . . . . . . gr. v.
Ol. eucalypti . . . . ♏iij.

Zinci sulph. . . . . . gr. 1/2.
Zinci oxidi . . . . . gr. j.
Hydrastis canad. . . gr. v.

Boroglyceridi . . . . gr. v.

Boroglyceridi . . . . gr. v.
Iodoformi . . . . . gr. ij.

Ergotini . . . . . . gr. iij.
Iodoformi . . . . . gr. iij.
Ext. opii aq. . . . . gr. j.

Bismuthi subnitrat. gr. iv.
Morphinæ sulph. . . gr. $\frac{1}{4}$.

Zinci sulph. . . . . gr. $\frac{1}{10}$.
Morphinæ sulph. . . gr. $\frac{1}{8}$.

Zinci sulph. . . . . gr. $\frac{1}{10}$.

Hydrastin. muriatis gr. $\frac{1}{4}$.

Hydrastin. muriatis gr. $\frac{1}{2}$.
Bismuth. subcarb. . gr. iij.

Plumbi acetatis . . . gr. $\frac{1}{2}$.
Ext. opii aq. . . . . gr. j.
Ext. belladonnæ . . gr. $\frac{1}{8}$.

Sanguinarinæ sulph. gr. $\frac{1}{100}$.

Cocain. hydrochlor. gr. j.

Cocain. hydrochlor. gr. $\frac{1}{2}$.
Morphinæ sulph. . gr. $\frac{1}{4}$.

Cocain. hydrochlor. gr. $\frac{1}{6}$.
Morphinæ sulph. . . gr. $\frac{1}{8}$.
Atropinæ sulph. . . . gr. $\frac{1}{100}$.

Iodoformi . . . . . . gr. j.
Morphinæ sulph. . . gr. $\frac{1}{8}$.

Iodoformi . . . . . . gr. j.
Thymol. . . . . . . gr. $\frac{1}{2}$.
Cocain. hydrochlor. gr. $\frac{1}{4}$.

Iodoformi . . . . gr. iij.
Hydrastin. muriat. . gr. $\frac{1}{2}$.

Potassii chlorat. . . gr. iij.
Thymol. . . . . . . gr. $\frac{1}{2}$.

Potassii chlorat. . . gr. iv.
Thymol. . . . . . . gr. $\frac{1}{2}$.

Bismuthi subnitrat. . gr. ij.
Eucalyptol. . . . . . ℳij.

Bismuthi subnitrat. . gr. iv.
Eucalyptol. . . . . . ℳij.

Iodoformi . . . . . . gr. ij.
Thymol. . . . . . . gr. $\frac{1}{2}$.

Iodoformi . . . . . . gr. ij.
Acidi tannici . . . . gr. ij.

Iodoformi . . . . . gr. ij.
Acidi tannici . . . . gr. iij.

Hydrarg. chlor. cor. . gr. $\frac{1}{10}$.
Potassii chlorat. . . . gr. j.

Hydrarg. chlor. cor. . gr. $\frac{1}{10}$.
Potassii chlorat. . . gr. ij.

Acidi borici . . . . gr. j.
Sodii biborat. . . . . gr. liss.
Thymol. . . . . . . gr. $\frac{1}{2}$.

Acidi borici . . . . gr. ij.
Sodii biborat. . . . gr. iv.
Thymol. . . . . . . gr. j.

Acidi benzoici . . . gr. j.
Iodoformi . . . . . . gr. j.
Hydrarg. chlor. cor. . gr. $\frac{1}{30}$.

Acidi benzoici . . . gr. ij.
Iodoformi . . . . . . gr. j.
Hydrarg. chlor. cor. gr. $\frac{1}{10}$.
Cocain. hydrochlor. gr. $\frac{1}{2}$.

Cocain. hydrochlor. gr. j.

Cocain. hydrochlor. gr. $\frac{1}{6}$.
Morphinæ sulph. . . gr. $\frac{1}{4}$.

Cocain. hydrochlor. gr. j.
Morphinæ sulph. . . gr. $\frac{1}{2}$.

Cocain. hydrochlor. gr. $\frac{1}{3}$.
Morphinæ sulph. . . gr. $\frac{1}{8}$.
Atropinæ sulph. . . gr. $\frac{1}{200}$.

Cocain. hydrochlor. gr. j.
Morphinæ sulph. . . gr. $\frac{1}{2}$.
Atropinæ sulph. . . gr. $\frac{1}{100}$.

Cocain. hydrochlor. gr. $\frac{1}{3}$.
Eucalyptol. . . . . ℳij.
Thymol. . . . . . . gr. $\frac{1}{2}$.

Cocain. hydrochlor. gr. j.
Eucalyptol. . . . . ℳiij.
Thymol. . . . . . . gr. j.

Morphinæ sulph. . . gr. $\frac{1}{8}$.
Zinci oxidi . . . . gr. ij.

Morphinæ sulph. . . gr. $\frac{1}{2}$.
Zinci oxidi . . . . gr. j.
Bismuthi subnitrat. . gr. iij.

Bismuthi subnitrat. . gr. iij.
Cocain. hydrochlor. gr. $\frac{1}{4}$.

Acidi tannici . . . gr. ij.
Iodoformi . . . . . gr. j.
Cocain. hydrochlor. . gr. $\frac{1}{4}$.

IV.

A Table of Formulæ for Hypodermic Medication.

Solutions of alkaloids usually undergo speedy alteration; they are not convenient to carry; and it is not always easy to secure by their use accuracy of dosage. For these reasons the soluble compressed tablets manufactured for hypodermic use are preferable. The tablet should be dissolved in a syringeful of water just boiled. The following alphabetical list contains the drugs available for use in this manner, in convenient doses.

Aconitinæ . . . . . . gr. $\frac{1}{50}$.	Morph. bi-mec. . . . gr. $\frac{1}{8}$.
Aconitinæ . . . . . . gr. $\frac{1}{120}$.	Morph. mur. . . . . . gr. $\frac{1}{6}$.
Aconitinæ . . . . . . gr. $\frac{1}{200}$.	Morph. mur. . . . . . gr. $\frac{1}{4}$.
Atrop. sulph. . . . . gr. $\frac{1}{60}$.	Morph. sulph. . . . . gr. $\frac{1}{2}$.
Atrop. sulph. . . . . gr. $\frac{1}{100}$.	Morph. sulph. . . . . gr. $\frac{1}{3}$.
Atrop. sulph. . . . . gr. $\frac{1}{150}$.	Morph. sulph. . . . . gr. $\frac{1}{4}$.
Atrop. sulph. . . . . gr. $\frac{1}{200}$.	Morph. sulph. . . . . gr. $\frac{1}{6}$.
Apomor. mur. . . . gr. $\frac{1}{10}$.	Morph. sulph. . . . . gr. $\frac{1}{8}$.
Apomor. mur. . . . . gr. $\frac{1}{20}$.	Morph. sulph. . . . . gr. $\frac{1}{12}$.
Caffeinæ . . . . . . gr. $\frac{1}{2}$.	Morph. sulph. . . . . gr. $\frac{1}{2}$.
Caffeinæ . . . . . . gr. i.	Atrop. sulph. . . . . gr. $\frac{1}{100}$.
Cocainæ mur. . . . gr. $\frac{1}{4}$.	Morph. sulph. . . . . gr. $\frac{1}{3}$.
Cocainæ mur. . . . gr. $\frac{1}{8}$.	Atrop. sulph. . . . . gr. $\frac{1}{130}$.
Cocainæ mur. . . . gr. $\frac{1}{10}$.	Morph. sulph. . . . . gr. $\frac{1}{4}$.
Conin. hydrob. . . gr. $\frac{1}{30}$.	Atrop. sulph. . . . . gr. $\frac{1}{150}$.
Conin. hydrob. . . gr. $\frac{1}{100}$.	Morph. sulph. . . . . gr. $\frac{1}{6}$.
Conin. hydrob. . . gr. $\frac{1}{100}$.	Atrop. sulph. . . . . gr. $\frac{1}{130}$.
Morph. sulph. . . . gr. $\frac{1}{6}$.	Morph. sulph. . . . . gr. $\frac{1}{2}$.
Curarin. sulph. . . gr. $\frac{1}{50}$.	Atrop. sulph. . . . . gr. $\frac{1}{200}$.
Curarin. sulph. . . gr. $\frac{1}{30}$.	Morph. sulph. . . . . gr. $\frac{1}{12}$.
Curarin. sulph. . . gr. $\frac{1}{100}$.	Atrop. sulph. . . . . gr. $\frac{1}{250}$.
Digitalin. . . . . . gr. $\frac{1}{100}$.	Physostyg. salic. . . gr. $\frac{1}{70}$.
Dubois. mur. . . . gr. $\frac{1}{50}$.	Physostyg. salic. . . gr. $\frac{1}{40}$.
Dubois. mur. . . . gr. $\frac{1}{100}$.	Picrotoxini . . . . . gr. $\frac{1}{10}$.
Dubois. mur. . . . gr. $\frac{1}{50}$.	Picrotoxini . . . . . gr. $\frac{1}{50}$.
Morph. sulph. . . . gr. $\frac{1}{4}$.	Picrotoxini . . . . . gr. $\frac{1}{80}$.
Dubois. mur. . . . gr. $\frac{1}{100}$.	Strych. sulph. . . . . gr. $\frac{1}{80}$.
Morph. sulph. . . . gr. $\frac{1}{8}$.	Pilocarp. mur. . . . gr. $\frac{1}{4}$.
Eserin. sulph. . . . gr. $\frac{1}{50}$.	Pilocarp. mur. . . . gr. $\frac{1}{6}$.
Eserin. sulph. . . . gr. $\frac{1}{30}$.	Pilocarp. mur. . . . gr. $\frac{1}{10}$.
Eserin. sulph. . . . gr. $\frac{1}{100}$.	Pilocarp. mur. . . . gr. $\frac{1}{2}$.
Eserin. sulph. . . . gr. $\frac{1}{100}$.	Pilocarp. mur. . . . gr. $\frac{1}{20}$.
Morph. sulph. . . . gr. $\frac{1}{6}$.	Pilocarp. mur. . . . gr. $\frac{1}{10}$.
Hyoscy. sulph. . . . gr. $\frac{1}{50}$.	Quin. carb. mur. . . gr. i.
Hyoscy. sulph. . . . gr. $\frac{1}{100}$.	Quin. carb. mur. . . gr. ij.
Hyoscy. sulph. . . . gr. $\frac{1}{50}$.	Quin. carb. mur. . . gr. iij.
Morph. sulph. . . . gr. $\frac{1}{4}$.	Spartein. sulph. . . gr. $\frac{1}{30}$.
Hyoscin. hydrobrom. gr. $\frac{1}{100}$.	Spartein. sulph. . . gr. $\frac{1}{50}$.
Hyoscin. hydrobrom. gr. $\frac{1}{50}$.	Strych. sulph. . . . . gr. $\frac{1}{50}$.
Hydrarg. chlor. cor. gr. $\frac{1}{30}$.	Strych. sulph. . . . . gr. $\frac{1}{100}$.
Hydrarg. chlor. cor. gr. $\frac{1}{50}$.	Strych. sulph. . . . . gr. $\frac{1}{150}$.
Morph. bi-mec. . . gr. $\frac{1}{3}$.	Trinitrin. . . . . . . gr. $\frac{1}{100}$.
Morph. bi-mec. . . gr. $\frac{1}{4}$.	Trinitrin. . . . . . . gr. $\frac{1}{50}$.
Morph. bi-mec. . . gr. $\frac{1}{6}$.	Trinitrin. . . . . . . gr. $\frac{1}{200}$.

The following substances are to be used in freshly-prepared solutions, etc.; they should be fully dissolved and carefully filtered:

Acidi Carbolici ʒii, Acidi Tannici ʒi, Alcoholis ʒiv, Glycerini ʒi. Dose, 1-5 m. for each hemorrhoid.

Acidi Chrysophanici gr. vi, Aq. Destil. fʒx: one minim = $\frac{1}{100}$ gr. Dose, 7½-15 m. = $\frac{1}{16}-\frac{1}{8}$ gr.

Acidi Osmici gr. vi, Aq. Destil. fʒx: one minim = $\frac{1}{100}$ gr. Dose, 7½-15 m. = $\frac{1}{16}-\frac{1}{8}$ gr.

Acidi Sclerotici ʒi, Aq. Destil. ʒv: one minim = $\frac{1}{4}$ gr. Dose, 15-30 m. = 3-6 gr.

Agaricin. gr. iii, Alcohol. Absol. fʒivss, Glycerini fʒvss: one minim = $\frac{1}{250}$ gr. Dose, 15-30 m. = $\frac{1}{16}-\frac{1}{8}$ gr.

Aloini gr. xii, Aq. Destil. ʒi: one minim = ⅛ gr. Dose, 10–15 m.

Aq. Ammoniæ ʒi, Aq. Destil. ʒiii. Dose, 20–30 m.

Antipyrin. gr. xxviiiss, Cocain. Mur. gr. iss, Aq. Bullicnt. f ʒii. Dose, 10 m. = Antipyrine 2½ gr. and Cocaine ¼ gr.

Antipyrin. Hydrochlor. ʒi, Aq. Destil. f ʒi. Heat in a test-tube. One minim = one gr. Dose, 15 m. = 15 gr.

Camphoræ gr. v, Alcohol. ʒi. Dose, 6–30 m.

Camphoræ gr. iii, Ol. Vaselini gr. c. Triturate and filter carefully. Dose, 20–60 m.

Chloral. Hydratis ʒi, Aq. Font. ʒii. Dose, 4–16 m.

Chloroformi ʒii. Dose, 5–15 m.

Chloroformi ʒi, Ol. Vaselini ʒiv. Dose, 15–30 m.

Cotoini Pur. gr. xv, Æther. Acetic. f ʒi : one minim = ¼ gr. Dose, 16–30 m. = 4–7½ gr.

Daturiæ gr. ss, Aq. Font. ʒi: one minim = ₁₅₀ gr. Dose, 4–10 m.

Ergotini gr. xv, Alcohol., Glycerini, āā ʒliss: one minim = ₂₀⁵ gr. Dose, 5–30 m.

Ext. Ergotæ Fl. q. s. Filter carefully. Dose, 10 m.

Eucalypti Ess. ℳxxv, Ol. Vaselini ʒv. Triturate and filter carefully. Dose, 15–30 m.

Eucalyptol. Pur. ℳlxxv, Iodoformi gr. iv. Triturate and dissolve, and add Ol. Vaselini ʒv, shake, and filter carefully. Dose, 15–30 m.

Helleborein. (Merck's) gr. xii, Aq. Destil. f ʒi: one minim = ₄₀¹ gr. Dose, 5–10 m.

Hydrarg. Chlorid. Corros., Ammonii Chlorid., āā gr. iii, Aq. Destil. f ʒiss; mix, dissolve and add Albuminis Ovi f ʒiss, Aq. Destil. f ʒv; filter, and add Aq. Destil. q. s. ad f ʒx. One minim = ₂₅₀ gr. Dose, 3–10 m. = ₈₀¹–₃₀¹ gr.

Hydrarg. Chlor. Mit. gr. iss, Glycerini ℳxv. Dose, 15 m.

Hydrarg. Chlor. Mit. gr. xv, Ol. Olivæ ʒiiss. Dose, 10–30 m.

Hydrarg. Chlor. Mit. gr. xii, Ol. Vaselini ℳccxxv. Dose, 20–30 m.

Hydrarg. Chlor. Mit., Sodii Chlorat., āā gr xv, Aq. Dest. ʒiiss. Dose, 10–30 m.

Hydrarg. Oxid. Flav. ʒiss, Hydrarg. Chlor. Corros. gr. ¾, Glycerini ʒxxv. Dose, 12½ m.

Hydrarg. et Sodii Iodidi gr. iii, Aq. Destil. f ʒiiiss, dissolve and filter: one minim = ₇₅¹ gr. Dose, 10 m. = ⅓ gr.

Hyoscyaminæ gr. i, Acid. Sulph. Dil. ℳv, Aq. Destil. f ʒi: one minim = ₄₈₀¹ gr. Dose, 5 m. = ₉₆¹ gr.

Iodi gr. i, Olei Vaselini gr. c. Triturate and filter carefully, and preserve in a yellow bottle. Dose, 15–30 m.

Iodoformi gr. i, Ol. Vaselini, gr. c. Triturate for a half-hour, adding the vaseline slowly. Filter carefully, and preserve in a yellow glass-stopped vial. Dose, 15–30 m.

Lobelinæ Hydrobrom. gr. i, Aq. Destil. f ʒv: one minim = ₅₀₀¹ gr. Dose, 3–15 m. = ₁₀₀¹–₂₀¹ gr.

Menthol Pur. gr. x, Ol. Vaselini ʒiss. Dissolve over a sand-bath at low heat, and filter carefully. Dose, 5–20 m.

Paraldehyde ʒiss, Aq. Laurocerasi f ʒiss, Aq. Destil. f ʒivss. Warm the solution before using. Dose, 30–60 m. = 6–12 gr.

Pareirin. Hydrochlor. gr. xv, Aq. Destil. f ʒv: one minim = ₂₀¹ gr. Dose, 2–10 m. = ₁₀¹–½ gr.

Phenol gr. i Ol. Vaselini gr. c. Dissolve over a sand-bath at low heat, and filter carefully. Dose, 5–30 m.

Physostigmatis Ext. gr. ii, Aq. Destil. ʒi. Dose, 10 m. = ⅓ gr.

Potassii Arsenitis Liq. Dose, 1–3 m.

Potassii Iodidi ʒi, Aq. Font. ʒiv. Dose, 6–20 m. = 1½–5 gr.

Potassii Permangan. ʒss, Aq. Destil. ʒiii: one minim = ⅛ gr. Dose, 25 m.

Quininæ Hydrobrom. gr. xlviii, Aq. Destil. f ʒiv: one minim = ½ gr. Dose, 20 m. = 4 gr.

Salol. ʒss, Ol. Vaselini ʒv: one minim = ₁₀¹ gr. Dose, 20–30 m.

Spartein. Sulph. gr. i, Aq. Destil. ʒi: one minim = ₆₀¹ gr. Dose, 10 m.

Terebinthinæ Olei gr. xxv, Ol. Vaselini gr. c. Triturate and filter carefully. Dose, 10–30 m.

Thallin. Sulph. ʒi, Aq. Destil. f ʒv: one minim = ⅛ gr. Warm the solution before using. Dose, 5–7½ m. = 1–1½ gr.

Thymol. gr. i. Ol. Vaselini gr. c. Dissolve over a sand bath at a low heat, and filter carefully. Dose, 10–30 m.

After drawing the fluid into the syringe, expel all the air, by pointing the syringe upwards and pressing the piston until a drop of the liquid appears at the point of the needle.

Draw the skin tense at the selected point, and thrust the needle through into the subcutaneous tissues, immediately but slowly injecting the fluid into them; after the needle has been withdrawn, place the finger over the puncture for a short time. Gentle circular friction with the finger-top serves to disperse the injected fluid and hasten absorption.

Avoid, in puncturing, large vessels, inflamed spots, and bony prominences.

Select for the injection the outer surfaces of the arms, thighs, the calves of the legs, the abdomen, or the back.

Hypodermic injections of the preparations of mercury should be made in the gluteal region and very deep, the needle being entered perpendicularly to the plane of the surface to the extent of one inch or more.

Hypodermic medication should be employed when immediate and decided results are required; when medicines otherwise administered fail of their effect; when medicines are indicated which the patient refuses or is unable to swallow; when there is an irritable state of the stomach precluding exhibition by the mouth.

Solutions intended for hypodermic use should be neutral, without acid or alkaline reaction, and non-irritating.

Indications for the Administration of Medicaments by the Hypodermic Method.

Arrest of Perspiration.—Pilocarpin.

Asthma.—Lobeline hydrobromate one two-hundredth to one-twentieth grain. Also in cardiac asthma and pseudo-angina.

Bubo has been aborted by injecting carbolic acid into the swelling.

Bowels, Obstruction of the.—Aloin, in doses of one-half to one grain.

Carcinoma.—Acetic acid, one part to three of water, injected into the cancer.

Chloroform Poisoning.—One-tenth grain of digitaline, followed an hour afterwards with one-tenth grain of atropine.

Chorea.—Curare, one-tenth to one-twentieth of a grain, daily, Liquor potassii arsenitis, one to three minims. Lobeline hydrobromate, one-hundredth to one-twentieth of a grain.

Congestive Chills.—Ten drops of tincture of belladonna every fifteen minutes, until the pulse becomes distinguishable, followed by hypodermics of quinine or dextro-quinine, brandy, or whiskey. Parcirine, one-tenth to one-half grain, also commended. Quinine muriate and hydrobromate may be used hypodermically.

Convulsions, Puerperal.—Chloral.

Convulsions, Infantile.—Morphine, with inhalations of five drops of nitrite of amyl, immediately following.

Convulsions.—Saturated tincture of gelsemium, ten to fifteen drops.

Croup.—Sulphate of atropine, one-per-cent. solution, three drops, repeated after four hours.

Diarrhœa.—Cotoin. four to seven and a half grains, hypodermically, every fifteen or twenty minutes, or every hour, except in intestinal ulceration, cirrhosis, and alcoholics. Also useful in cholera, night-sweats, and ptyalism.

Dysentery.—Morphine, in one-third grain doses.

Dysmenorrhœa.—Antipyrine, two and one-third grains, and cocaine, one-eighth grain, in combination.

Eczema.—Arseniate of sodium, in solutions of one-fifth, one-half, and one per cent., commencing with ten minims of the weaker, and gradually increasing. Chrysophanic acid, one-fifteenth to one-seventh grain, highly recommended in eczema, lichen, prurigo, and psoriasis. Pilocarpin is also of use.

Enuresis, Nocturnal.—Very small doses of the nitrate of strychnine, injected in the vicinity of the rectum at intervals.

Epilepsy.—Curare, in solution, seven grains in seventy-five minims of water, with two drops of hydrochloric acid. About once a week inject eight drops beneath the skin. Also lobeline hydrobromate, one-hundredth to one-twentieth grain.

Erysipelas.—Carbolic acid, three-per-cent. solution, eight or ten injections at the same time, so as to surround and cover the inflamed regions. Also salicylic acid in the same manner.

240

Fevers.—Antipyrine, hypodermically, is very valuable as an antipyretic in doses of ten or fifteen grains. Cocaine, one-eighth grain, may be added. Thallin sulphate, one to one and a half grains, is also useful.

Fractures, Ununited.—Glacial acetic acid, five to ten minims between the ends of the bones. Iodine also used in the same way.

Foreign Body in the Œsophagus.—Threatened strangulation from impaction of the gullet has been promptly relieved by inducing vomiting; apomorphine, one-tenth grain. Emetia also suggested.

Goitre.—Ergotine, one-third grain, gradually increased to one grain.

Hæmoptysis.—Sclerotinic acid, five-per-cent. solution, injected in the neck or arm.

Heart-Failure.—Tincture of digitalis, ten to thirty minims. Digitaline and helleborein (Merck's); brandy and whiskey also.

Hemorrhages (Hæmoptysis, Hæmatemesis, and Uterine Hemorrhages).—Ergotine. In pain, add morphine.

Hemorrhoids.—Iodine, carbolic acid, perchloride of iron, a few drops of either injected into each pile, usually operating on only one at a time, waiting several days before repeating.

Hernia.—Morphine, with or without atropine.

Hiccough.—Three-eighths of a grain of hydrochlorate of pilocarpin.

Hydrophobia.—Curare.

Mania and Melancholia.—Paraldehyde, six to twelve minims in solution. Hyoscyamia, one-ninety-sixth grain, and hyoscine hydrobromate, one-two-hundredth to one-ninetieth grain, also useful.

Nasal Polypus.—Carbolic acid, one part, glycerin, four parts; twenty drops injected into the tumor.

Neuralgias.—Osmic acid, one-fifteenth to one-seventh grain. Also chloroform and antipyrine.

Night Sweats.—Atropine, one-fortieth grain at bedtime. Agaricin, one-tenth grain.

Opium Habit.—Sparteine sulphate.

Opium Poisoning.—Fluid extract of coffee in thirty-minim doses. Caffeine citrate and atropine sulphate.

Paralysis.—Strychnine.

Peritonitis.—Morphine and conium.

Sciatica.—Chloroform and salol.

Sepsis.—Iodoform, turpentine, menthol, thymol, phenol, iodine, and camphor, dissolved in liquid vaseline.

Skin-Diseases (mycotic).—Sulphuric, carbolic, salicylic, or sclerotinic acid, hypodermically, as in erysipelas.

Snake-Bites.—Ammonia, brandy, carbolic or salicylic acid. Also permanganate of potassium.

Strychnine Poisoning.—Caffeine, one grain; alcohol; chloral.

Surgical Shock.—Quinine, six grains, with one-third grain of morphine. Also quinine hydrobromate, four grains.

Suspension of Salivary Secretion.—Pilocarpin.

Syphilis.—Mercurials.

Tetanus.—Curare, physostigmine, morphine, and cocaine; also pilocarpin.

Trichinosis.—Tincture of ergot and ergotine.

Urticaria.—Saturated solution of bisulphide of sodium into the part affected. Chrysophanic acid, one-fifteenth to one-seventh grain.

Varicose Veins.—Ergot or ergotine, injected near the affected veins.

V.

A List of Drugs for Inhalation.

The doses are calculated for an ordinary steam-atomizer, and are to be added to one ounce of water.

Acidi carbolici, gtt. iij to x. In phthisis.

Acidi tannici, gr. j to xx. In chronic catarrhal affections and laryngeal ulcerations.

Aluminis, gr. v to xxx. In cases of excessive secretions from bronchi.

Ammonii chloridi, gr. ij to 3ij. To promote expectoration in acute and chronic catarrh.

Aquæ amygdulæ amaræ 3j. (Add no water.) In painful affections of the upper air-passages and paroxysmal cough.

Aquæ ferventis. In acute inflammations of the mucous membrane, as in laryngitis.

Argenti nitratis, gr. j to x. In ulcerations and follicular pharyngitis. A face-shield should be worn.

Calcis liquoris, 3j. (Add no water.) In diphtheria and croup.

Cannabis indicæ ext., gr. ¼ to j. In chronic catarrh and emphysema.

Conii ext., gr. j to vj. In irritative coughs and asthma.

Cupri sulphatis, gr. j to xx. In chronic inflammations and coughs.

Hyoscyami ext., gr. ½. In whooping-cough and spasmodic coughs.

Iodi tinct., gtt. j to xx. In inflammatory affections of the larynx and pharynx.

Morphinæ acetatis, gr. ⅛ to ½. In irritative cough and its constitutional effect.

Opii ext. aquosi, gr. ⅛ to ½. In irritative cough.

Picis liq. infus., 3j to 3ij. In offensive bronchial secretions.

Plumbi acetatis, gr. iij to v. In advanced stages of acute catarrhs. Astringent and sedative.

Potassii carbonatis, gr. x to 3ij. In follicular pharyngitis.

Potassii chloratis, gr. x to xx. In chronic and subacute catarrhal affections

Potassii bromidi, gr. j to x. In spasmodic laryngeal affections.

Potassii iodidi, gr. ij to xx. In granular inflammations, and chronic bronchitis with emphysema.

Sodæ chloratæ liq., 3½ to j. In offensive bronchial secretions.

Terebinthinæ ol., gtt. j to ij. In chronic bronchitis with offensive secretions.

Zinci sulphatis, gr. j to vj. In bronchorrhœa, etc.

VI

A List of Common Poisons and their Antidotes.

In cases of poisoning when the substance has been taken by way of the mouth, the stomach must be emptied before proceeding to administer the antidote. This can be done by means of—

(a) *Emetics:*

Large draughts of lukewarm water; mustard-water, a teaspoonful of powdered mustard to the tumblerful of water; alum-water, a dessertspoonful of powdered alum to the tumblerful of water; sulphate of zinc, 10 to 30 grains; powdered ipecac, 10 grains; or—

(b) *The stomach-pump.*

Where the stomach-pump cannot be promptly obtained, a rubber tube may be used for the purpose of washing out the stomach.

The only exceptions to the above rule are: first, when a considerable period of time—several hours—has elapsed after the ingestion of a small amount of highly poisonous substance; and, second, when highly corrosive substances have been taken which are likely to have partially dissolved the wall of the stomach.

POISONS.	ANTIDOTES.

ACIDS.

Acids. *Sulphuric.* *Hydrochloric.* *Nitric.* *Phosphoric.*	*Alkalies.* Bicarbonate of sodium or potassium. Magnesia. Chalk or whiting. Plaster from the wall; soap, to be followed by copious draughts of tepid water or flaxseed tea; milk; eggs beaten up; olive or almond oil.
Oxalic. *Binoxalate of Potassium.* *Tartaric.* *Acetic.*	Chalk or whiting, or plaster from the wall, with water.
Hydrocyanic.	Alternate hot and cold affusion; artificial respiration; atropine hypodermically; ammonia.
Carbolic.	Saccharated lime: Glauber's or Epsom salts; stimulants; white of egg, milk, or wheat flour.

ALKALIES.

Caustic Potash.	Vinegar, or other dilute acids.
Caustic Soda.	Lemon juice.
Caustic Lime.	Milk.
Caustic Ammonia. *Carbonate of Sodium or of Potassium,*	Castor, linseed, almond, or other oil, freely.

MINERAL POISONS.

Antimony.	If vomiting does not occur, wash out the stomach with water. Follow with astringent infusions, as of galls, oak bark, very strong green tea, or tannic or gallic acid. Follow this by white of egg.

MINERAL POISONS (Continued).

Arsenic.	Administer freshly-precipitated hydrated oxide of iron freely.

[To make hydrated oxide of iron: "Take of solution of tersulphate of iron a pint; water of ammonia, water, each a sufficient quantity. To the solution of tersulphate of iron, previously mixed with three pints of water, add water of ammonia with constant stirring until in slight excess. Then pour the whole on a wet muslin strainer, wash the precipitate with water, pressing the strainer forcibly with the hands until no more liquid passes. Lastly, mix the precipitate with sufficient water to bring the mixture to the measure of a pint and a half, and transfer it to a wide-mouthed bottle, which must be well stopped."—*U.S.P.*]

or—

Dialyzed iron in tablespoonful doses, followed by 15-grain doses of chloride of sodium, repeated every ten or fifteen minutes.

In the absence of the above, magnesia or oils or fats, as sweet oil, butter, milk, should be freely administered.

Barium Salts.	Epsom or Glauber's salts, or dilute sulphuric acid.
Copper. *Corrosive Sublimate.*	} See *Metallic Salts.*
Cyanide of Potassium.	} See *Hydrocyanic Acid.*
Insect Powder.	See *Arsenic.*
Iodine. *Iodide of Potassium.*	} Starch, wheat flour, or arrow-root, well boiled with water, very freely. Afterwards, vinegar and water.
Lead.	See *Metallic Salts.*
Metallic Salts.	White of egg, freely, to form insoluble albuminate. Then wash out stomach and follow by demulcents, poultices to epigastrium, and opium by suppository, or morphine hypodermically.
Phosphorus.	Sulphate of copper; magnesia; copious draughts of water and mucilaginous drinks; oil of turpentine (old); animal charcoal. Avoid oils and fats.
Rat Paste.	See *Phosphorus.*

ALKALOIDS, ETC.

Aconite.	Alcohol, whiskey, brandy, etc.; ammonia; artificial heat; digitalis; atropine.
Alcohol.	Coffee; cold affusion to head; artificial heat to head and feet; strychnine hypodermically.
Atropine.	Coffee and stimulants; hypodermic injections of caffeine; artificial respiration; physostigma, cautiously.
Belladonna.	See *Atropine.*
Calabar Bean.	Stimulants; atropine; artificial respiration.
Cannabis Indica.	See *Morphine.*
Cantharides.	Demulcents, freely. Avoid fats and oils.
Cherry-Laurel Water.	} See *Hydrocyanic Acid.*
Chloral.	External warmth; strong, hot coffee per rectum; strychnine hypodermically, repeated at intervals of fifteen or twenty minutes. Keep the patient roused.
Codeine.	See *Morphine.*
Colchicum.	Tannic or gallic acid; stimulants; opium.
Conium.	Tannic acid; stimulants; coffee.
Creasote.	See *Carbolic Acid.*
Croton Oil.	Demulcents; stimulants; opium.

ALKALOIDS, ETC. (Continued).

Curare.	Artificial respiration: if the poison has been introduced by a weapon, incise the wound freely and suck it. If the wound is upon a limb, tie a bandage above the wound. The bandage should be from time to time loosened for a moment, in order to allow the unremoved poison to pass into the system by degrees.
Digitalis.	Strong tea; tannin; stimulants; aconite; absolute quiet.
Ergot.	Stimulants.
Gelsemium.	Atropine; stimulants; artificial respiration.
Hyoscyamus.	See *Atropine.*
Lobelia.	Tannin; stimulants; strychnine hypodermically.
Morphine.	Keep the patient aroused and moving: cold affusion; general faradization; alcohol; atropine hypodermically; artificial respiration.
Mushrooms.	Atropine hypodermically; castor oil; stimulants.
Nitrite of Amyl.	Stimulants; alternate cold and hot douches; artificial respiration.
Nitroglycerin.	Cold to the head; ergotine; atropine hypodermically.
Oil of Bitter Almonds.	See *Hydrocyanic Acid.*
Opium.	See *Morphine.*
Quinine.	Tannic or gallic acid; strong tea or coffee; alcohol; ammonia; artificial respiration.
Physostigma.	Stimulants; atropine; chloral; strychnine; artificial respiration.
Picrotoxine.	Chloral; bromide of potassium.
Pilocarpine.	Atropine.
Snake-Bite.	A bandage around the limb; fresh incision and sucking of the wound; actual cautery or permanganate of potassium, locally; alcoholic stimulants freely; ammonia; artificial respiration; strychnine hypodermically.
Stramonium.	See *Atropine.*
Strychnine.	Chloroform; tannin; bromide of potassium; chloral.
Tobacco.	Tannin; diffusible stimulants; strychnine.
Turpentine.	Demulcents; sulphate of magnesia.
Veratrine.	Diffusible stimulants; hot coffee; absolute rest in a recumbent posture.

AERIAL POISONS.

Anæsthetics. *Chloroform.* *Ether.* *Nitrous Oxide.* *Bromide of Ethyl, etc.*	Artificial respiration; inversion of the body; flagellation, etc.
Chlorine. *Bromine.* *Iodine Vapor.*	Steam inhalations.
Coal Gas. *Charcoal Fumes.* *Carbonic Acid Gas.* *Choke Damp.* *Marsh Gas.* *Fire Damp.*	Artificial respiration; alternate warm and cold douches; frictions; sinapisms; venesection; inhalations of oxygen.
Carbon Monoxide.	Fresh air; artificial respiration; transfusion.

VII

A Posological Table.

For hypodermic use the dose should be half that used by the mouth.
For use by the rectum the dose should be twice that by the mouth.

Doses for Different Ages.

GAUBIUS'S RULE:

Regulating the Ordinary Proportion of Doses according to the Age of the Patient.

For an adult, suppose the dose to be . . . . . . 1, or 1 drachm.
Under 1 year will require . . . . $\frac{1}{12}$ " 5 grains.
" 2 years " " . . . . $\frac{1}{8}$ " 8 "
" 3 " " " . . . . $\frac{1}{6}$ " 10 "
" 4 " " " . . . . $\frac{1}{4}$ " 15 "
" 7 " " " . . . . $\frac{1}{3}$ " 1 scruple.
" 14 " " " . . . . $\frac{1}{2}$ " $\frac{1}{2}$ drachm.
" 20 " " " . . . . $\frac{2}{3}$ " 2 scruples.
From 21 years to 60 years, the full dose . . . . 1 " 1 drachm.
Above 60 years an inverse gradation should be observed.

YOUNG'S RULE:

For children under 12 years the doses of most medicines must be diminished in the proportion of the age to the age increased by 12. Thus, at 2 years the dose will be $\frac{1}{7}$ of that for an adult, viz.:

$$\frac{2}{2 + 12} = \frac{1}{7}.$$

Sex, temperament, constitutional strength, and the habits and idiosyncrasies of individuals must be taken into account. Nor does the same rule apply to all medicines. Calomel, for instance, is generally borne better by children than by adults; while opium affects them more powerfully, and requires the dose to be diminished considerably below that indicated in the table.

Table for the Administration of Laudanum.

For a child at birth, or one month old . . . . . . $\frac{1}{10}$ to $\frac{1}{4}$ drop.
Under a year old . . . . $\frac{1}{4}$ to 1 "
From one to two years . . . . 1 to 3 drops.
" two to five years . . . . 2 to 5 "
" five to ten years . . . . 5 to 10 "
" ten to fifteen years . . . . 10 to 20 "
At fifteen years . . . . 15 to 20 "
For an adult . . . . 20 to 30 "

It is important, in the employment of laudanum, that it should be of the proper strength and perfectly clear. Thirteen minims represent one grain of opium. Laudanum becomes stronger with age, especially if the bottle be not tightly corked.

A POSOLOGICAL TABLE.

Drug or Preparation.	Dose.
Abstract. belladonnæ	$\frac{1}{2}$ grain.
cannabis ind.	1 grain.
conii	1 to 3 grs.
gelsemii	1 grain.
hyoscyami	2 grains.
nuc. vom.	1 grain.
podophylli	4 grains.
Acetphenetidine	3 to 10 grs.
Acet. opii	5 minims
scillæ	10 to 30 min.
Acid. acet. dil.	60 minims.
arsenios	$\frac{1}{32}$ to $\frac{1}{12}$ gr.
benzoic	5 to 15 grs.
boric	5 to 10 grs.
carbolic	1 to 3 grs.
folicis	5 to 15 grs.
gallic	3 to 15 grs.
hydrobrom. 34 per cent.	10 to 15 grs.
hydrobrom. dil.	15 to 60 min.
hydrochlor.	3 to 10 min.
hydrochlor. dil.	10 to 30 min.
hydrocyan. dil.	2 to 6 min.
lactic.	15 to 60 grs.
nitric.	3 to 10 min.
nitr. dil.	10 to 30 min.
nitrohydrochlor.	3 to 10 min.
nitrohydrochlor. dil.	5 to 20 min.
oxalic.	$\frac{1}{2}$ to 2 grs.
phosphoric. 50 per cent.	3 to 15 grs.
phosphoric. dil.	10 to 20 min.
salicylic.	5 to 15 grs.
sulphuric.	5 to 10 min.
sulphuric. dil.	10 to 20 min.
sulphuric. arom.	5 to 30 min.
sulphuros.	30 to 60 min.
tannic.	2 to 15 grs.
Aconitina (white cryst.).	$\frac{1}{400}$ to $\frac{1}{200}$ gr.
Adonidine	$\frac{1}{16}$ to $\frac{1}{3}$ gr.
Agaricin.	$\frac{1}{24}$ to $\frac{1}{6}$ gr.
Airol	2 to 5 grs.
Alantol	$\frac{1}{6}$ to 10 min.
Aletris cordial	1 to 4 drs
Aloe	2 to 5 grs.
Aloinum	1 to 3 grs.
Alumen	5 to 15 grs.
Ammonii benzoas	10 to 20 grs.
bromid.	5 to 30 grs.
carb.	3 to 10 grs.
Ammonii chlorid.	5 to 30 grs.
iodid.	3 to 15 grs.
phosp.	5 to 20 grs.
picras	$\frac{1}{8}$ to $1\frac{1}{2}$ grs.
valer.	3 to 15 grs.
Ammonol	5 to 20 grs.
Amyl. hydras	15 to 75 min.
nitris	2 to 5 min.
Antifebrin (acetanilide)	2 to 15 grs.
Ant. et pot. tart.: diaphoretic	$\frac{1}{16}$ to $\frac{1}{8}$ gr.
emetic	1 to 2 grs.
Antikamnia	5 to 15 grs.
Antimonii oxysulphuret.	$\frac{1}{2}$ to 2 grs.
Antipyrin.	5 to 30 grs.
Apiol	5 to 10 min.
Apomorph. hydrochlor.	$\frac{1}{30}$ to $\frac{1}{8}$ gr.
Aqua ammoniæ	5 to 30 min.
amygd. amar.	2 fl. drs.
camphoræ	1 to 4 fl.drs.
chlori	1 to 4 fl drs.
creasoti	1 to 4 fl.drs.
Aqua laurocerasi	6 to 30 min.
Arbutin	8 to 15 grs.
Argenti nitras	$\frac{1}{6}$ to $\frac{1}{4}$ gr.
Arsenauro	5 to 15 min.
Arsen-hemol	$1\frac{1}{2}$ grs.
Arsenii iodidum	$\frac{1}{64}$ to $\frac{1}{10}$ gr.
Asafœtida	5 to 20 grs.
Asaprol	8 to 15 grs.
Atropina	$\frac{1}{120}$ to $\frac{1}{60}$ gr.
Atropinæ sulph.	$\frac{1}{120}$ to $\frac{1}{60}$ gr.
Auri et sodii chlorid.	$\frac{1}{32}$ to $\frac{1}{16}$ gr.
Balsamum gurjunæ	15 to 40 grs.
peruviani	20 to 30 min.
Beberiæ sulphas: tonic	1 to 3 grs.
antiperiodic	3 to 10 grs.
Belladonnæ fol.	1 to 10 grs.
Belladonnæ rad.	1 to 5 grs.
Benzanilide	4 to 30 grs.
Benzosol	3 to 15 grs.
Berberina	1 to 15 grs.
Bismal	3 to 15 grs.
Bismuthi citras	3 to 15 grs.
et ammonii citr.	1 to 15 grs.
salicylas	2 to 8 grs.
subnitr.	3 to 15 grs.
valer.	1 to 3 grs.
Borolyptol	$\frac{1}{2}$ to 1 dr.
Bromo-hemol	15 to 30 grs.
Caffeina	1 to 5 grs.
Calcii chloridum	10 to 20 grs.
hippuras	5 to 10 grs.
hypophosphis	3 to 15 grs.
iodidum	1 to 3 grs.
phosphas	15 to 30 grs.
santoninas	$\frac{1}{4}$ to $\frac{3}{4}$ gr.
Calx sulphurata	$\frac{1}{3}$ to 1 gr.
Cambogium	1 to 4 grs.
Camphora	3 to 10 grs.
monobrom.	2 to 5 grs.
Cannabinon	$\frac{3}{4}$ to $1\frac{1}{2}$ grs.
Cannabin. tannas	4 to 15 grs.
Cantharis	$\frac{1}{2}$ to 2 grs.
Capsicum	1 to 3 grs.
Carnogen	2 to 4 drs.
Castoreum	6 to 15 grs.
Catechu	15 to 30 grs.
Celerina	1 to 2 drs.
Cerii nitras	1 to 3 grs.
oxalas	1 to 3 grs.
Chinoidinum	3 to 30 grs.
Chinoline	8 to 30 grs.
Chloral	10 to 30 grs.
Chloroformum	1 to 5 min.
Chrysarobinum	3 to 15 grs.
Cinchona	15 to 60 grs.
Cinchonidina	1 to 30 grs.
Cinchonina	1 to 30 grs.
Cinnamomum	6 to 30 grs.
Cocæ fol.	$\frac{1}{2}$ to 2 drs.
Cocainæ hydrochlor.	$\frac{1}{6}$ to 1 gr.
Codeina	$\frac{1}{2}$ to 2 grs.
Colchicin.	$\frac{1}{120}$ to $\frac{1}{16}$ gr.
Colocynthin.	$\frac{1}{6}$ to $\frac{2}{3}$ gr.
Confectio sennæ	1 to 2 grs.
Coniina and its salts	$\frac{1}{64}$ to $\frac{1}{32}$ gr.
Convallamarin.	$\frac{1}{2}$ to 4 grs.
Copaiba	15 to 60 min.
Cotoinum	$\frac{1}{2}$ to 1 gr.
Creasotum	1 to 3 min.
Creta præpar.	15 to 75 grs.
Croton chloral.	1 to 10 grs.
Cubeba	15 to 60 grs.
Cupri acetas	$\frac{1}{2}$ to 6 grs.
sulphas	$\frac{1}{2}$ to 10 grs.
Cupro-hemol	1 to 3 grs.
Cuprum ammon.	$\frac{1}{6}$ to 1 gr.
Curare	$\frac{1}{32}$ to $\frac{1}{2}$ gr.

Drug or Preparation.	Dose.
Decoct. aloes comp. .	$\frac{1}{2}$ to 2 fl. oz.
sarsap. comp. . .	2 to 6 fl. oz.
Dermatol	4 to 8 grs.
Diastase	5 to 15 grs.
Digitalinum	$\frac{1}{60}$ to $\frac{1}{30}$ gr.
Digitalis	$\frac{1}{2}$ to 3 grs.
Duboisina and its salts	$\frac{1}{120}$ to $\frac{1}{60}$ gr.
Elaterinum, U. S. P. 1880	$\frac{1}{60}$ to $\frac{1}{16}$ gr.
Elaterinum, U. S. P. 1870	$\frac{1}{16}$ to $\frac{1}{2}$ gr.
Ergota	15 to 60 grs.
Ergotinum	2 to 8 grs.
Ergotole	5 to 20 min. (hypoderm.)
Eserina and its salts	$\frac{1}{64}$ to $\frac{1}{20}$ gr.
Ethoxycaffeina . .	1 to 3 grs.
Eucalyptol	5 to 16 min.
Euonymin.	2 to 4 grs.
Europhen	$\frac{1}{2}$ to $1\frac{1}{2}$ grs. (hypoderm.)
Ext. aconiti rad., U. S. P. 1880 . .	$\frac{1}{12}$ to $\frac{1}{4}$ gr.
aconiti [rad.] fl. .	1 to 5 min.
aloes aquos. . . .	$\frac{1}{2}$ to 3 grs.
angusturæ fl. . .	15 to 45 min.
angelicæ rad. fl. .	30 to 60 min.
anthemidis . . .	2 to 10 grs.
anthemidis fl. . .	30 to 60 min.
apocyni cannab. fl.	8 to 30 min.
arecæ fl.	45 to 75 min.
arnicæ flor. . . .	3 to 8 grs.
arnicæ fl.	5 to 15 min.
arnicæ rad. . . .	2 to 5 grs.
arnicæ rad. fl. . .	5 to 15 min.
aromat. fl.	30 to 60 min.
aspidospermæ fl. .	15 to 45 min.
aurantii cort. fl. .	$\frac{1}{2}$ to $2\frac{1}{2}$ fl. drs.
azedarach fl. . . .	15 to 75 min.
baptisiæ fl.	7 to 30 min.
bellad. fol. fl. . .	3 to 7 min.
bellad. rad. . . .	$\frac{1}{8}$ to $\frac{1}{4}$ gr.
bellad. rad. fl. . .	1 to 6 min.
brayeræ fl.	2 to 4 fl. drs.
bryoniæ fl. . . .	15 to 60 min.
buchu fl.	$\frac{1}{2}$ to $2\frac{1}{2}$ fl. drs.
calami fl.	15 to 60 min.
calend. fl.	15 to 60 min.
calumbæ	3 to 10 grs.
calumbæ fl. . . .	15 to 60 min.
canellæ fl.	15 to 60 min.
cannab. amer. fl. .	3 to 15 min.
cannab. ind. . . .	$\frac{1}{6}$ to 2 grs.
cannab. ind. fl. . .	3 to 6 min.
cantharidis fl. . .	1 to 3 min.
capsici fl.	1 to 3 min.
cardam. comp. fl. .	15 to 45 min.
cascarillæ fl. . . .	$\frac{1}{2}$ to $2\frac{1}{2}$ fl. drs.
caulophylli fl. . .	15 to 30 min.
chimaph. fl. . . .	$\frac{3}{4}$ to $1\frac{1}{4}$ fl. drs.
cimicifugæ fl. . .	8 to 30 min.
cinchonæ	15 to 30 grs.
cinchonæ fl. . . .	30 to 60 min.
cinchonæ arom. fl.	30 to 60 min.
cinchonæ comp fl.	$\frac{1}{2}$ to $1\frac{1}{4}$ fl drs.
cocæ	10 to 25 grs.
cocæ fl.	1 to 2 drs.
cocculi fl.	1 to 3 min.
colch. rad.	$\frac{1}{3}$ to $1\frac{1}{2}$ grs.
colch. rad. fl. . .	3 to 15 min.
colch. sem. fl. . .	$1\frac{1}{2}$ to 10 min.
colocynth.	1 to 5 grs.
colocynth. comp. .	1 to 5 grs.
conii fol. fl. . . .	3 to 15 min.
convallariæ rad. fl.	15 to 30 min.
corn. flor. fl. . . .	30 to 60 min.
coto fl.	5 to 15 min.
Ext. cubebæ fl. . . .	15 to 30 min.
cypripedii fl. . . .	15 to 60 min.
damianæ fl. . . .	$\frac{1}{2}$ to 2 fl. drs.
digitalis	$\frac{1}{6}$ to $\frac{1}{2}$ gr.
digitalis fl.	1 to 6 min.
droseræ fl.	5 to 10 min.
dulcamaræ . . .	5 to 15 grs.
dulcamaræ fl. . .	1 to 2 fl. drs.
ergotæ	1 to 8 grs.
ergotæ fl.	15 to 60 min.
erythroxyli fl. . .	$\frac{1}{2}$ to 2 fl. drs.
eucalypti fl. . . .	15 to 60 min.
euonymi fl. . . .	15 to 60 min.
eupatorii fl. . . .	30 to 60 min.
euphorbiæ pil. fl. .	10 to 30 min.
gallæ fl.	$\frac{3}{4}$ to 2 fl. drs.
gelsemii	2 to 8 min.
gelsemii fl. . . .	1 to 8 min.
gentianæ fl. . . .	30 to 60 min.
gent. comp. fl. . .	30 to 60 min.
geranii fl.	15 to 90 min.
gilleniæ fl.	15 to 30 min.
gossypii fl.	15 to 45 min.
granati rad. co. fl.	$\frac{3}{4}$ to 2 fl drs.
grind. rob. fl. . .	30 to 60 min.
grind. squarr. fl. .	30 to 60 min.
guaiaci ligni fl. .	30 to 60 min.
guaranæ fl. . . .	15 to 30 min.
hæmatoxyli . . .	8 to 30 grs.
hæmatoxyli fl. . .	30 to 60 min.
hamamelidis fl. .	60 to 90 min.
hellob. nigris .	$\frac{1}{2}$ to 3 grs.
helleb. nigris fl. .	5 to 15 min.
heloniæ fl.	8 to 30 min.
hepaticæ fl. . . .	30 to 60 min.
humuli	3 to 15 grs.
humuli fl.	30 to 60 min.
hydrangeæ fl. . .	30 to 60 min.
hydrastis	3 to 10 grs.
hydrastis fl. . . .	8 to 30 min.
hyoscyami fol. fl. .	3 to 30 min.
hyoscyami sem. fl.	3 to 8 min.
ignatiæ	$\frac{1}{3}$ to $1\frac{1}{4}$ grs.
ignatiæ fl.	1 to 6 min.
ipecac. fl.	3 to 60 min.
iridis versicol. . .	3 to 6 grs.
iridis versicol. fl. .	15 to 30 min.
jalapæ, U. S. P. 1870	5 to 10 grs.
jalapæ fl.	15 to 60 min.
juglandis . . .	15 to 30 grs.
juglandis fl. . . .	$\frac{3}{4}$ to 2 fl. drs.
junip. fl.	30 to 60 min.
kino fl.	15 to 30 min.
krameriæ	5 to 15 grs.
krameriæ fl. . . .	30 to 60 min.
lactucæ	5 to 15 grs.
lactucæ fl.	15 to 60 min.
lactucarii fl. . . .	8 to 30 min.
leptandræ	3 to 10 grs.
leptandræ fl. . . .	30 to 60 min.
lobeliæ fl.	$\frac{1}{4}$ to 1 fl. dr.
lobeliæ sem. fl. . .	$\frac{1}{8}$ to $\frac{1}{2}$ fl. dr.
lupulini fl. . . .	10 to 30 min.
lycopi fl.	5 to 30 min.
malti	1 to $2\frac{1}{2}$ drs.
matico fl.	30 to 60 min.
mezerei	$\frac{1}{2}$ to 1 gr.
mezerei fl.	3 to 10 min.
nectandræ fl. . .	1 to 4 fl drs.
nuc. vom.	$\frac{1}{3}$ to 1 gr.
nuc. vom. fl. . . .	1 to 5 min.
opii	$\frac{1}{4}$ to $\frac{1}{2}$ gr.
papaveris	$\frac{1}{2}$ to 2 grs.
papaveris fl. . . .	15 to 45 min.
pareiræ fl.	30 to 60 min.
petroselini fl. . .	1 to 2 fl. drs.
physostigmæ . .	$\frac{1}{16}$ to $\frac{1}{6}$ gr.

Drug or Preparation.	Dose.
Ext. physostigmæ fl.	1 to 3 min.
phytolaccæ bac. fl.	5 to 30 min.
phytolaccæ rad.	1 to 3 grs.
phytolaccæ rad. fl.	5 to 30 min.
pilocarpi fl.	15 to 60 min.
piper niger fl.	15 to 45 min.
piscidiæ fl.	15 to 60 min.
podophylli	1/2 to 1 1/2 grs.
podophylli fl.	8 to 30 min.
prun. virg. fl.	30 to 60 min.
pulsatillæ fl.	2 to 10 min.
quassiæ	1 to 5 grs.
quassiæ fl.	30 to 60 min.
quebracho fl.	20 to 60 min.
quercus fl.	30 to 60 min.
rhamnus purshian. fl.	5 to 90 min.
rhei	5 to 15 grs.
rhei fl.	15 to 45 min.
rhois arom. fl.	15 to 60 min.
rhois glabr. co. fl.	30 to 60 min.
rhois glab. frct. fl.	30 to 60 min.
rhois toxicod. fl.	1 to 6 min.
ricini fol. fl.	1/2 to 2 fl. drs.
rosæ fl.	1/2 to 2 fl. drs.
rubi fl.	15 to 50 min.
sabinæ fl.	5 to 15 min.
salicis fl.	1/2 to 2 fl. drs.
salviæ fl.	1/2 to 2 fl. drs.
sanguin. fl.	5 to 15 min.
santali cit. fl.	1 to 2 fl. drs.
santonicæ fl.	15 to 60 min.
sarsap. fl.	1/2 to 2 fl. drs.
sassafras fl.	1/2 to 2 fl. drs.
scillæ fl.	1 to 5 min.
scillæ comp. fl.	1 to 5 min.
scoparii fl.	1/2 to 1 fl. dr.
senegæ fl.	8 to 15 min.
sennæ fl.	1 to 4 fl. drs.
serpent. fl.	30 to 60 min.
simarubæ fl.	15 to 30 min.
spigeliæ fl.	15 to 60 min.
spigeliæ et sennæ fl.	1/2 to 2 fl. drs.
stigmatæ maid. fl.	1 to 2 fl. drs.
stillingiæ fl.	1/2 to 2 fl. drs.
stillingiæ comp. fl.	1/2 to 2 fl. drs.
stramonii fol. alc.	1/3 to 2/3 gr.
stramonii sem.	1/6 to 1/2 gr.
stramonii fl.	1 to 6 min.
sumbul fl.	15 to 6' min.
taraxaci	5 to 15 grs.
taraxaci fl.	1/2 to 2 fl. drs.
trit. rep. fl.	1 to 4 fl. drs.
urticæ rad. fl.	5 to 15 min.
ustilag. maid. fl.	15 to 60 min.
uvæ ursi fl.	30 to 60 min.
valerianæ	5 to 15 grs.
valer. fl.	30 to 60 min.
veratr. vir. fl.	2 to 8 min.
viburni [prunif.] fl.	1 to 2 fl. drs.
xanthoxyli cort. fl.	15 to 30 min.
xanthoxyli frct. fl.	15 to 30 min.
zingiberis fl.	8 to 30 min.
Fel bovis purif.	3 to 6 grs.
Ferri arsen.	1/20 to 1/2 gr.
benzoas	1 to 5 grs.
bromid.	1 to 5 grs.
carb. sacch.	4 to 15 grs.
chlorid.	1 to 3 grs.
citr.	5 to 10 grs.
et ammon. citr.	5 to 10 grs.
et ammon. sulph.	5 to 10 grs.
et ammon. tartr.	5 to 15 grs.
et cinchonid. citr.	5 to 10 grs.
et pot. tartr.	5 to 30 grs.
et quin. citr.	5 to 10 grs.
et strychn. citr.	1 to 5 grs.
Ferri hypophosphis.	5 to 10 grs.
iodidum	1 to 5 grs.
iodidum sacch.	2 to 10 grs.
lactas	1 to 3 grs.
oxalas	1 to 3 grs.
oxid. hydrat.	1/2 to 2 oz.
phosphas	1 to 5 grs.
pyrophosphas	1 to 5 grs.
subcarb.	5 to 30 grs.
sulphas	1 to 3 grs.
sulphas exsiccat.	1 to 3 grs.
valer.	1 to 3 grs.
Ferrum dialysatum	5 to 15 min.
redactum	1 to 5 grs.
Globon	1/2 to 1 dr.
Glycozone	1 to 2 fl. drs.
Guarana	10 to 30 grs.
Helleborein (Merck's)	1/10 to 1/4 gr.
Hemoglobin	75 to 150 grs.
Hemol	2 to 8 grs.
Hydrarg. chlorid. corr.	1/64 to 1/16 gr.
chlorid. mite	1/20 to 10 grs.
cyanid.	1/16 to 1/2 gr.
iodid. flav.	1/6 to 1 gr.
iodid. rubr.	1/16 to 1/2 gr.
iodid. vir.	1/6 to 1 gr.
oxid. flav.	1/16 to 1/2 gr.
oxid. nigr.	1/10 to 1 gr.
oxid. rubr.	1/10 to 1/2 gr.
salicylas	1/10 to 1/8 gr.
subsulphas flav.	1/4 to 1 gr.
tannas	1/2 to 1 1/2 grs.
cum creta	1 to 8 grs.
Hydrochinon	5 to 30 grs.
Hydroleine	2 dr. to 1 oz.
Hyoscin hydrobrom.	1/200 to 1/50 gr.
Hyoscyamina and salts	1/60 to 1/24 gr.
Hypnone	3/4 to 2 grs.
Ichthyol	3 to 5 grs.
Infusum digitalis	2 to 4 fl. drs.
sennæ comp.	1 to 2 fl. oz.
Ingluvin	5 to 20 grs.
Iodoformum	1 to 3 grs.
Iodol	1/4 to 2 grs.
Iodothyrine	15 to 40 grs.
Iodum	1/8 to 1/2 gr.
Ipecacuanhæ: expectorant	1/6 to 1 gr.
emetic	15 to 30 grs.
Iridin	2 to 4 grs.
Jalapa	15 to 30 grs.
Kairine	4 to 15 grs.
Kamala	1 to 2 drs.
Kino	8 to 30 grs.
Kosin	10 to 40 grs.
Kyrofine	8 to 15 grs.
Lactopeptine	10 to 20 grs.
Lactucarium	8 to 15 grs.
Liq. ammon. acet.	2 to 4 fl. drs.
acidi arseniosi	2 to 7 min.
arsen. et hydr. iod.	2 to 7 min.
calcii chloridi	30 to 60 min.
ferri chloridi	2 to 10 min.
ferri dialys.	10 to 15 min.
ferri nitrat.	8 to 15 min.
hydrog. perox. (10 vol.)	1/2 to 4 drs.
pepsini	1 to 4 fl. drs.
potassii arsenit.	3 to 7 min.
potassii citrat.	2 to 4 fl. drs.
sodæ	5 to 30 min.
sodii arseniatis	3 to 7 min.
Listerine	1 dr. (diluted).
Lithii benzoas	2 to 5 grs.

A POSOLOGICAL TABLE (Continued).

Drug or Preparation.	Dose.	Drug or Preparation.	Dose.
Lithii bromid. . . .	1 to 3 grs.	Physostigminæ sali-	
carb.	2 to 6 grs.	cyl.	1/120 to 1/24 gr.
citr.	2 to 5 grs.	sulphas	1/125 to 1/24 gr.
salicylas	2 to 8 grs.	Picrotoxinum . .	1/24 to 1/8 gr.
Lobeliinæ hydrobro.	1/25 to 1/10 gr.	Pilocarpina and salts	1/4 to 1/2 gr.
Lupulinum	5 to 10 grs.	Pil. aloes	1 to 3 pills.
Lycetol	4 to 10 grs.	aloes et asafœt..	2 to 5 pills.
Magnesia	15 to 60 grs.	aloes et ferri .	1 to 3 pills.
Magnesii carb. . . .	15 to 60 grs.	aloes et mast..	1 to 3 pills.
citr. gran. . . .	2 to 4 drs.	aloes et myrrhæ .	2 to 5 pills.
sulphas	2 to 8 drs.	antim. comp. .	1 to 3 pills.
sulphis	8 to 30 grs.	asafœtidæ . .	1 to 6 pills.
Maltzyme	1/2 to 1 oz.	cathart. comp. .	1 to 4 pills.
Mangani oxidum		ferri comp. . . .	2 to 5 pills.
nig.	2 to 10 grs.	ferri iodidi .	1 to 4 pills.
sulphas	2 to 10 grs.	opii	1 to 2 pills.
Manna	1 to 2 oz.	phosphori . .	1 to 4 pills.
Massa copaibæ . . .	5 to 30 grs.	rhei	2 to 5 pills.
ferri carb. . . .	5 to 15 grs.	rhei comp. . .	2 to 5 pills.
hydrarg.	1 to 10 grs.	Piperazin . . .	10 to 15 grs.
Menthol	1/2 to 1 1/2 grs.	Piperinum	1 to 8 grs.
Mercauro . . .	5 to 15 min.	Plumbi acetas . .	1/2 to 3 grs.
Methelene blue . .	2 to 5 grs.	iodidum . . .	1/2 to 3 grs.
Methylal	1 to 4 drs.	Potassa sulphurata	1 to 10 grs.
Mist ammoniaci . .	4 to 8 fl. drs.	Potassii acetas .	15 to 60 grs.
asafœtidæ . .	2 to 4 fl. drs.	bicarb. . . .	8 to 60 grs.
chloroformi . . .	2 to 4 fl. drs.	bitartr. . . .	1 to 2 drs.
cretæ . . .	1 to 4 fl. drs.	bromid. . . .	8 to 60 grs.
ferri comp. . .	1/2 to 2 fl. oz.	carb. . . .	8 to 30 grs.
ferri et anim. acet.	1 to 4 fl. drs.	chloras . . .	5 to 30 grs.
glycyrrh. comp. .	1 to 4 fl. drs.	citras . . .	15 to 60 grs.
magnes. et asa-		cyanid. . . .	1/8 to 1/3 gr.
fœt. . . .	1 to 4 fl. drs.	et sodii tartr. .	1/2 to 1 oz.
potassii citr. . .	1/2 to 1 fl. oz.	hypophosphis .	5 to 15 grs.
rhei et sodæ . .	1/2 to 1 fl. oz.	iodid. . . .	5 to 60 grs.
Morrhuol	4 to 12 grs.	nitras . .:..	8 to 15 grs.
·Morphina and its		permangauas . .	1/4 to 1 gr.
salts	1/8 to 1/2 gr.	sulphis . . .	15 to 30 grs.
Naphthalinum . .	2 to 10 grs.	tartras. . .	1 to 8 drs.
Naphthol . . .	5 to 15 grs.	Propylamina. . .	2 to 15 grs.
Narceina	1/6 to 2 grs.	Prostaden . . .	10 to 40 grs.
Nitroglycerinum .	1/100 to 1/8 gr.	Protonuclein . .	3 to 10 grs.
Nux vomica . . .	1 to 5 grs.	Ptyalin . . .	10 to 30 grs.
Oleoresina aspidii	20 to 40 min.	Pulv. antimonialis	3 to 10 grs.
capsici	1/6 to 1/2 gr.	aromat. . . .	5 to 30 grs.
cubebæ	5 to 30 grs.	cretæ comp. .	8 to 30 grs.
piperis	1 to 3 grs.	glycyrrh. comp.	30 to 60 grs.
zingiberis . . .	1 to 3 grs.	ipecac. et opii	5 to 15 grs.
Oleum copaibæ . .	8 to 15 min.	jalapæ comp . .	30 to 60 grs.
cubebæ . . .	15 to 30 min.	morphinæ comp.	8 to 15 grs.
erigerontis . .	5 to 15 min.	rhei comp. . .	30 to 60 grs.
eucalypti . . .	10 to 30 min.	Pyridin . . .	2 to 5 drops.
gaultheriæ . .	2 to 10 min.	Quinalgen . . .	5 to 15 grs.
phosphoratum . .	1 to 3 min.	Quinidina and salts	1 to 30 grs.
sabinæ . . .	1 to 3 min.	Quinina and salts	1 to 30 grs.
terebinthinæ .	5 to 60 min.	Quininæ arsenias.	1/8 to 1 gr.
tiglii	1 to 4 drops.	Resina copaibæ .	2 to 10 grs.
Opium (14 per cent.		guaiaci . . .	10 to 30 grs.
morphine) . . .	1/4 to 1 1/2 grs.	jalapæ . . .	2 to 5 grs.
Orthoform	8 to 15 grs.	podophylli . .	1/4 to 1/2 gr.
Ovariin	8 to 24 grs.	scammonii . .	2 to 10 grs.
Pancreatin . . .	5 to 15 grs.	Resorcin . . .	5 to 30 grs.
Papayotin . . .	1 to 5 grs.	Rheum	2 to 30 grs.
Paracotoin . . .	1 1/2 to 3 grs.	Saccharin . . .	1/4 to 2 grs.
Paraldehyde . . .	30 to 90 min.	Salicinum . . .	8 to 30 grs.
	(diluted).	Salol	5 to 30 grs.
Pareirin hydrochlor.	1/12 to 1 gr.	Salophen . . .	15 to 20 grs.
Pelletierine sulphas	3 to 6 grs.	Santonica . . .	8 to 60 grs.
tannas . . .	12 to 24 grs.	Santoninum . . .	1 to 5 grs.
Pepsin	5 to 15 grs.	Scammonium . .	3 to 15 grs.
Pepsinum purum. .	15 grains.	Scoparine . . .	1/2 to 1 gr.
saccharatum . .	30 gmins.	Seng	1 fl. dr.
Peptenzyme . . .	3 to 10 grs.	Senna	8 to 60 grs.
Pepto-mangan		Sodii acetas . .	15 to 60 grs.
(Gude)	1 to 4 drs.	arsenias . .	1/30 to 1/10 gr.
Phenacetin . . .	.7 to 11 grs.	benzoas . . .	5 to 15 grs.
Phenalgin . . .	5 to 15 grs.	bicarb. . . .	8 to 30 grs.
Phosphorus . . .	1/25 to 1/10 gr.	bisulphis . . .	8 to 30 grs.

Drug or Preparation.	Dose.	Drug or Preparation.	Dose.
Sodii boras	8 to 30 grs.	Tinct. cocæ (1–5) . .	2 to 30 min.
bromid	8 to 30 grs.	colchici rad. . .	5 to 20 min.
carb.	8 to 30 grs.	colchici sem. . .	15 to 60 min.
hypophosphis . .	8 to 15 grs.	conii	5 to 30 min.
hyposulphis . . .	8 to 30 grs.	cubebæ	1 to 2 fl. drs.
iodidim	5 to 15 grs.	digitalis . . .	5 to 15 min.
phosphas . . .	2 to 15 grs.	ferri acet. . . .	15 to 30 min.
salicylas	5 to 30 grs.	ferri chloridi . . .	15 to 60 min.
santoninas . . .	2 to 10 grs.	ferri chloridi	
sulphas	1 to 2 drs.	æther. . .	15 to 30 min.
sulphis	8 to 30 grs.	gallæ . . .	$\frac{1}{2}$ to 2 fl. dre.
Spartein, sulphas . .	$\frac{1}{10}$ to 1$\frac{1}{2}$ grs.	gelsemii . . .	5 to 10 min.
Spermine, essence	10 to 30 min.	guaiaci	30 to 60 min.
Spir. æther . . .	30 to 60 min.	guaiaci ammon. .	30 to 60 min.
æther, nitrosi .	$\frac{1}{2}$ to 2 fl. drs.	hellebori . . .	10 to 15 min.
ammoniæ . . .	8 to 30 min.	humuli . .	1 to 4 fl. drs.
ammoniæ arom .	15 to 60 min.	hydrastis . .	30 to 90 min.
camphoræ . . .	8 to 30 min.	hyoscyami fol. . .	15 to 60 min.
chloroformi . .	15 to 60 min.	hyoscyami sem. .	15 to 30 min.
lavand. comp. .	30 to 60 min.	ignatiæ . . .	5 to 15 min.
menth. pip. . .	30 to 60 min.	iodi	5 to 15 min.
Strophanthin		ipecac. et opii . .	5 to 15 min.
(Merck's)	$\frac{1}{320}$ to $\frac{1}{160}$ gr.	jalapæ	$\frac{1}{2}$ to 2 fl. drs.
Strychnina (and salts)	$\frac{1}{24}$ to $\frac{1}{12}$ gr.	kino	$\frac{1}{2}$ to 2 fl. drs.
Sulphonal	15 to 30 grs.	krameriæ . . .	$\frac{1}{2}$ to 2 fl. drs.
Sulphur	$\frac{1}{2}$ to 4 drs.	lavand. comp. .	$\frac{1}{2}$ to 2 fl. drs.
Syrup acidi hydriodici	1 to 4 fl. drs	lobeliæ . . .	15 to 45 min.
allii	1 to 4 fl. drs.	lupulini . . .	$\frac{1}{2}$ to 2 fl. drs.
calcii lactophos. .	1 to 2 fl. drs.	matico . . .	$\frac{1}{2}$ to 2 fl. drs.
calcis . . .	15 to 30 min.	nucis vomicæ . .	5 to 30 min.
ferri bromidi . .	15 to 60 min.	opii	5 to 25 min.
ferri iodidi . .	15 to 60 min.	opii camph. . .	1 to 4 fl. drs.
ferri oxidi . .	1 fl. dr.	physostigmatis .	5 to 15 min.
ferri hypophosph.	1 fl. dr.	quassiæ . . .	$\frac{1}{2}$ to 2 fl. drs.
fer. quin. et stryc. phos. .	1 fl. dr.	rhei	1 to 8 fl. drs.
hypophosphit. .	1 fl. dr.	rhei arom. . . .	30 to 75 min.
ipecac. . . .	$\frac{1}{2}$ to 4 fl. drs.	rhei dulc. . . .	1 to 4 fl. drs.
krameriæ . . .	$\frac{1}{2}$ to 4 fl. drs.	sanguinariæ . .	15 to 60 min.
lactucarii . . .	1 to 3 fl. drs.	scillæ . . .	8 to 60 min.
rhei	1 to 4 fl. drs.	serpentariæ . .	$\frac{1}{2}$ to 2 fl. drs.
rhei arom. . . .	1 to 4 fl. drs.	stramon. fol. . .	8 to 15 min.
rosæ	1 to 2 fl. drs.	stramon. sem. .	6 to 15 min.
rubi	1 to 2 fl. drs.	strophanthi (1–20) .	5 to 10 min.
sarsap. comp. .	1 to 4 fl. drs.	sumbul . . .	8 to 30 min.
scillæ . . .	$\frac{1}{2}$ to 1 fl dr.	valerianæ . . .	$\frac{1}{2}$ to 2 fl. drs.
scillæ comp. .	15 to 60 min.	valer. ammon. .	$\frac{1}{2}$ to 2 fl. drs.
senegæ . . .	1 to 2 fl. drs.	veratri viridis .	1 to 10 min.
sennæ . . .	1 to 4 fl. drs.	zingiberis . . .	15 to 60 min.
Taka-diastase . .	1 to 5 grs.	Tongaline . . .	1 to 2 fl. drs.
Terebene . . .	5 to 15 drops.	Trimethylamina .	2 to 15 grs.
Terpene hydrate .	3 to 20 grs.	Tritur. elaterii .	$\frac{1}{4}$ to $\frac{1}{2}$ gr.
Testadin . . .	30 grains.	Urea	50 to 100 grs.
Thallin. sulph. . .	1 to 5 grs.	Urethano . . .	15 to 60 grs.
Thymol . . .	$\frac{1}{2}$ to 5 grs.	Urotropin . . .	15 to 30 grs.
Thyradin . . .	5 to 10 grs.	Veratrina . . .	$\frac{1}{60}$ to $\frac{1}{5}$ gr.
Tinct. aconiti fol. . .	5 to 16 min.	Vinum aloes . . .	1 to 2 fl. drs.
aconiti rad. . .	1 to 5 min.	antim. { expect. & alt. . .	1 to 8 min.
aconiti rad., Fleming's	$\frac{3}{4}$ to 2$\frac{1}{2}$ min.	{ emet. . .	30 to 75 min.
aloes (1880) . .	$\frac{1}{2}$ to 2 fl. drs.	cocæ . . .	2 to 4 drs.
aloes et myrrhæ .	1 to 2 fl. drs.	colch. rad. . .	8 to 45 min.
arnicæ flor. . .	8 to 30 min.	colch. sem. . .	5 to 30 min.
arnicæ rad. . .	15 to 30 min.	ergotæ . . .	1 to 4 fl. drs.
asafœtidæ . . .	30 to 60 min.	ferri amarum .	1 fl. dr.
belladonnæ . .	5 to 15 min.	ferri citrat. . .	1 fl. dr.
bryoniæ . . .	15 to 30 min.	ipecac. { expector. .	5 to 15 min.
calendulæ . .	15 to 30 min.	{ emetic .	2 to 4 fl. drs.
calumbæ . .	1 to 4 fl. drs.	opii . . .	5 to 10 min.
cannabis ind. .	15 to 30 min.	rhei . . .	1 to 2 fl. drs.
cantharidis . .	5 to 15 min.	Xylolum . . .	5 to 15 grs.
capsici. . .	8 to 15 min.	Zinci acet. . .	1 to 2 grs.
catechu comp. .	$\frac{1}{2}$ to 2 fl. drs.	bromid. . . .	$\frac{1}{2}$ to 2 grs.
cimicifugæ . . .	30 to 60 min.	cyanid . . .	$\frac{1}{8}$ to $\frac{1}{4}$ gr.
cinchonæ . . .	$\frac{1}{2}$ to 2 fl. drs.	iodid . . .	$\frac{1}{2}$ to 3 grs.
cinchonæ comp.	$\frac{1}{2}$ to 2 fl. drs.	oxid. . . .	1 to 10 grs.
		phosphid. . .	$\frac{1}{16}$ to $\frac{1}{4}$ gr.
		sulphas, emetic .	15 to 30 grs.
		valerianas . . .	1 to 6 grs.

VIII.

A List of Incompatibles.

Those substances are incompatible—

I. Between which chemical reaction may occur, destroying the properties of both. The reaction may or may not occasion the formation of a precipitate.

II. Which introduce a solution of a substance in a certain menstruum into a large quantity of another menstruum in which the substance is insoluble.

III. Besides such mixtures, those must be avoided in which oxidizing agents, or iodine, or bromine, would come in contact with combustible substances.

Acids must not be compounded with alkalies nor alkaline carbonates.

Liquids containing mucilaginous matters are precipitated by salts of iron, lead, and other heavy metals ; also by alcohol, ether, and mineral acids.

Tinctures and fluid extracts containing resins are precipitated by water.

Liquids containing tannin or bitter substances are precipitated by salts of iron and other heavy metals. ☞ Chiretta does not contain tannin.

Salts of the alkaloids are usually precipitated by ammonia and other alkalies, the alkaloid being thrown down ; they are also precipitated by tannic acid, and many of them by iodine and iodides.

Chromic acid, potassium chromate, potassium permanganate, must not be compounded with organic or combustible matters, such as sugar, glycerin, starch, alcohol, sulphur, sulphides, phosphorus. Neither potassium chlorate nor potassium nitrate must be triturated with any of the preceding substances, and iodine and bromine must not come in contact with oil of turpentine, nor phosphorus, nor sulphur.

The medicinal metallic salts, excepting those of potassium, sodium, lithium, magnesium, and calcium, are precipitated by ammonia and alkalies, and, not excepting the last two, by alkaline carbonates.

Chlorides are decomposed by salts of lead and silver.

Iodides and bromides are decomposed by nitric and by nitromuriatic acid ; also by soluble salts of silver, lead, and mercury (☞ the precipitated mercuric iodide, formed by the action of corrosive sublimate on potassium iodide, dissolves in excess of the latter); also by strong sulphuric acid, by potassium permanganate, and by other energetic oxidizing agents.

Sulphides are decomposed by salts of heavy metals generally.

Sulphates are decomposed by lead solutions.

Carbonates are decomposed by acids and acid salts.

Phosphates are precipitated when phosphoric acid is introduced into alkaline solutions containing magnesium or calcium.

Hydrogen peroxide is decomposed by most substances; it may be mixed with ether or glycerin.

Chloral hydrate is decomposed by alkalies.

Arsenious acid and arsenites are incompatible with magnesia, lime water, tannin, and ferric hydroxide.

Antimonial preparations are incompatible with acids, especially tannic acid, and alkalies.

Cocaine solutions are precipitated by borax.

Antipyrine is incompatible with calomel and with sweet spirit of nitre.

IX

Tables of Approximate Relative Weights and Measures in the Metric and Apothecaries' Systems.

Approximate Equivalents of Milligrammes in Grains.

Milligramme.	Grain.	Milligrammes.	Grain.	Milligrammes.	Grain.
0.1	= $\frac{1}{600}$	1	= $\frac{1}{60}$	8	= $\frac{1}{8}$
0.2	= $\frac{1}{300}$	1.2	= $\frac{1}{50}$	9	= $\frac{1}{7}$
0.3	= $\frac{1}{200}$	1.6	= $\frac{1}{40}$	10	= $\frac{1}{6}$
0.4	= $\frac{1}{150}$	2	= $\frac{1}{30}$	12	= $\frac{1}{5}$
0.5	= $\frac{1}{120}$	3	= $\frac{1}{20}$	16	= $\frac{1}{4}$
0.6	= $\frac{1}{100}$	4	= $\frac{1}{15}$	20	= $\frac{1}{3}$
0.7	= $\frac{1}{90}$	5	= $\frac{1}{12}$	30	= $\frac{1}{2}$
0.8	= $\frac{1}{80}$	6	= $\frac{1}{10}$	60	= 1
0.9	= $\frac{1}{70}$	7	= $\frac{1}{8}$		

Approximate Equivalents of Centigrammes in Grains.

Centigrammes.	Grain.	Centigrammes.	Grains.	Centigrammes.	Grains.
1	= $\frac{1}{6}$	6	= 1	18	= 3
2	= $\frac{1}{3}$	7	= $1\frac{1}{6}$	25	= 4
3	= $\frac{1}{2}$	9	= $1\frac{1}{2}$	50	= 8
4	= $\frac{2}{3}$	10	= $1\frac{2}{3}$	75	= 12
5	= $\frac{4}{5}$	12	= 2	100	= 16

Approximate Equivalents of Grammes in Grains.

Grammes.	Grains.	Grammes.	Grains.	Grammes.	Grains.
0.001	= $\frac{1}{60}$	11	= 176	27	= 432
0.010	= $\frac{1}{6}$	12	= 192	28	= 448
0.100	= $1\frac{2}{3}$	13	= 208	29	= 464
0.250	= 4	14	= 224	30	= 480
0 500	= 8	15	= 240	31	= 496
0.750	= 12	16	= 256	32	= 512
1	= 16	17	= 272	33	= 528
1.50	= 24	18	= 288	34	= 544
2	= 32	19	= 304	35	= 560
3	= 48	20	= 320	36	= 576
4	= 64	21	= 336	37	= 592
5	= 80	22	= 352	38	= 608
6	= 96	23	= 368	39	= 624
7	= 112	24	= 384	40	= 640
8	= 128	25	= 400	50	= 800
9	= 144	26	= 416	100	= 1600
10	= 160				

Approximate Equivalents of Cubic Centimetres in U. S. Apothecaries' Fluidrachms.

Cubic Centimetres.	U. S. Fluid-drachms.	Cubic Centimetres.	U. S. Fluid-drachms.	Cubic Centimetres.	U. S. Fluid-drachms.
1	= $\frac{1}{4}$	9	= $2\frac{1}{4}$	16	= 4
2	= $\frac{1}{2}$	10	= $2\frac{1}{2}$	20	= 5
3	= $\frac{3}{4}$	11	= $2\frac{3}{4}$	24	= 6
4	= 1	12	= 3	28	= 7
5	= $1\frac{1}{4}$	13	= $3\frac{1}{4}$	32	= 8
6	= $1\frac{1}{2}$	14	= $3\frac{1}{2}$	48	= 12
7	= $1\frac{3}{4}$	15	= $3\frac{3}{4}$	64	= 16
8	= 2				

X.

External Antipyretics.

a. COLD SPONGING.—The water may be of the temperature of the room or cooled with ice. A little alcohol or vinegar may be added to it, or Labarraque's solution. A sponge or wash-cloth may be used, and more or less moderate friction, according to the sensations of the patient. In all use of water great care must be taken to protect the bed.

Every part of the body is in turn bared, washed, dried, and again covered. The spongings may be repeated at intervals of two or three hours. They not only add greatly to the comfort of the patient, but also exert a favorable influence upon the nervous system and circulation of the blood, by causing it to flow more freely in the vessels directly under the skin. They lower the temperature only slightly, unless the water be very cold and the spongings frequently repeated.

b. COLD COMPRESSES.—For this purpose three or four thicknesses of old table linen or towelling, which is porous enough to hold a good deal of water, is most useful. The compress is wrung out of water of the required temperature and reapplied as it becomes warm. Or two compresses may be used alternately, each being cooled in turn by placing it on a block of ice in a basin or pan at the bedside. Cold compresses are often used for the head, and are commonly very acceptable to patients. They are without appreciable effect upon the general temperature. Very large cold compresses extending over the entire thorax and abdomen and frequently renewed exert a decided effect upon the internal fever. The compresses are sometimes allowed to remain continuously in position, a small quantity of cold water being from time to time added to replace that lost by evaporation.

Leiter's coils, which may be fitted to the head or applied over the heart or to other regions of the body in such a manner as to reduce local temperature by means of cold water flowing through them from a reservoir over the bed, exert an influence analogous to but not exactly the same as that exerted by the cold compress.

c. THE APPLICATION OF ICE.—Ice is commonly applied by means of a bladder or gum ice-bag. It must be cracked into pieces the size of a walnut and introduced into the bag with a little water, the bag being about half or two-thirds full. The air is then squeezed out and the stopper adjusted. If the bag be filled, or air enough left in it to distend it, it will not conform itself to the part to which it is applied. A much more effectual method of applying ice to the abdomen or over the heart is by spreading out a thick layer of finely-cracked ice between the folds of a coarse towel, which is then placed directly over the skin. This method requires constant watching, and is almost sure to wet the bedding. It is not available for prolonged use.

d. THE COLD PACK.—A blanket is spread evenly over a couch or bed; over this blanket is laid a coarse sheet wrung lightly out of water of the prescribed temperature and folded once. The patient is lifted upon the bed thus prepared and quickly wrapped in the wet sheet by the attendant in such a manner that it lies as smoothly as possible over every part of the body except the head. If the extremities feel cold before the packing, they must be warmed by friction, or else not included in the packing.

As soon as the damp linen is everywhere in contact with the body, the attendant folds the blanket over the patient in the same way, first drawing over and tucking one side smoothly under, and then the other, seeing that the chin is free and that the blanket is folded evenly, but without tension at the neck. Finally, the long end is drawn down and folded smoothly under the feet.

Three or even four thicknesses of wet sheets spread upon the blanket are necessary to reduce the temperature effectively.

The reduction of temperature from a single pack is usually transient, and repeated packings, even to the number of five or six, are often administered, the rise of temperature being slower after each. When the temperature does not rise above normal, or when shivering takes place, the packing must not again be renewed. When repeated packings are necessary, two couches are used side by side, and the patient is lifted directly from one pack on to the other. The same effect is produced, but less completely, by unfolding the blanket and sprinkling the sheet afresh with cold water.

The patient is allowed to remain in the last pack from three-quarters of an hour to an hour and a half: at the expiration of this time the skin generally becomes pleasantly warm, and in many cases outbreaks of perspiration take place.

During the packing the pulse is felt at the carotid or temporal artery and the temperature taken in the mouth.

e. THE COLD OR GRADUALLY-COOLED BATH.—The quantity of water used should be sufficient to wholly immerse the body of the patient. The tub must stand at the bedside. During the bath the skin should be gently rubbed. The temperature of the water should be about 90° F., or even higher than this, at the first bath. As the patient becomes accustomed to the bath it is gradually cooled by the addition of cold water to 80° F., or lower. Under no circumstances should it be cooled below 65° F. The average duration of the bath is fifteen minutes. But if shivering or great uneasiness occur, the patient is at once lifted into bed, placed upon a sheet previously made ready, and wiped dry, with brisk rubbing of the extremities and back. The moist sheet is then removed. The patient is covered up, and some hot soup or wine, or brandy and water, administered. The temperature is not always immediately reduced, but—as measured in the rectum—usually falls within an hour from one and a half to four or five degrees. In the course of some hours it rises again, and the bath is then repeated. If cold baths are not not well borne, good results in lowering the temperature often follow prolonged luke-warm baths. Sometimes it becomes necessary to repeat the bath four or five times in the course of twenty-four hours. A patient who is quietly sleeping, even if his temperature be high, should not be roused and immediately placed in the bath.

When young children are treated by this method, the temperature of the bath at the beginning should be warm, and a blanket spread over the tub, in which the little patient is gradually lowered into the water.

Not only is the temperature lowered by this means, but also a very favorable influence is exerted upon the state of the nervous system. The intellect clears up, the dulness diminishes.

f. COLD AFFUSION.—While the patient is in the tub, cold water —60° F.—is thrown by means of a sponge over his head, face, neck, shoulders, and chest. This is repeated once or twice just before he is removed from the tub. It is done rather for the sake of its good effects upon the nervous system in cases of great stupor and other evidences of serious nervous derangement than merely as a means of reducing high temperature. Cold affusions may be practised in bed, the mattress being suitably protected by water-proof sheets.

g. ICED-WATER ENEMAS.—Large rectal injections of iced water are sometimes followed by a fall of temperature. They are, when carefully administered, rather grateful than otherwise to patients. They are best given by means of the fountain syringe, the water being introduced into the bowel slowly, and the flow stopped for a few minutes by pressure upon the tube without withdrawing the nozzle, whenever a sense of pain or of desire to evacuate the bowel is experienced. In this way a large quantity of fluid may be injected. It is not often necessary to exceed three pints. This method of applying cold constitutes a useful addition to those in ordinary use, and may be advantageously employed in connection with them under suitable circumstances.

The patient's head and face must always be well bathed with cold water just before and during applications of cold to the general surface of the body. The occurrence of chill or rigor may be delayed by more or less vigorous rubbing or chafing of the body.

XI

Disinfectants.

The following list includes the disinfectants available for general purposes:

Dry and Moist Heat.
Formaldehyde Fumes.
Fumes of Sulphur (Sulphur Dioxide).
Chloride of Lime (Calcium Hypochlorite).
Labarraque's Solution (Solution of Chlorinated Soda).
Corrosive Sublimate (Mercuric Chloride).
Sulphate of Copper (Cupric Sulphate).
Carbolic Acid.

DISINFECTION OF THE SICK-ROOM.—In the sick-room no disinfection can take the place of thorough ventilation and cleanliness. Complete disinfection of a room while it is occupied is impracticable. Much, however, can be done by washing the floor, window-ledges, and other surfaces with a solution of corrosive sublimate of the strength of one part in one thousand (1 : 1000), or a solution of carbolic acid, two parts in one hundred (2 : 100), or of chloride of lime, one part in one hundred (1 : 100), or formaldehyde (2 : 100). Among the manufactured articles sold in the shops for this purpose Platt's Chlorides is unequalled. It is to be diluted in the proportion of from one part in four to one part in ten of water. Compressed tablets of corrosive sublimate are sold by the chemists for the purpose of making the disinfectant solution. Each tablet contains seven and three-tenths grains, and the solution formed by dissolving one tablet in a pint of water is of about the strength of one part to one thousand (1 : 1000).*

Care must be taken to keep chemical disinfectants in large bottles or demijohns suitably and conspicuously labelled and marked POISON, and in a place entirely apart and away from all medicines, food, and beverages.

DISINFECTION OF APARTMENTS.—At the close of an infectious disease the rooms may be effectually disinfected. For this purpose the more reliable gaseous disinfectants are formaldehyde, the fumes of sulphur (sulphur dioxide), and chlorine. Formaldehyde is the best. It is evaporated in the closed room over a lamp made for this purpose. From a practical point of view sulphur is the best, and is commonly used, being cheap and easy to procure. The fireplace, windows, and doors are closed, the cracks packed with paper, or covered with paper pasted on. Roll sulphur, broken fine, or the flowers of sulphur (sulphur sublimatum) may be used. A little sawdust mixed with the latter causes it to burn more freely. It may be placed in a shallow iron vessel or earthenware dish, which, to avoid the danger of fire, should be placed in the bottom of a high tin wash-boiler, or on tongs laid across a tub of water. It is ignited by a live coal or by first pouring over it a little alcohol. Three pounds of sulphur is the quantity to be used for every thousand cubic feet. A room fifteen feet long by twelve broad, with a ceiling ten feet high, contains eighteen hundred cubic feet ($15 \times 12 \times 10 = 1800$). As the fumes cannot be breathed even in a diluted form, the doors must be immediately and tightly closed. The day following the windows are widely opened and are allowed to remain so for twenty-four hours. Whitewashed walls are to be scraped and rewashed in addition to the disinfection.

DISINFECTION OF CLOTHING.—Boiling for half an hour will destroy the vitality of all known disease-germs, and there is no better way of disinfecting clothing that can be washed than to subject it to the ordinary operations of the laundry. Clothing may be disinfected by immersion for two hours in a solution of corrosive sublimate of the strength of 1 : 1000, or of formaldehyde, 1 : 100, or of carbolic acid, 1 : 50, or of chloride of lime, 1 : 100. The bleaching properties of chloride of lime must not be forgotten. The clothing of the sick-room should not be allowed

---

* As suggested by Dr. C. M. Wilson.

to accumulate, but should go to the laundry as promptly as can be arranged. As an additional measure, and to lessen the risks of the laundry-women, it should be at once freely sprinkled with one of the above solutions. Articles of clothing that would be injured by boiling or by immersion in a disinfectant solution may be disinfected by exposure to dry heat in a properly-constructed "oven," such as are arranged in the hospitals of our large cities, and which may be used by the public. The separate articles must be freely spread out, as the penetrating power of dry heat is feeble. A temperature of 230° to 284° F. and an exposure of three hours are necessary. This heat is injurious to woollen fabrics. Finally, we must not forget the purifying effects of fire. Articles not readily disinfected by ordinary measures can be destroyed by burning.

DISINFECTION OF THE PERSON.—The hands of those who nurse persons sick of infectious diseases should be occasionally washed in a solution of corrosive sublimate, 1 : 2000, or of carbolic acid, 1 : 50, or of Labarraque's solution, 1 : 10. This should invariably be done before taking food. If a solution of corrosive sublimate be employed, the hands must be afterwards rinsed with fresh water as a safeguard against mercurial poisoning, of which an early sign is soreness of the mouth and gums.

The above solutions are to be used for washing instruments and utensils that are exposed in the sick-room, except such as are used for eating and drinking purposes.

For bathing the patient's body weaker solutions must be employed,—corrosive sublimate, 1 : 5000; carbolic acid, 1 : 250; Labarraque's solution, 1 : 30. The dead should be wrapped in a sheet wet with strong disinfectant solutions,—corrosive sublimate, 1 : 500; carbolic acid, 1 : 20; or chloride of lime, 1 : 25.

DISINFECTION OF THE DISCHARGES, ETC.—Dissolve chloride of lime in water in the proportion of four ounces to the gallon; use one quart of this solution for the disinfection of each liquid stool in typhoid fever or cholera. If the discharge be very copious, it will be advisable to use even a larger amount. For the disinfection of solid fecal matter the above solution should be of double the strength. The matter to be disinfected must be exposed to the action of the solution for four hours, and solid masses are to be broken up by agitation of the vessel. Solutions of carbolic acid, 1 : 20, or of formaldehyde, 1 : 25, may also be used for this purpose. But the best of all is a solution of corrosive sublimate of the strength of 1 : 500. This fluid should, on account of its highly poisonous properties, be colored red by the addition of potassium permanganate.

DISINFECTION OF WATER-CLOSETS, PRIVY-VAULTS, ETC.—No stool from a case of typhoid fever should be thrown into a closet without having been previously disinfected as above. Great care must be taken to prevent the contact of the discharges with the wood-work of the seat. The closet is to be thoroughly flushed several times a day, and in the intervals of its use a quantity of carbolic acid or chloride of lime solution should be allowed to remain in the hopper.

A privy-vault requiring disinfection may be treated with two or three pounds of corrosive sublimate dissolved in a large quantity of water and slowly poured into the vault. During an epidemic chloride of lime should be freely sprinkled over the surface of the contents of the vault every day.

XII

Medical Thermometry.

The art of taking and recording the temperature of the body is called Medical Thermometry. The instruments used are known as Clinical Thermometers. They are marked off into degrees upon the glass, and each degree is subdivided into fifths, so that the readings may conveniently be recorded in fractions of the decimal system.

The thermometers commonly used in the United States and Great Britain are marked in degrees of *Fahrenheit's* scale: those used in Europe are graduated according to the *Centigrade* scale. The scale of *Réaumur* is rapidly going out of use, but is still employed in some parts of Europe. On the scale of Fahrenheit the distance through which the mercury rises from zero to the boiling-point of water is divided into two hundred and twelve degrees, of which the thirty-second marks the melting-point of ice. Between the melting-point of ice and the boiling-point of water there are one hundred and eighty degrees ($32^\circ + 180^\circ = 212^\circ$ F.). The melting-point of ice is taken as zero in the Centigrade scale and in that of Réaumur, but in the Centigrade the boiling-point of water is at one hundred (100° C.), while in Réaumur's it is at eighty (80° R.).

The relation of the three scales to one another is, therefore,

F.	C.	R.
9	5	4

To convert recordings of the Fahrenheit scale into Centigrade degrees:

Subtract 32, multiply by 5, and divide by 9: thus, $98.6 - 32 = 66.6 \times 5 = 333.0 \div 9 = 37$. That is, 98.6° F. $= 37^\circ$ C.

To convert Centigrade degrees into Fahrenheit degrees:

Multiply by 9, divide by 5, and add 32: thus, $37 \times 9 = 333 \div 5 = 66.6 + 32 = 98.6$. That is, 37° C. $= 98.6^\circ$ F.

The Centigrade scale is better than that of Fahrenheit, and many physicians in this country prefer to use it. The following table of equivalents may therefore prove of use:

F.	C.	F.	C.	F.	C.
$96.0^\circ = 35.55^\circ$		$101.3^\circ = 38.5^\circ$		$106.7^\circ = 41.5^\circ$	
$96.8^\circ = 36.00^\circ$		$102.0^\circ = 38.88^\circ$		$107.0^\circ = 41.66^\circ$	
$97.0^\circ = 36.11^\circ$		$102.2^\circ = 39.00^\circ$		$107.6^\circ = 42.00^\circ$	
$98.0^\circ = 36.66^\circ$		$103.0^\circ = 39.44^\circ$		$108.0^\circ = 42.22^\circ$	
$98.6^\circ = 37.00^\circ$		$103.1^\circ = 39.5^\circ$		$108.5^\circ = 42.5^\circ$	
$99.0^\circ = 37.22^\circ$		$104.0^\circ = 40.00^\circ$		$109.0^\circ = 42.77^\circ$	
$99.5^\circ = 37.5^\circ$		$104.9^\circ = 40.5^\circ$		$109.4^\circ = 43.00^\circ$	
$100.0^\circ = 37.77^\circ$		$105.0^\circ = 40.55^\circ$		$110.0^\circ = 43.33^\circ$	
$100.4^\circ = 38.00^\circ$		$105.8^\circ = 41.00^\circ$		$111.2^\circ = 44.00^\circ$	
$101.0^\circ = 38.33^\circ$		$106.0^\circ = 41.11^\circ$			

As thermometers are liable after a time to give readings that are slightly too high, in consequence of the gradual contraction of the glass of which they are formed, it is necessary at intervals to compare them carefully with a standard instrument. This is done at the public observatories, to which any instrument-maker will send them.

This contraction of the glass is called "seasoning," and goes on slowly. After two or three years it practically comes to an end, and the thermometer is then seasoned.

Clinical thermometers are maximum, or self-registering; that is, a small portion of the mercury is separated from the main bulk of it, or separates itself from it as it contracts, by reason of a device in the twist of the tube, in such a way that it remains in position in the tube, when the temperature falls, until shaken down, and thus indicates the highest temperature reached during the observation. The separated portion of the mercury is known as the "index." The reading is taken from the upper end of the index, which is then shaken down by a quick motion of the wrist, such as is made in cracking a whip, the thermometer being held by its upper end. Before taking the temperature the index should be below 95°. The best clinical thermometers are now made with a curved surface, which, acting as a lens, magnifies the width of the mercury; and with a flattened back, which lessens the danger of breakage from rolling.

Surface thermometers are clinical thermometers of a special shape, designed for measuring surface temperatures.

The object being to measure the internal temperature, the thermometer must be placed in such a position that the tissues of the body completely surround its bulb. The positions available are the armpit, or axilla, the mouth, the vagina, and the rectum. The fold of the groin, when the thigh is bent up or flexed over the abdomen, is in infants also occasionally used.

The axilla is usually selected. If very moist, it should be dried with a towel before the instrument is introduced; or if dry and harsh, it must be bathed with warm water and then dried. There is no difference in the temperature of the two armpits under ordinary circumstances. The bulb of the instrument must be placed deeply in the hollow, and the arm brought well across the chest. Care must be taken that no fold of clothing interfere with the contact of the instrument with the skin. The mercury rises rapidly at first, then more slowly. Allow five minutes for the taking of the temperature in the axilla or mouth. In the rectum or vagina less time is required,—not more than three or three and a half minutes. Time may be saved by rolling the bulb of the thermometer briskly between the palms of the hands, or with a piece of cloth or flannel, until the mercury reaches 95° or 96°.

In taking the temperature in the mouth, the bulb must be placed under the tongue and the lips closed about the stem, the patient breathing through his nose. Dip the instrument in water and wipe it with a clean napkin in the presence of the patient both before and after using it in the mouth. It is not safe to take the temperature in the mouth either in young children or in conditions of delirium. When the patient is in an insensible state, or when doubts arise as to the correctness of an axillary observation, the rectum or vagina may be used for applying the thermometer, and with self-registering instruments this plan involves no exposure of the person.

In restless children care must be taken to prevent the instruments from being broken, and in all cases to prevent a small thermometer from slipping entirely into the bowel. The temperature may be rapidly taken in unmanageable children by means of an old-fashioned thermometer which is not self-registering, by cautiously warming it until the mercury reaches a very high point, say 108°, and then quickly placing it in the armpit. The mercury falls rapidly to the temperature of the patient's body and then stops. After remaining stationary for half a minute, it may be read off.

The human body in health, like that of all warm-blooded animals, has a temperature of its own, which is nearly constant at all periods of life, in all seasons, and in every climate. This is known as the Normal Temperature, and as measured in the axilla is about 98.6° F. (37° C.) In the mouth it is about the same, but in the vagina and rectum it is fully half a degree F. higher. The surface temperature, being influenced by external causes, is lower, and varies in different parts of the body, the exposed and distant parts being coolest. The temperature of infants and children is a fraction of a degree higher and much more easily disturbed than that of adults, and after middle life the average temperature is somewhat lower than before that period. A diurnal variation independent of food or exercise, and amounting to one or one and a half degrees F., is observed in health,—the minimum being reached between 2 A.M. and 6 A.M., and the maximum being attained, after a gradual rise, between 5 P.M. and 8 P.M. This daily rhythmical fluctuation of temperature takes place not only in health, but also when in disease the whole range of the temperature is either abnormally depressed or elevated.

The temperature is usually elevated a fraction of a degree after taking food. Alcoholic drinks have a tendency to lower it. Very active exercise causes it to rise a degree or more, but when muscular exercise is carried to exhaustion a fall below the normal may be noted.

It is desirable to take the temperature at least twice daily, the best times being between seven and eight in the morning and about eight in the evening. The observations must be repeated at the same hours each day. In cases characterized by great or sudden variations of temperature or by very high temperature, or when the influence of treatment upon the fever is being closely watched, observations must be made at shorter intervals of time, and it may become necessary to take the temperature as often as every hour.

The temperature in disease may range below or above the normal. Sudden falls of temperature in fever are very significant; just as are abrupt rises from the temperature of health. The following terms are used to indicate the general condition of the patient in abnormal ranges of temperature:

Below the Normal		
	a. Temperature of Collapse	Below 96·5° F.
	b. Subnormal Temperature	96.5° – 98° F.

	c. Normal Temperature . . . . 98° – 99.5° F.

<table>
<tr><td rowspan="8">Above the Normal.</td><td>d. Subfebrile Temperature . . . . 99.5°–100.5° F.</td></tr>
</table>

| | c. Normal Temperature . . . . 98° – 99.5° F. |

Above the Normal.
{
d. Subfebrile Temperature . . . . 99.5°–100.5° F.
e. Moderate Febrile Temperature ⎰ 100.5°–102° F., A.M.
   (Mild Pyrexia) ⎱ 102.2°–103° F., P.M.
f. High Febrile Temperature ⎰ 102° – 104° F., A.M.
   (Severe Pyrexia) ⎱ 104° – 105.8° F., P.M.
g. Intense Febrile Temperature
   (Hyperpyrexia) . . . . 105.8° – 110° F.
}

The range of deviation from the normal within the limits of which life can be well maintained is comprised between 92° F. and 110° F. A temperature of 95° on the one hand, or of 106° F. on the other, indicates great danger, especially if it be prolonged, and beyond these limits in both directions the danger to life speedily becomes extreme.

a. TEMPERATURE OF COLLAPSE, OR SHOCK.—A considerable and rapid fall of temperature attends the collapse which sometimes occurs during or towards the close of some of the essential fevers. In typhoid fever this condition may be produced by hemorrhage from the bowels, or by sudden peritonitis due to perforation of the wall of the bowel at some point of ulceration, or in consequence of sudden failure of the heart. The last of these accidents is liable to occur in any very grave case of fever, and occasionally follows the critical fall of temperature which occurs in pneumonia, in relapsing fever, and more rarely in other febrile diseases.

Very low axillary temperatures are met with in the stage of collapse in the algid or cold stage of cholera, the internal temperature as indicated by the vagina or rectum remaining extremely high. Great depression of the general temperature occurs in the collapse produced by various poisons, and especially by large quantities of alcohol. The temperature is apt to fall considerably below the normal in ordinary deep alcoholic intoxication, especially if the patients have been exposed to cold and wet.

b. SUBNORMAL TEMPERATURE.—This condition attends considerable losses of blood, starvation from any cause, the wasting of certain of the chronic diseases, such as cancer of various organs, some diseases of the brain and spinal cord, and the later stages of chronic diseases of the lungs and heart, especially when attended by dropsy.

The temperature is very apt to reach subnormal ranges in the morning for a few days at the termination of febrile disorders.

c. NORMAL TEMPERATURE.—If in the course of a continued fever, as typhoid, the temperature, which has been elevated, *suddenly* falls to normal or near it, though not below, this in itself is significant of something wrong, and may even acquire the importance of the "temperature of collapse," as indicating internal hemorrhage, perforation, or failure of the heart.

d. SUBFEBRILE TEMPERATURE.—Slight elevations of temperature often accompany trifling and transient disturbances of the general health, especially in children. They are also observed at the beginning of gradually-developing fevers, as typhoid, and at the close of slowly-subsiding febrile conditions.

e. MODERATE FEBRILE TEMPERATURE.—When the morning temperature reaches 101°–102° F. and the evening shows a further increase of one or two degrees, we have to do with actual fever.

f. HIGH FEBRILE TEMPERATURE.—When the temperature in the morning is above 102°–104° F., and in the evening reaches or ranges higher than 104.5°, the case becomes serious from the intensity of the fever alone. High fever is unattended by immediate danger to life if it be transient, but when prolonged it is ominous.

g. HYPERPYREXIA, OR INTENSE FEBRILE TEMPERATURE.—The temperature reaches 105.8° and continues to rise, or at all events does not fall. The condition is one of extreme and imminent danger to life. Hyperpyrexia often supervenes with great suddenness. It has been encountered after injuries to the brain and to the upper part of the spinal cord, in lockjaw, in sunstroke, and very often in the infectious diseases, especially scarlet fever and pneumonia. It sometimes occurs in rheumatic fever, especially after the intensity of the symptoms has begun to subside, or even when the patient is apparently almost well. Hyperpyrexia is often one of the indications of approaching death. In such cases a temperature of 110° to 112° is sometimes seen. The temperature sometimes continues to rise slowly for an hour or two after death.

The thermometer may be made to indicate a temperature much higher than that of the patient's body, by friction, or by being slipped against a poultice or hot-water bag, or into a cup of tea, when the attention of the nurse is given to other duties. These tricks are sometimes played by hysterical girls.

The temperature of a patient may be somewhat affected by excitement, fatigue, or exposure. Hence hospital patients often show for a few hours after admission a temperature higher than subsequently, or, if they have been exposed to cold, lower than really corresponds to their condition.

It is a peculiarity of the state of convalescence from the acute fevers that the temperature, though normal, is disturbed by trifling causes, and may be made to rise two or three degrees by the first visit of a friend, the first solid food, or even by sitting up. Such rises are usually very brief, the temperature quickly falling again to normal. They occasion uneasiness lest they be the beginning of a relapse. On the other hand, it occasionally happens that, though all the other symptoms have disappeared and the patient is almost well, the temperature remains subfebrile, and the patient is for that reason alone kept in bed. In more than one such case I have seen all traces of fever vanish upon cautiously allowing the patient to sit up an hour or so each day.

The attack of fever may begin suddenly, as in pneumonia, in which the temperature often rises rapidly and continuously to 104° F. or more. Such diseases are apt to begin with a more or less violent rigor or chill. Or it may be gradual, as in typhoid fever, in which the temperature rises little by little from the normal until the fourth or fifth day, when it attains about the height which, in the absence of complications, would be characteristic of the attack, 103°–105° F.

The fever having attained its height, remissions or falls of temperature follow. If these are not more than one or two degrees in extent, conforming to the diurnal variation in health, but at a higher range, the temperature is said to be continuous, or, more properly, subcontinuous, and the fever is a Continued Fever; if, however, the decline is greater than in health, the remissions being marked as compared with the rises or exacerbations, the fever is said to be of Remittent type; and, thirdly, when the remissions reach the normal or fall below it, we speak of the fever as being of the Intermittent type.

Remittent and Intermittent Fevers are grouped with the Periodical Fevers. When acute, they are usually of malarial origin. The symptomatic fever which accompanies chronic inflammatory diseases, especially those of a tuberculous character, as pulmonary consumption, is of well-marked remittent or of intermittent type.

The daily exacerbation or increase of fever occurs, as a rule to which there are very few exceptions, in the afternoon or evening; the remissions or falls, in the morning. In rare cases of general tuberculosis, and still less frequently in typhoid fever, this order is reversed, the rise occurring in the morning and the decline in the evening. The fever is then said to be of "Inverse type."

The range of the temperature after it has reached its height is called the *fastigium*.

The decline of the fever is known as the *defervescence*. It is usually gradual, the remissions between the evening and morning exceeding the evening exacerbations until the normal is again established. This form of defervescence constitutes *lysis*. On the other hand, the decline of the temperature is sometimes abrupt, the temperature falling in the course of a single night or in a few hours from a considerable height to the normal or below it. This is known as a *critical defervescence*, or *crisis*. It is very often attended by some critical discharge, as of sweat or diarrhœa, and is liable to be followed by collapse.

Marked irregularity of the temperature-course of a fever usually indicates some disturbance or complication.

A gradual fall of temperature often precedes death; in some cases of fever, however, the temperature rises as death draws near (*preagonistic rise*), and it may even continue to rise for a short time after dissolution has taken place.

A transient rise in temperature after defervescence has taken place is called a *recrudescence;* a recurrence of fever with the other symptoms of the original attack, lasting several days or weeks, constitutes a *relapse.* Recrudescences are due to accidental causes, relapses to reinfection; the former are usually of trifling importance, the latter always serious. In order to detect at once these occasional recurrences of fever, the temperature ought to be systematically taken for at least a week after it has fallen to the normal range.

261

XIII.

Urinary Tests.

(QUALITATIVE.)

Albumin.

1. *Heat Test.*

The following sources of error occur:

(a) The phosphates are precipitated, but are redissolved by the addition of dilute acid, whilst albumin is not.

(b) In highly alkaline urine the serum albumin may be converted into alkaline albumin not coagulated by heat. This error is avoided by acidulating the urine.

(c) In highly acid urine the albumin is converted into acid albumin not coagulated by heat. The addition of a drop of liquor potassæ converts the acid albumin into serum albumin, and coagulation occurs.

(d) There is occasionally a precipitate of uric acid. This precipitate may be recognized by its deep-brown color, and by the facts that it is never flocculent, and that it does not occur until the specimen begins to cool.

(e) When the urine contains resinous acids in considerable amounts, a precipitate is formed upon the application of heat. This precipitate is soluble in alcohol.

2. *Nitric Acid Test.* (*Heller's Test.*)

A small quantity of strong nitric acid is placed in the bottom of a test-tube, and then, by means of a pipette, an equal quantity of urine is floated gently upon the surface of the acid. If albumin be present, there will be formed at the line of junction a disk of coagulated albumin, not disappearing upon the application of heat.

Sources of error:

(a) In highly acid urines a disk of hydrated uric acid is formed, or

(b) A crystalline disk of nitrate of urea may be formed.

(c) In neutral urines a precipitate of amorphous urates is formed.

These precipitates disappear upon the application of heat.

(d) After the use of balsam of copaiba, a similar disk may be formed at the line of juncture.

3. *Acetic Acid and Ferrocyanide of Potassium Test.*

The urine is filtered. To the clear filtrate a large quantity of acetic acid (sp. gr. 1064) and a few drops of a ten-per-cent. solution of ferrocyanide of potassium are added. If serum albumin be present, a flocculent precipitate will form; if merely a trace, slight opalescence.

4. *The Biuret Test.*

The urine is treated with caustic potash, and a dilute solution of sulphate of copper is added, drop by drop. If albumin be present, a reddish-violet color will be developed; if peptones, the coloration will be red.

5. *Potassio - Mercuric Iodide Test.*

The solution employed in this test is made by mixing 1.35 grammes of perchloride of mercury, 3.32 grammes of iodide of potassium, 20 cubic centimetres of acetic acid, and 64 cubic centimetres of water. It is used by overlaying it with urine previously acidulated. If upon the application of heat the precipitate redissolves, it consists either of peptones, alkaloids, or urates.

6. *The Picric Acid Test.*

A saturated solution of picric acid precipitates serum, alkaline and acid albumins, peptones, urates, alkaloids, oleoresins. The latter four are redissolved by heat.

Albumin (Continued).

7. The Brine Test. The solution is made by adding a drachm of dilute hydrochloric acid to a pint of water and saturating the solution with common salt. It is employed by the overlaying process.

8. The Sodium Tungstate Test. The solution consists of a mixture of equal volumes of a saturated solution of sodium tungstate and a saturated solution of citric acid, with a volume of water equivalent to the united bulk of these solutions. Overlaying process.

9. The Terchloracetic Acid Test. If urine containing albumin be overlaid with a solution of terchloracetic acid, a precipitate without coloration will form at the line of junction. A delicate test, not precipitating peptones.

Blood.

One part in two thousand gives urine a smoky tint, and one in five hundred produces a bright cherry color.

The presence of blood gives characteristic reaction for proteids, as serum albumin and serum globulin, which are always present.

Spectroscopic Examination.

Microscopic Examination.

Chemical Examination.

The Guaiac Test. Freshly-prepared tincture of guaiac; ozonic ether. The test is performed by placing a drachm of urine in a test-tube. Add a drop of the guaiac tincture, thoroughly mixing them, and gently shaking with as much ozonic ether as will equal the quantity of urine. If blood be present, the ozonic ether which separates will acquire a bright-blue color.

Sources of error:

(a) Saliva and nasal mucus produce the same blue line.

(b) Iodide of potassium in the urine gives a similar reaction.

Hæmoglobin.

The presence of hæmoglobin in the urine is established by the presence of blood coloring matter as determined by the spectroscope and the guaiac test, when at the same time the microscope reveals masses of brown pigment and very few or no red corpuscles.

Bile

Gives the urine various shades of color from dark green to reddish brown. Bile pigments are recognized by the play of colors, in which green is distinctive. This play of colors is produced by several reagents:

1. Nitric Acid Test. A small quantity of the urine to be examined should be placed on a white porcelain dish, and near it a few drops of fuming nitric acid. The two fluids are gently brought into contact. If bile pigment be present, there will result a play of colors in which the green tint predominates.

2. Nitric and Sulphuric Acid Test. Equal volumes of the suspected urine and nitric acid are mixed in a test-tube. This mixture, upon being underlaid with sulphuric acid, shows, if bile pigment be present, the green tint and play of colors at the line of junction.

3. The Hydrochloric Acid and Nitric Acid Test. If a mixture of equal bulks of urine and hydrochloric acid be underlaid with strong nitric acid, the presence of bile pigment will give the play of colors as above.

4. The Iodine Test. If a small quantity of urine be floated upon the surface of tincture of iodine in a test-tube, the presence of bile pigment will develop a beautiful green color at the line of contact.

Glucose.

1. The Liquor Potassæ Test. (Moore's Test.)

This consists in a mixture of equal parts of the suspected urine and liquor potassæ in a test-tube, the upper layer of which is to be boiled. The presence of glucose develops a red-brown color in the heated portion, from the formation of glucic and mellisic acids.

2. The Liquor Potassæ and Sulphate of Copper Test. (Trommer's Test.)

A drop or two of a weak solution of sulphate of copper is added to the urine, and then a volume of solution of potash equal to that of urine. Upon the addition of the potash solution, a blue precipitate of hydrated cupric oxide is thrown down. If sugar is present, this is dissolved on shaking the tube; a clear blue fluid results: on boiling the mixture a dense yellow precipitate of hydrated cuprous oxide is produced by the reduction of the cupric oxide by the sugar. This yellow precipitate afterwards undergoes a change to red.

3. Fehling's Test.

This is a modification of that of Trommer. The reagent employed is composed of—
(a) Cupric sulphate, 34.64 grammes, dissolved in 500 cubic centimetres of distilled water:
(b) Neutral potassium tartrate, 173 grammes, dissolved in 500 cubic centimetres of solution of caustic soda (specific gravity 1.12).
These should be kept in separate bottles, and mixed, when required, in equal proportions.
The strength of this solution is so adapted that 10 cubic centimetres are reduced by 0.05 gramme of glucose. The test is therefore of use in the quantitative estimation of sugar in the urine.

5. The Bismuth Test. (Böttger's Test.)

Equal volumes of urine and liquor potassæ are mixed in a test-tube. To this mixture is added a small quantity of bismuth subnitrate. If glucose be present, a precipitate of metallic bismuth will be thrown down upon the addition of heat. This precipitate will be gray if sugar be present in only small amount, and black if in larger quantity.

6. Fermentation Test.

Four ounces of urine are placed in an eight-ounce vial with a small fragment of yeast. In another similar bottle the same quantity of urine is placed without the yeast. The specific gravity is then taken. The two bottles are now set aside in a warm place for twenty-four hours, and the specific gravity of each is again taken. Each degree of specific gravity lost in the urine which contains the yeast indicates the presence of one grain of sugar in every fluidounce of urine. If metric measures are employed, each degree of specific gravity lost represents 0.22 gramme of sugar in every 100 cubic centimetres of urine.

Enteric Fever, Measles, Acute Tuberculosis.

The Diazo Reaction. (Ehrlich's Test.)

It is said to be characteristic of the urine in enteric or typhoid fever, measles, and acute tuberculosis to yield a deep-red color with diazo-benzol-sulphonic acid.
Ehrlich uses as a test not the diazo-benzol-sulphonic acid, but sulphanilic acid.
The procedure is as follows:
50 cubic centimetres of hydrochloric acid are made up to 1000 cubic centimetres with water, and sulphanilic acid added to saturation. To 200 cubic centimetres of the mixture 5 cubic centimetres of a half-per-cent. solution of sodium nitrite are added, and the resulting fluid is added to the urine in equal parts; or five or six times the volume of absolute alcohol is added to the fluid to be tested, and the reagent prepared as above is discharged, drop by drop, into the filtrate. Normal urine gives a yellow color, while the urine of fever patients turns scarlet.

XIV

Miscellaneous Tables.

A TABLE OF THE NUMBER OF DROPS IN A FLUIDRACHM.

The size of drops varies greatly, not only in different liquids, but also in the same liquid, according as it comes from different bottles. A bottle with a thick lip gives a larger drop than one with a thin lip, especially if the liquid be allowed to diffuse itself over the lip. "Droppers," as usually made, give a drop much smaller than that from a bottle, the size of the drop being dependent upon the size and bore of the point of the dropper. A dropper with a thick tip may give a very large drop. The average drop of watery solutions, *waters* or *liquors*, is about 60 to the fluidrachm; of *syrups*, except some which are very thick, about 60 to the fluidrachm; of alcoholic solutions, *tinctures*, 120 to the fluidrachm; of *volatile oils*, 110 to 120; of *wines*, 75; of *vinegars*, 75; of *ether*, 150; of *chloroform*, 200. *Deodorized laudanum* (*tinctura opii deodorata*) is really a watery preparation: hence, whilst laudanum averages 120 drops, deodorized laudanum averages 100 to the fluidrachm.

Acetum colchici	75	Oleum chenopodii	97
" destillatum	78	" cinnamomi	100
" opii	90	" cubebæ	86
" scillæ	78	" fœniculi	103
Acidum aceticum	73	" gaultheriæ	102
" hydrocyan. dilut.	45	" menthæ piperitæ	103
" muriaticum	54	" olivæ	76
" nitricum	84	" rosmarini	104
" " dilutum	62	" sabinæ	102
" sulphuricum	90	" sassafras	102
" " aromat.	116	" tiglii	80
" " dilutum	54	Spiritus ætheris nitrosi	90
Alcohol	118	" " compositus	90
" dilutum	98	Syrupus acaciæ	58
Aqua	64	" scillæ	85
" ammoniæ	49	Tinctura aconiti	118
Creasotum	91	" asafœtidæ	120
Chloroformum	180	" digitalis	120
Ether	150	" ferri chloridi	106
Glycerina	55	" guaiaci	120
Liquor iodi compositus	75	" iodi	144
" hydrarg. et ars. iod.	52	" opii	147
" potassii arsenitis	60	" opii camphorata	110
Oleum amygdalæ dulcis	120	" tolu	138
" anisi	85	Vinum antimonii	87
" carui	106	" colchici	75
" caryophylli	103	" opii	92

A glassful or cupful is estimated to contain about 4-6 fluid-ounces.

A wineglassful, about 1½-2 fluidounces.

A tablespoonful of liquid, about ½ ounce; of powder, about 2 drachms.

A teaspoonful of liquid, about 1 drachm; of powder, about 2½ scruples.

A teaspoonful of magnesia, 10 grains; of powdered herbs, 1 scruple.

A teaspoonful of salts, sugar, sulphur, ½ drachm.

A teaspoonful of metallic oxides, 1-1½ drachms.

A drop of water and watery fluids, about 1℔.

A drop of oils and tinctures, about ½℔.

A drop of chloroform, about ¼℔.

THE PULSE.

AVERAGE FREQUENCY AT DIFFERENT AGES—IN HEALTH.

Ages.	Beats per minute.		
In the fœtus *in utero*	between 150	and	140
New-born infants	" 140	"	130
During 1st year	from 130	down to	115
" 2d year	" 115	"	100
" 3d year	" 105	"	95
From 7th to 14th year	" 90	"	80
" 14th to 21st year	" 85	"	75
" 21st to 60th year	between 75	and	79
In old age	" 75	"	80

The pulse is generally more frequent *in females*, by 10–14 beats per minute; *during* and *after exertion*, unless long continued; *during digestion* or *mental excitement*; generally, more frequent *in the morning*; and less frequent, in health, *in the nervous* as well as in the *phlegmatic* temperament. It is temporarily accelerated after sudden change of posture from the recumbent to the sitting, and from either to the standing position, especially during convalescence and in other states where the action of the heart is feeble.

RESPIRATIONS AT VARIOUS AGES.

	Number of respirations per minute.
First year	35
Second year	25
At puberty	20
Adult age	18

THE ORDER OF THE ERUPTION OF THE TEETH.

FIRST DENTITION.

As a rule, the teeth of the lower jaw precede those of the upper, except in the case of the lateral incisors.

Central incisors	5th to 8th month.
Lateral incisors	7th to 9th month.
First molars	12th to 16th month.
Canines	16th to 20th month.
Second molars	20th to 36th month.

SECOND DENTITION.

First molars	5th to 7th year.
Central incisors	7th to 8th year.
Lateral incisors	8th to 9th year.
First bicuspids	9th to 10th year.
Second bicuspids	10th to 11th year.
Canines	11th to 12th year.
Second molars	12th to 13th year.
Third molars	17th to 21st year.

A TABLE OF THE APPROXIMATE RELATION BETWEEN THE HEIGHT AND WEIGHT UNDER NORMAL CIRCUMSTANCES.

A man of 4 ft. 6 in. to 5 ft. 0 in.	ought to weigh about	92.26 lbs.
" 5 ft. 0 in. to 5 ft. 1 in.	" " "	115.52 "
" 5 ft. 2 in. to 5 ft. 3 in.	" " "	127.86 "
" 5 ft. 4 in. to 5 ft. 5 in.	" " "	139.17 "
" 5 ft. 6 in. to 5 ft. 7 in.	" " "	144.29 "
" 5 ft. 8 in. to 5 ft. 9 in.	" " "	157.76 "
" 5 ft. 10 in. to 5 ft. 11 in.	" " "	170.86 "
" 5 ft. 11 in. to 6 ft. 0 in.	" " "	177.25 "
" 6 ft. 0 in.	" " "	218.66 "

(HUTCHINSON.)

STATURE.	Capacity of Healthy Male.	Early Stage of Consumption.	Advanced Stage of Consumption.
	Cubic ins.	Cubic ins.	Cubic ins.
m 5 ft. to 5 ft. 1 in. . .	174	117	82
5 ft. 1 in. to 5 ft. 2 in. . .	182	122	86
5 ft. 2 in. to 5 ft. 3 in. . .	190	127	89
5 ft. 3 in. to 5 ft. 4 in. . .	198	133	93
5 ft. 4 in. to 5 ft. 5 in. . .	206	138	97
5 ft. 5 in. to 5 ft. 6 in. . .	214	143	100
5 ft. 6 in. to 5 ft. 7 in. . .	222	149	104
5 ft. 7 in. to 5 ft. 8 in. . .	230	154	108
5 ft. 8 in. to 5 ft. 9 in. . .	238	159	112
5 ft. 9 in. to 5 ft. 10 in. . .	246	165	116
5 ft. 10 in. to 5 ft. 11 in. . .	254	170	119
5 ft. 11 in. to 6 ft.	262	176	123

(HUTCHINSON.)

OBSTETRIC CALENDAR.

The date in the upper line of each section 1, 1' being that of the first day of the last menstruation before conception, that corresponding to the lower line 3, 3' indicates approximately the commencement of labor; while the corresponding date in the midd. line 2, 2' in⎯⎯tes the ave⎯ but v⎯⎯ vr ⎯⎯ time of the "quickening."

The altern⎯te days only are given, to sa⎯ ⎯ace.